T0336136

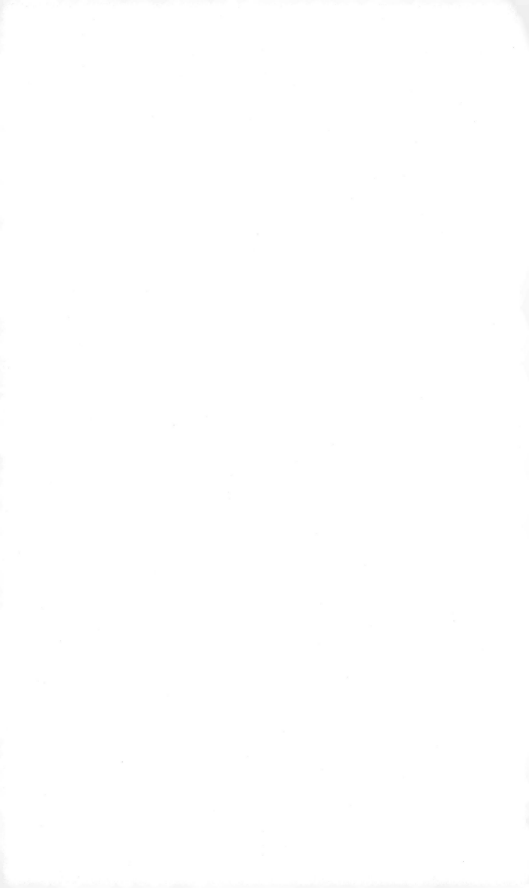

Cancer Genetics

More information about this series at http://www.springer.com/series/7706

Carlos A. Torres-Cabala • Jonathan L. Curry
Editors

Genetics of Melanoma

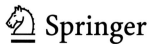 Springer

Editors
Carlos A. Torres-Cabala
MD Anderson Cancer Center
The University of Texas
Houston, TX, USA

Jonathan L. Curry
MD Anderson Cancer Center
The University of Texas
Houston, TX, USA

ISBN 978-1-4939-3552-9   ISBN 978-1-4939-3554-3   (eBook)
DOI 10.1007/978-1-4939-3554-3

Library of Congress Control Number: 2016936786

Printed on acid-free paper

This Springer imprint is published by Springer Nature
The registered company is Springer Science+Business Media LLC New York

Dedication by Carlos A. Torres-Cabala

To E. Maria Luisa, my wife, and Adriana, my beautiful daughter, whom I love and admire.

To Luis and Consuelo, my parents, to whom I owe everything that I am and want to be.

To Carmen, Eliana, and José Luis, my siblings, and their families, who are always there for me.

Dedication by Jonathan L. Curry

To my amazing wife Choladda and our beautiful children Rachel and Nathanial, I am blessed to have a loving family.

To my parents James and Carol, without their love, sacrifice, and support my dreams would not have been possible.

To my sister Elizabeth and her family Paul and Jennifer, who have always given me their love and support.

Preface

Advances in molecular technologies and high-throughput sequencing testing platforms have brought an impressive amount of discoveries in the field of melanoma genetics that have changed our approach in understanding the pathogenesis and treatment of this lethal disease. Knowledge of the genetic aberrations in melanoma is essential for the diagnosis and appropriate selection of patients who may benefit from personalized targeted therapeutic agents.

This book is intended to span the basic molecular, genetic, epigenetic, pathological, immunological, and clinical aspects of melanoma, focusing on the practical application of this large volume of knowledge to the management of patients. A multidisciplinary team of experts have contributed with the most updated view of the basic mechanisms and therapeutic approach of the disease, making this book a valuable source of information as well as a practical guide on the genetics of melanoma and its relevance in the clinical setting. Our intention is that this book will serve as a practical resource to pathologists, dermatologists, oncologists, and other physicians and scientists whose primary interest is melanoma.

We hope the readers of *Genetics of Melanoma* will glean a further understanding of melanoma that will translate into the delivery of the best health care to these patients.

Houston, TX, USA

Carlos A. Torres-Cabala
Jonathan L. Curry

Acknowledgments

We would like to thank all the contributors as well as Faculty and staff members in our melanoma program at the University of Texas MD Anderson Cancer Center. It is with teamwork from all specialties that allow us to deliver the best patient care to those afflicted with melanoma.

Dr. Torres-Cabala would like to thank the following mentors who influenced his training in science, pathology, and dermatopathology: Drs. Sixto Recavarren, Francisco Bravo, Mehrdad Nadji, W. Marston Linehan, Maria J. Merino, Elaine S. Jaffe, and Victor G. Prieto, who among many others made his education a fascinating experience.

Dr. Curry would like express his sincere gratitude to his mentors Dr. Brian J. Nickoloff and Dr. Jon A. Reed, both of whom have provided indispensible support, guidance, and knowledge to his scientific and medical education in dermatopathology.

He also would like to acknowledge Dr. Kenneth D. McClatchey for his tremendous contribution and legacy to Pathology and Laboratory Medicine. His mentorship was immense to Dr. Curry's career in pathology.

Finally, we would also like to express our great appreciation to the publishers for their support in this endeavor and to the fruition of this book.

Contents

Contributors

Yeorim Ahn Ritz Dermatology Clinic, Seoul, South Korea

Phyu P. Aung Department of Pathology, The University of Texas, MD Anderson Cancer Center, Houston, TX, USA

Leomar Y. Ballester Department of Pathology and Genomic Medicine, Houston Methodist Hospital, Houston, TX, USA

Chantale Bernatchez Department of Melanoma Medical Oncology, The University of Texas, MD Anderson Cancer Center, Houston, TX, USA

Young Kwang Chae Division of Hematology and Oncology, Department of Medicine, Northwestern University, Robert H. Lurie Comprehensive Cancer Center, Chicago, IL, USA

Marjan Champine University of Utah Health Sciences, Salt Lake City, UT, USA

Jie Qing Chen Department of Melanoma Medical Oncology, The University of Texas, MD Anderson Cancer Center, Houston, TX, USA
Lion Biotechnologies, Tampa, FL, USA

Ana Ciurea Department of Dermatology, The University of Texas, MD Anderson Cancer Center, Houston, TX, USA

Jonathan L. Curry Department of Pathology and Department of Dermatology, The University of Texas, MD Anderson Cancer Center, Houston, TX, USA

Michael A. Davies Departments of Melanoma Medical Oncology & Systems Biology, The University of Texas MD Anderson Cancer Center, Houston, TX, USA

Marie-Andree Forget Department of Melanoma Medical Oncology, The University of Texas, MD Anderson Cancer Center, Houston, TX, USA

Isabella C. Glitza Department of Melanoma Medical Oncology, The University of Texas, MD Anderson Cancer Center, Houston, TX, USA

Cara Haymaker Department of Melanoma Medical Oncology, The University of Texas, MD Anderson Cancer Center, Houston, TX, USA

Wen-Jen Hwu Department of Melanoma Medical Oncology, The University of Texas, MD Anderson Cancer Center, Houston, TX, USA

Dae Won Kim Moffitt Cancer Center, Tampa, FL, USA

Kevin B. Kim Department of Melanoma Medical Oncology, The University of Texas MD Anderson Cancer Center, Houston, TX, USA

California Pacific Medical Center, San Francisco, CA, USA

Wendy Kohlmann University of Utah Health Sciences, Salt Lake City, UT, USA

Alexander J. Lazar Departments of Pathology & Translational Molecular Pathology, The University of Texas MD Anderson Cancer Center, Houston, TX, USA

Sancy A. Leachman Oregon Health and Science University, Portland, OR, USA

Chyi-Chia R. Lee Laboratory of Pathology, National Cancer Institute, National Institutes of Health, Bethesda, MD, USA

Priyadharsini Nagarajan Department of Pathology, The University of Texas, MD Anderson Cancer Center, Houston, TX, USA

Keyur Pravinchandra Patel Department of Hematopathology, The University of Texas MD Anderson Cancer Center, Houston, TX, USA

Lana N. Pho University of Utah Health Sciences, Salt Lake City, UT, USA

Victor G. Prieto Department of Pathology and Department of Dermatology, The University of Texas, MD Anderson Cancer Center, Houston, TX, USA

Laszlo Radvanyi Department of Melanoma Medical Oncology, The University of Texas, MD Anderson Cancer Center, Houston, TX, USA

EMD Serono Research and Development Institute, Billerica, MA, USA

Alaa A. Salim Department of Hematopathology, The University of Texas MD Anderson Cancer Center, Houston, TX, USA

Christopher R. Shea Department of Medicine, University of Chicago, Chicago, IL, USA

Geok Choo Sim Department of Melanoma Medical Oncology, The University of Texas, MD Anderson Cancer Center, Houston, TX, USA

Moffit Cancer Center, Tampa, FL, USA

Alan E. Siroy Departments of Pathology & Translational Molecular Pathology, The University of Texas MD Anderson Cancer Center, Houston, TX, USA

Michael T. Tetzlaff Department of Pathology, The University of Texas, MD Anderson Cancer Center, Houston, TX, USA

Carlos A. Torres-Cabala Department of Pathology and Department of Dermatology, The University of Texas, MD Anderson Cancer Center, Houston, TX, USA

Van A. Trinh Pharmacy Clinical Programs, The University of Texas MD Anderson Cancer Center, Houston, TX, USA

Tao Wang Division of Biotechnology Products Research and Review IV, Laboratory of Immunobiology, OBP/OPQ/CDER, Food and Drug Administration, MD, USA

Xiaowei Xu Department of Pathology and Laboratory Medicine, University of Pennsylvania, Philadelphia, PA, USA

Sook Jung Yun Department of Pathology and Laboratory Medicine, University of Pennsylvania, Philadelphia, PA, USA

Department of Dermatology, Chonnam National University Medical School, Gwangju, South Korea

Part I
Pathogenesis of Melanoma

Chapter 1
The Biology of Melanoma

Tao Wang, Sook Jung Yun, and Xiaowei Xu

Abstract Melanoma is the most deadly form of skin cancer. Currently, the incidence of melanoma in the USA has been extrapolated to 76,690 per year and the incidence is rising. Although somatic mutations such as *BRAF* and *NRAS* mutations are crucial for melanomagenesis, the host and tumor microenvironmental factors are also critical to regulate melanoma initiation, melanoma cell intravasation, colonization of distant sites, and formation of macrometastasis. Targeting the tumor microenvironment may increase the antitumor activity of current therapies for melanoma.

Keywords Melanoma • Tumor microenvironment • Macrophage • Fibroblast Hypoxia

1.1 Introduction

Melanoma is the fifth leading cancer in men and the seventh in women in the USA. The incidence is substantially increased in recent years, especially in women. Melanoma is the most aggressive skin cancer, and most of the advanced melanoma patients die of disseminated metastasis which usually occurs several months to years after resection of the primary melanoma. Until recently, treatment of advanced

T. Wang (✉)
Division of Biotechnology Products Research and Review IV, Laboratory
of Immunobiology, OBP/OPQ/CDER, Food and Drug Administration,
WO72, 2329, 10903, New Hampshire Avenue, Silver Spring, MD 20993-0002, USA
e-mail: tao.wang@fda.hhs.gov

S.J. Yun
Department of Pathology and Laboratory Medicine,
University of Pennsylvania, Philadelphia, PA, USA

Department of Dermatology, Chonnam National University Medical School,
Gwangju, South Korea

X. Xu (✉)
Department of Pathology and Laboratory Medicine,
University of Pennsylvania, Philadelphia, PA, USA
e-mail: xug@mail.med.upenn.edu

© Springer Science+Business Media New York 2016
C.A. Torres-Cabala, J.L. Curry (eds.), *Genetics of Melanoma*, Cancer Genetics,
DOI 10.1007/978-1-4939-3554-3_1

melanoma produced cure rates of less than 3 %, and overall 5-year survival rates were ~15 %. Fortunately, this paradigm is changing with the development of targeted therapy and immunotherapy for melanoma. Although a major breakthrough in treatment of metastatic melanoma has been achieved with several newly approved drugs, such as vemurafenib and ipilimumab, both therapies have their limitations. Vemurafenib, which targets melanomas harboring BRAFV600E mutation, achieves rapid tumor regression, but patients inevitably develop resistance within 6 months. Ipilimumab, which blocks the immune suppression of T cells induced by cytotoxic T lymphocyte antigen 4 (CTLA-4), achieves durable benefits, but most patients (80–85 %) do not respond. Consequently, better understanding of the biology of melanomas is essential to develop novel strategies for melanoma therapy. While genetic and epigenetic changes in melanoma cells are crucial for tumor development and progression, recent studies have shown that tumor microenvironment has an equally profound influence on the growth and metastasis of melanoma than was previously appreciated. Accumulating evidences indicate that tumor microenvironment plays an essential role in all stages of melanoma development, including melanoma initiation, progression, metastasis, angiogenesis, and immunosuppression. In this chapter, we discuss how the complex network of melanoma microenvironment affects melanoma development with focus on the effects of stromal fibroblasts, macrophages, and tissue hypoxia. However, other components of tumor microenvironment, such as immune cells, endothelial cells, keratinocytes, etc., are also critical for melanoma development. A better understanding of how tumor microenvironment affects melanoma progression will open up new strategies for diagnosis, prognosis, and therapy of melanoma.

1.1.1 Complexity of Melanoma Microenvironment

The skin is the largest organ of the human body and accounts for about 16 % of total body weight in adult humans. The normal skin consists of two distinct layers: the epidermis and the dermis. Keratinocytes are the most abundant cell type in the epidermis, and melanocytes and Langerhans cells are interspersed in the epidermis layer. One melanocyte is normally surrounded by 5–8 keratinocytes, forming the "epidermal-melanocytes unit." Keratinocytes produce the major structural protein of the skin, keratin, and many growth factors to maintain normal skin homeostasis. Keratinocytes also regulate melanocyte proliferation through E-cadherin, desmoglein-1, and connexins [1]. Melanocytes produce pigment granules called melanosomes containing melanin. Upon ultraviolet (UV) radiation, a major risk factor of melanoma, the melanosomes are transferred from the melanocytes to the keratinocytes, thus providing a mechanism to protect against UVR-induced DNA damages [2]. Langerhans cells are dendritic-like immune cells that are the antigen-presenting cells of the skin. The dermis is composed of fibroblasts, macrophages, adipocytes, vascular endothelial cells, and pericytes. The major structural components of the dermis are fibroblast-produced collagens, as well as other extracellular proteins, such as elastin, which maintain a tight connection to the epidermis through a basement membrane.

The conditions within the melanoma microenvironment differ significantly from those in normal skin, which is often altered as the melanoma progresses from early-stage radial growth phase (RGP) to vertical growth phase (VGP) and then to a metastatic stage. The melanoma microenvironment is also highly heterogeneous, containing many different types of noncancerous cells, such as keratinocytes, fibroblasts, inflammatory cells, and a variety of extracellular matrix (ECM) and growth factors produced by cancer cells and stromal cells. The interaction between melanoma cells and their surrounding stromal cells promotes tumor progression and metastasis despite fluctuations in nutrient and oxygen supply within tumors. The interplay between cancer cells and the surrounding stromal cells is extremely complex. Melanoma cells produce growth factors and cytokines to recruit many types of stromal cells and activate stromal cells within the tumor microenvironment, which in turn either directly promotes melanoma growth or indirectly affects functions of other types of stromal cells, facilitating melanoma initiation, progression, and metastasis. In addition, the hypoxic dermal microenvironment is a host factor that promotes melanomagenesis [3]. As a tumor grows, it rapidly outgrows its blood supply, resulting in an uneven distribution of vasculature [4]. As a consequence, tumors contain pockets of hypoxic regions which can be visualized by immunohistochemistry [5]. The development of hypoxic regions in a tumor is clinically important because hypoxic tumor cells have different metabolic rates and biological properties, compared to well-oxygenated tumor cells [4]. In addition, hypoxic tumor cells are associated with worse prognosis and are more resistant to chemo- and radiation therapies [6]. The link between hypoxia and tumor aggressiveness is further illustrated by recent studies in which mouse tumors that were treated with antiangiogenic agents which induce more tumor hypoxia displayed enhanced migration and invasion properties [7, 8].

Thus, tumor-stromal cells and hypoxic tumor microenvironment are crucial for melanoma initiation, progression, and treatment resistance.

1.2 Fibroblasts

The major function of normal skin fibroblasts is to maintain the integrity of the basement membrane and dermal collagens. Skin fibroblasts produce ECM components, such as type I and type IV collagens. They also produce matrix metalloproteinases (MMPs), which are involved in remodeling ECM. Fibroblasts also play critical roles in other skin functions, such as melanocyte proliferation and pigmentation, which are both dependent on the growth factors secreted by fibroblasts. Studies by Hearing's group and others have identified many factors involved in the regulation of skin pigmentation after UV exposure and melanocyte proliferation, such as Dickkopf-related protein 1 (DKK1), neuregulin-1, stem cell factor (SCF), hepatocyte growth factor (HGF), interferon-γ (IFN-γ), endothelin-1 (ET-1), basic fibroblast growth factor (bFGF), interleukin-1 (IL-1), and granulocyte-macrophage colony-stimulating factor (GM-CSF) [2, 9]. Importantly, it appears that some of these factors have been reported to promote melanoma growth and metastasis, as well as modulate other components of tumor-stromal cells that facilitate tumor progression.

Melanoma-associated fibroblasts (MAFs) have profound effects in many aspects of melanoma development, including melanoma growth, invasion, and metastasis, as well as immune functions, though the mechanisms underlying these functions remain poorly understood. In the following section, we will systemically summarize recent progress in the ontogeny of MAFs, the roles of MAFs in melanoma development, and the potential therapeutic implications for targeting MAFs in melanomas.

1.2.1 Markers of Melanoma-Associated Fibroblasts

During tumor development, fibroblasts are activated by tumor cells or other types of stromal cells and play a critical role in tumor growth and progression. The activated fibroblasts in the tumor site are designated as cancer-associated fibroblasts (CAFs). CAFs are highly heterogeneous in terms of their markers and functions. The most commonly used and most specific marker of CAFs is fibroblast-specific protein 1 (FSP1, also called S100A4). In addition, fibroblast activation protein (FAP), vimentin, α-smooth muscle actin (αSMA), platelet-derived growth factor receptors α and β (PDGFRα, PDGFRβ), and $\alpha1\beta1$ integrin are also frequently used as the markers of CAFs. However, there is no definite marker for CAFs and none of these markers are specific. In addition, other types of cells also express nearly all markers currently used for CAFs, reducing specificity of these markers. For example, some invasive cancer cells also express FSP1 and activated melanocytes express FAP.

Like other types of cancers, the markers of melanoma-associated fibroblasts (MAFs) are not well defined. FSP1, a commonly used marker in other cancers, is also expressed in melanoma cells [10]. It seems that FSP1 is a good MAF marker because it is induced by melanoma cells and cannot be detected in normal skin fibroblasts [11]. Another possible marker for MAFs is PDGFRα, which is expressed by activated MAFs and melanocytes, but is significantly downregulated in melanoma cells [12]. αSMA has been reported to be expressed by MAFs, but is also expressed by vascular smooth muscle cells and pericytes [13, 14].

1.2.2 The Ontogeny of Melanoma-Associated Fibroblasts

The origin of CAFs remains controversial. It has been proposed that CAFs are derived from four different compartments. First, CAFs are the resident fibroblasts activated by factors produced by tumor cells or other types of stromal cells. Second, other types of cells in the tumor, including epithelial cells and endothelial cells, can be transdifferentiated into CAFs. Third, mesenchymal cells in the tumor, such as vascular smooth muscle cells, pericytes, and adipocytes, can also be transdifferentiated into CAFs. Last is the recruitment of bone marrow-derived progenitor cells and mesenchymal cells into tumors, where these cells can be transdifferentiated into CAFs [15–17]. Although many studies have shown that tumor cells can activate normal fibroblast to CAFs, again, there is no unique marker that can be used for CAFs. Of note, most data of proposed sources of CAFs is studied using either in vitro cell-culture systems or using mouse systems, and most markers of CAFs have not been validated in human tumors.

Studies from several laboratories suggested that MAFs are mainly derived from resident fibroblasts activated by tumor cells. Early study by Halaban et al. showed that melanoma cells produce PDGF that activates fibroblasts to produce several growth factors, including insulin-like growth factor-1 (IGF-1), HGF, bFGF, and endothelin-1 (ET-1). Ulmer et al. showed that the increased activity of cathepsin B in fibroblasts isolated from primary melanoma has increased activity in comparison to that from normal skin fibroblasts. Wandel et al. showed that fibroblasts derived from surrounding melanomas express higher levels of MMP-1 and intercellular adhesion molecule-1 (ICAM-1) than fibroblasts derived from benign melanocytic nevi [18, 19]. Further studies indicated that MMP-1 is induced by interleukin-1α (IL-1α) and bFGF produced by highly invasive melanoma cell lines [20].

In addition to activation of fibroblasts by secreted factors, melanoma cells may also activate fibroblasts by direct cell-cell contact. It has been reported that expression of CD147 on melanoma cells induces fibroblasts to produce MMPs, which is attributed to the proinvasive phenotypes of melanoma [21]. Melanoma cells also increase expression of tenascin in fibroblasts by direct cell-cell contact, which promotes melanoma progression [22].

MAFs may also be derived from circulating blood cells. Using a B16 mouse melanoma model, Anderberg et al. found that melanoma cells produced platelet-derived growth factor-CC (PDGF-CC) that recruited blood fibroblast to the tumor-stromal cells and then activated fibroblasts to the MAFs [23]. It has also been reported that PDGF-BB promotes dermal fibroblast migration by activation of the MAPK and PI3K pathways through two SH2-/SH3-containing adapter proteins, Nckα and Nckβ [24]. There is no report that other types of stromal cells or bone marrow-derived progenitor cells and mesenchymal cells can be transdifferentiated into MAFs.

The effects of melanoma cells on activation of the fibroblasts are also dependent on the stage of melanoma. Gene expression array analysis indicated there is a significant difference in gene expression between fibroblasts cocultured with late-stage melanoma and those cocultured with earlier-stage melanoma [25].

In summary, it seems that MAFs are primarily derived from resident fibroblasts, which can be activated by melanoma cells through direct cell-cell contact or via growth factors produced by melanoma cells. It is possible that circulation fibroblasts are another source of MAFs.

1.2.3 Fibroblasts Promote Melanoma Growth and Survival

MAFs have profound effects on melanoma cell growth and survival. Early studies by Gartner et al. provided direct evidences that MAFs can increase melanoma growth in vivo. Co-injection of melanoma cells with fibroblasts increases tumor growth in a xenograft model [26]. Coculturing normal dermal fibroblasts with melanoma cells promotes tumor cell growth mainly in earlier-stage melanoma cells, but has little effect on metastatic melanoma cells [27]. Supporting this, Satyamoorthy et al. also found that overexpression of insulin-like growth factor-1 (IGF-1) in fibroblasts induces survival and growth of biologically early-stage melanoma cell lines through activation of both mitogen-activated protein kinase (MAPK) and beta-catenin pathways [28]. Other fibroblast-produced growth factors, such as bFGF, HGF [29], epithelial growth factor (EGF), and vascular endothelial growth factor (VEGF), are potent mitogens for melanoma cells.

In addition to the growth factors, MAFs also promote melanoma growth through glycosaminoglycan hyaluronan (also called hyaluronic acid, hyaluronate, or HA). The induction of HA in MAFs is enhanced by melanoma-produced PDGF-AA and PDGF-CC through activation of two HA synthases: HAS1 and HAS2. HA is a major component of the ECM and has been demonstrated to promote tumor growth, angiogenesis, and metastasis [30]. Consistent with this, Pasonen-Seppänen et al. reported that melanoma cell-derived factors stimulate hyaluronan synthesis in dermal fibroblasts by upregulating HAS2 through PDGFR-PI3K-AKT and p38 signaling [31].

It also has been shown that stromal fibroblast-specific expression of ADAM-9 modulates proliferation and apoptosis in melanoma cells both in vitro and in vivo. However, whether it exerts a pro-tumor growth or tumor growth inhibitory effect remains controversial [32, 33]. ADAM-9 is a member of a family of proteases with a disintegrin and metalloprotease domain (ADAM). It is upregulated in melanomas and is expressed at the tumor-stromal border. ADAM-9 interacts with several integrins to regulate melanoma growth and apoptosis.

Fibroblasts also promote melanoma growth and survival by direct cell-cell contact. Loss of E-cadherin in melanocytes and increased expression of N-cadherin is an early event of melanoma transformation. Fibroblasts express N-cadherin, which cause homotypic aggregation, forming a gap junction between melanoma cells and fibroblasts. This unique structure allows communication between melanoma cells and fibroblasts and in turn promotes melanoma cell proliferation [1]. Further study indicates that glycogen synthase kinase (GSK)-3β is one of the major regulators of N-cadherin expression. Inhibition of GSK-3β through chemical and genetic approaches significantly downregulates N-cadherin expression and disrupts the interaction between melanoma cells and fibroblasts [34].

Interestingly, it has been shown that cancer cells can suppress expression of tumor suppressor p53 in adjacent fibroblasts. Thus, tumor cells may overcome the non-cell-autonomous tumor suppressor function of p53 in stromal fibroblasts [35]. Further studies indicate that p53 status in stromal fibroblasts modulates tumor growth in a stromal cell-derived factor 1 (SDF1)-dependent manner [36]. In liver cancer, proliferating p53-deficient liver fibroblasts secrete factors that enhance the proliferation of premalignant cells through modulating differentiation of macrophages [37]. In melanoma, in which dysfunction of p53 occurs in more than 90 % of cases, it will be interesting to see whether non-cell-autonomous tumor suppressor function of p53 in stromal fibroblasts occurs [38].

1.2.4 Fibroblasts Promote Melanoma Cell Invasion and Metastasis

Most cancer deaths are caused by spread of the primary cancer to distant sites. Melanoma metastasis, like other cancers, includes multiple sequential steps: primary tumor cells acquire an invasive phenotype that separates tumor cells from the basement membranes; tumor cells then reach the regional site or distant organs through lymphatic or hematogenous dissemination; and ultimately tumor cells survive in new metastatic organs, such as the brain, lungs, liver, bone, etc. [39, 40]. In melanoma, the invasive potential of human melanoma cell lines has been shown to correlate with their ability to alter fibroblast gene expression, suggesting that MAFs may play critical roles in metastasis [41]. The increased invasive activity of melanoma cells by fibroblasts is carried out primarily through proteinases, such as MMPs, urokinase-type plasminogen activator (uPA), and cathepsins. These proteinases degrade and process ECM and the basement membrane, therefore providing an environment that promotes tumor cell invasion. In addition, melanoma invasion is enhanced by dermal fibroblast through upregulating expression of matrix metalloproteinase-2 (MMP-2) in a cell-cell contact-dependent manner [42]. Other MMPs, such as MMP-1 and MMP-13, have been shown to increase melanoma invasion as well. Expression of MMPs appears to be regulated by invasive tumor cell-derived cytokines or growth factors, such as IL-1alpha and bFGF [18, 19, 43].

Another important type of proteinase, cysteine cathepsin B, has also been reported to increase melanoma invasion. Cathepsin B is highly expressed in MAFs and is an endopeptidase that modulates many proteases, such as MMPs, that facilitates tumor cell invasion and metastasis. Cathepsin B also mediates proteolytic breakdown of ECMs, therefore releasing ECM-bound growth factors such as bFGF, EGF, TGF-β, IGF-1, and VEGF, which has been shown to increase melanoma invasion [44]. In contrast, Yin et al. demonstrated that fibroblasts express cathepsin L, but not cathepsin B, which is expressed in melanoma cells. It is not clear what causes this discrepancy. Nonetheless, Yin et al. found that upregulation of TGF-beta expression by cathepsin B is required for melanoma cell invasion [45].

Formation of new blood vessels is termed angiogenesis, which is a critical step for tumor cell metastasis. Fibroblasts also play a critical role in melanoma angiogenesis. Goldstein et al. reported that normal human fibroblasts enable melanoma cells to induce angiogenesis in a three-dimensional collagen gel embedded with melanoma cells alone and a fibroblast type I collagen model [46]. Mechanistically, bFGF-induced host stromal reaction during initial tumor growth promotes progression of mouse melanoma via VEGF-dependent neovascularization [47].

In summary, MAFs enhance melanoma invasion and angiogenesis to promote melanoma metastasis. Whether MAFs play a role in other steps of metastasis, such as lymphatic metastasis or metastasis to specific organs, remains poorly understood. Future studies on how fibroblasts affect different steps of metastasis process are warranted.

1.2.5   Fibroblasts Inhibit Antitumor Immunity

The studies on how MAFs affect antitumor immunity remain poorly defined. It has been found that fibroblasts derived from metastatic melanomas significantly suppress NK cell-mediated antitumor activity including cytotoxicity and cytokine production, but fibroblasts from normal tissues do not exert this function. Mechanistically, melanoma-derived fibroblasts inhibit the IL-2-induced upregulation of the surface expression of activated NK cell receptors including NKp44, NKp30, and DNAM1, as well as the increased production of cytolytic granules. Induction of DNAM is cell-to-cell contact dependent, and induction of expression of NKp44 and NKp30 is dependent on prostaglandin E2 (PGE2) produced by fibroblasts [48]. It has been reported that fibroblasts produce immune-suppressing factors, such as COX-2, PD-L1, and PD-L2, which are upregulated by BRAF-mutant melanoma cell-produced interleukin-1 (IL-1) [49]. Because many tumor cells also express PD-L1, whether fibroblast-produced PD-L1 and/or PD-L2 play a dominant role remains to be determined.

1.2.6   Targeting MAFs

Because MAFs play an important role in promoting tumor growth, survival, angiogenesis, immune suppression, and metastasis, MAFs have become a legitimate target for melanoma therapy. Many strategies have been developed for targeting MAFs. The ideal targets might be the molecules that are specifically expressed by both tumor cells and MAFs. Below are some strategies that have been developed in recent years.

1. *Small molecular inhibitor*: Hyaluronan, produced by both melanoma cells and fibroblasts, promotes melanoma growth and metastasis. Therefore, targeting hyaluronan should inhibit tumor growth and metastasis. Indeed, 4-methylumbelliferone (4-MU), a compound that inhibits hyaluronan synthesis in both fibroblasts and melanoma cells, inhibits melanoma cell growth [50]. However, the inhibitory effect on tumor growth by 4-MU is not striking.

A combination with current targeted therapy or immune therapy may increase the anti-melanoma activity of 4-MU.

2. *Oncolytic adenovirus*: The conditionally replicative oncolytic adenovirus (CRAd) has been shown to have antitumor activity when used alone or in combination with chemotherapy or radiotherapy. This type of virus also shows a favorable safety profile [51, 52]. Viale and colleagues reported that a new construction of CRAd can target both fibroblasts and melanoma cells. The CRAd showed potent antitumor activity and eliminated all tumors in a xenograft model of tumor cells cocultured with fibroblasts [53].

3. *Immune therapy*: The aforementioned FSP1 is a specific marker for MAFs, and FSP1 is also expressed in tumor cells including melanoma cells, but at very low levels in normal fibroblasts and other nonmalignant cells. FSP1 can enhance tumor growth and metastasis, as well as suppress immune functions [54]. Therefore, FSP1 appears an attractive target for MAFs. Targeting FSP1 with immunization against FSP1 using dendritic cells transfected with FSP1 mRNA significantly inhibits melanoma cell growth in a mouse model. Side effects appear mild with a small delay in wound healing in immunized mice [55]. In agreement with this finding, an oral DNA vaccine specifically targeting FSP1 suppresses tumor growth and metastasis in murine colon and breast carcinoma through induction of CD8+ T cell-mediated killing of tumor-associated fibroblasts. More importantly, this vaccine markedly enhances antitumor activity of chemotherapy, providing a rationale for the combination of chemotherapy with targeting tumor-associated fibroblasts [56]. Targeting FSP1 using T cells genetically engineered with FAP-reactive chimeric antigen receptors (CARs) only has a moderate inhibitory effect on tumor growth in mice, but causes severe side effects with induction of significant cachexia and lethal bone toxicities. Further studies indicated that bone marrow stromal cells express high level of FSP, and elimination of these cells accounts for the side effect caused by FSP1-specific CAR T cells [57].

Early phase clinical trials with a humanized antibody (sibrotuzumab) targeting FSP1 [58] in colorectal cancer or an FSP1 enzyme inhibitor in several cancers including lung cancer and colorectal cancer have not shown clinical efficacy [59, 60]. Therefore, it appears that targeting FSP1 alone in melanomas will not achieve meaningful clinical responses in metastatic melanoma patients. More specific targets for fibroblasts should be identified in the future studies. Whether combination of targeting fibroblast therapy with targeted therapy or anti-immune checkpoint will increase the antitumor effect remains unknown. A preclinical experiment will be instructive to test the possibility of using these combinations in melanoma patients. The detailed information of current clinical trials on targeting fibroblasts or both fibroblasts and cancer cells is summarized in Table 1.1.

In summary, MAFs have a profound biological consequence on melanoma growth and metastasis. Targeting fibroblasts might be an option to increase the efficacy of current anti-melanoma therapies.

Table 1.1 Summary of drugs that target fibroblasts

Name	Pathways	Clinical indication	Therapy combination	ClinicalTrials.gov identifier	Phase
N/A	FGF5	Kidney cancer	IL-2	NCT00089778	II
Debio 1347	FGFR1-3	Advanced solid tumors	No	NCT01948297	I
JNJ-42756493	FGFRs	Advanced or refractory solid tumors or lymphoma	No	NCT01703481	I
GSK3052230	FGFR1	Solid tumors	Paclitaxel, carboplatin, or docetaxel	NCT01868022	I
BIBH-1	FAP	Advanced solid tumors	Radiation	NCT00004042	I
Dovitinib	FGFR2	Unresectable gastric cancer with FGFR2 amplification	No	NCT01719549	I
Dovitinib (TKI258)	FGFR3	BCG refractory urothelial carcinoma with FGFR3 mutations or overexpression	No	NCT01732107	II
Dovitinib (TKI258)		Castration-resistant prostate cancer	No	NCT01741116	II
BIBF 1120	FGFRs, VEGFR, PDGFR	Second-line treatment for patients with small cell lung cancer	No	NCT01441297	II
BIBF 1120		Metastatic colorectal cancer		NCT00904839	II
AZD4547	FGFR1	Breast cancer	No	NCT01791985	II
Adoptive T cell transfer	FAP	Malignant pleural mesothelioma	No	NCT01722149	I

Note: FGFRs are also highly expressed in tumor cells. Therefore, above listed agents that are targeting FGFR(s) have dual effects on inhibition of tumor cells, as well as fibroblasts

1.3 Macrophages

Melanoma tumor microenvironment contains all types of inflammatory cells, including macrophages, neutrophils, mast cells, myeloid-derived suppressor cells, dendritic cells, and natural killer cells, T and B cells. Tumor-associated macrophages (TAMs) are another major component of tumor stroma and are the most abundant cell type among the immune cells. TAMs modulate the tumor microenvironment by increasing tumor initiation and growth, remodeling the ECM, promoting angiogenesis, and suppressing antitumor immunity through producing cytokines, chemokines, growth factors, and reactive oxygen and nitrogen species (NOS) [61–64]. TAMs are also attributable to cancer cell resistance to anticancer therapies, such as chemotherapy, immune therapy, radiotherapy, and targeted therapy. The number of macrophages is a prognostic marker for predicting patient responses to antitumor therapies. High numbers of infiltrating macrophages are associated with a poor prognosis in a variety of cancers, including breast cancer and colon cancer, among others [63–65].

Recent studies have indicated that melanomas are highly inflamed tumors and TAMs also provide an inflammatory microenvironment, which plays an essential role in every step of melanoma development. In the following section, we discuss the definition of TAMs, the clinical implications of TAMs, the roles of TAMs in melanoma development, and the potential therapeutic implications for targeting TAMs in melanomas.

1.3.1 Differentiation of Melanoma-Associated Macrophages

Macrophages have been classified as "activated macrophages" (M1 macrophages) and "alternatively activated macrophages" (M2 macrophages), largely based on the microenvironment cue. M1 macrophages are polarized by microbial agents such as bacterial lipopolysaccharide (LPS), as well as pro-inflammatory factors such as IFN-γ. M1 macrophages produce a lower level of immunosuppressive cytokine IL-10 and higher levels of IL-12, IL-6, TNF-α, nitric oxide (NO), and reactive oxygen species (ROS). Conversely, M2 macrophages are polarized by anti-inflammatory molecules, such as glucocorticoid hormones, IL-4, IL-10, and IL-13. M2 macrophages produce higher levels of IL-10, TGF-β, IL-1 receptor antagonist (IL-1ra), CCL-1, CCL-18, and CCL-22 and lower levels of IL-12. It is generally accepted that TAMs resemble M2 macrophages and exert pro-tumor activity. However, recent studies indicated that many growth factors produced by M1 macrophages have potent effects on promoting tumor growth and metastasis, such as TNF-α and IL-6. Therefore, this characterization of M1 and M2 macrophages is oversimplified and does not reflect the complexity of TAMs.

TAMs are differentiated from monocytes. Tumor cells produce chemokines, cytokines, and growth factors to recruit blood monocytes to the tumor site, where monocytes are stimulated by tumor-derived growth factors and cytokines to differentiate into TAMs [66–68]. Experimentally, TAMs can be differentiated from peripheral blood monocytes by factors secreted from tumor cells and stromal cells [61]. A major factor that differentiates monocytes to TAMs is M-CSF. Solinas et al. reported that pancreatic cancer-conditioned medium (PCM) was able to differentiate monocytes to PCM-induced macrophages (PCMI-Mϕ), which depends on the tumor-produced M-CSF. Neutralization of M-CSF totally inhibited PCMI-Mϕ differentiation [69]. However, other tumor-produced cytokines, chemokines, and growth factors, such as VEGFA, CCL-2, IL-6, leukocyte inhibitory factor (LIF), and GM-CSF, have also been reported to involve the differentiation of monocytes to macrophages [66, 70–73].

In order to better characterize TAMs in melanoma, we have developed a highly efficient in vitro model to differentiate monocytes to macrophages with modified melanoma-conditioned medium (MCM). This effect appears not only dependent on M-CSF, since neutralization of M-CSF signaling with a monoclonal antibody only partially affects the differentiation of macrophages, but also dependent on melanoma cell-produced cytokines and growth factors, such as VEGF, GM-CSF, IL-6, LIF, etc. Characterization of these macrophages indicated that they express both M1 and M2 macrophage markers. Functionally, they suppress antigen-specific T cell immune responses and increase tumor cell invasion. Supporting this, several studies indicated that melanoma-associated macrophages (MAMs) are highly heterogeneous and have mixed phenotypes of M1 and M2 macrophages [74]. Microarray analysis revealed that many genes associated with melanoma cell invasion and metastasis are upregulated, such as CCL-2 and MMP-9. Blockade of both CCL-2 and MMP-9 is necessary to reverse macrophage-mediated melanoma cell invasion. Finally, we validated several less studied or unknown markers of TAMs in human melanoma tissues, such as the proinvasion gene, glycoprotein nonmetastatic melanoma protein B (GPNMB), CD7, deafness, autosomal dominant 5 (DFNA5), and metallothionein ([75] and unpublished data). These data indicated our model is highly relevant to TAMs in melanomas and provides a valuable tool to further understand the roles of interaction between melanoma cells and TAMs in melanoma progression and metastasis.

1.3.2   TAMs as a Biomarker for Melanoma Prognosis

Macrophages are the most abundant leukocytes in melanoma lesions [76]. Although early reports suggested that infiltrating macrophages result in tumor regression [76], later studies demonstrated that the increased number of TAMs infiltrating in melanoma was associated with poor prognosis [77–80]. Jessen et al. reported that the number of macrophages in melanoma tissues has been reported to correlate with poor prognosis in early-stage melanomas (stage I or II) [81]. In addition, high macrophage counts were significantly associated with markers of aggressive disease, such as Breslow thickness, ulceration and mitotic rate, lymphatic vessel invasion, and high microvessel density [82]. In accordance with this, other studies support the potential roles of macrophages in melanoma invasion and metastasis. Varney et al. reported that the level of TAM density was significantly higher in thick than thin melanomas and positively correlated with melanoma invasiveness and metastasis [80]. Additionally, the presence of CD163-positive infiltrating macrophages correlates with metastasis formation [83]. Of note, macrophages are also present in nevi tissues in addition to primary and metastatic melanomas [84]. Therefore, TAMs appear to be involved in every stage of melanoma development and metastasis, and the amount of TAMs can be used as a prognostic marker for melanomas.

1.3.3 TAMs Promote Melanomagenesis

Ultraviolet radiation (UVR) is one of the major risk factors for melanoma development, particularly during childhood. However, the mechanisms by which UVR leads to the development of melanoma are not fully understood. Several reports indicate that macrophages are essential for UV radiation-induced melanomagenesis. A notable study by Zaidi et al. in neonatal mice using the HGF/scatter factor transgenic mouse model indicated a single dose treatment of UVB significantly increases recruitment of macrophages to the skin in a CCR2-dependent manner. Macrophages then activate IFN-γ-related signaling in melanocytes to increase the numbers of melanocytes; blockade of IFN-γ signaling with an anti-IFN-γ antibody diminishes macrophage-mediated activation of melanocytes [85]. In support of this study, Handoko et al. indicated that a single dose of UVB treatment on neonatal mice results in an increase in the number of melanocytes in the epidermis, as well as F4/80-positive macrophages in the epidermal layer. Depletion of macrophages with clodronate liposome treatment reversed macrophage-mediated increase in melanocyte numbers. However, unlike Zaidi's study, Handoko et al. found that recruitment of macrophages by UVB treatment is not dependent on CCR2 signaling and IL-17 is one of the factors that confers macrophage-mediated activation of melanocytes upon UVB treatment [86]. The discrepancy is likely attributable to the differences in postnatal timing of UVB treatment, the time between UVB exposure and melanocyte counting, mouse strains, and the methods used to block IFN-γ signaling. Importantly, UVR exposure was found to induce an increase in macrophages in the human skin, which may result in an increase in melanocytes and contribute to the immunosuppressive phenotype [87]. Our own study demonstrates that macrophages also protect UVA-induced apoptosis of human melanocytes by activation of the MAPK pathway (unpublished data). Collectively, these studies provide a strong link between macrophages and melanocyte response, suggesting that macrophages might be a target for preventing UVR-induced melanoma [88].

1.3.4 Macrophages Promote Angiogenesis and Metastasis

Like CAFs, TAMs also produce a plethora of proteinases, such as urokinase-type plasminogen activator receptor (uPAR) and MMP-9, which play critical roles in melanoma invasion and metastasis through degradation of ECM and modulation of tissue remodeling [89]. TAMs also produce many growth factors, cytokines, and chemokines to promote melanoma angiogenesis, including TNF-α, IL-1α, and CCL-2, among others. Targeting TAMs by blockade of these cytokines and chemokines inhibits melanoma angiogenesis and growth in a mouse xenograft model [65, 90].

1.3.5 Immunosuppression

The number of TAMs is negatively correlated with antitumor immune responses in melanoma. It has been reported that high numbers of CD64-positive macrophages in tumor biopsies had a statistically significant association with poor response to IL-2-based immunotherapy [91]. Furthermore, macrophages isolated from metastatic lymph nodes of patients with malignant melanoma downregulate levels of CD3 zeta and CD16 zeta expression in autologous peripheral blood T cells and NK cells, respectively. Coculturing activated monocytes impairs calcium mobilization in peripheral blood-derived T cells when stimulated with monoclonal antibodies to CD3 and also strongly inhibits melanoma-specific cytotoxic T lymphocyte (CTL) activity and NK activity [92]. Our study has demonstrated that macrophages produce CCL-17 and CCL-22, which increase recruitment of T regulatory cells (Tregs, formerly known as suppressor T cells) through CCR4 expressed on Tregs [93]. Macrophage-derived TNF-α is attributable to melanoma resistance to adoptive T cell transfer therapies (ACT) through downregulation of T cell-specific antigens recognized by T cells [94]. Finally, macrophages produce high amounts of immune checkpoint molecule, PD-L1, which inhibits anticancer T cell responses through PD-1, a co-inhibitory receptor expressed on activated T cells. Several clinical trials indicated targeting PD-1 significantly increases patient survival in melanoma patients.

1.3.6 Humanized Mouse Model to Study Biology of Macrophages

Macrophages promote melanoma development by multiple mechanisms. However, studies on interaction between macrophages and tumor cells were hammered by the difference between mouse and human macrophages, especially for preclinical mouse tumor xenograft model, in which tumor cells were implanted into immunodeficient mice. For example, mouse macrophages have high NO synthase (NOS) activity, while human macrophages have relative lower activity of NOS [95]. To overcome this, a humanized mouse model has been developed, which shows promise to study the human immune system in vivo. However, macrophages that differentiated from human CD34-positive hematopoietic stem cells in the mouse bone marrow environment are poorly developed and do not have functions of human macrophages. Dr. Flavell's group has developed two novel humanized models to study the functions of human macrophages. Using knockin technology, human M-CSF and IL-3/GM-CSF were introduced into Rag2$^{-/-}$/IL-2rg$^{-/-}$ immunodeficient mice. Mice were then injected with human CD34+ hematopoietic stem cells. Both models demonstrated high yield of human macrophages. Macrophages from humanized IL-3/GM-CSF knockin mice are mainly present in the lung tissues and can mount human macrophage responses against human influenza virus infection. Macrophages from humanized M-CSF mice are present in multiple tissues, including the bone marrow, spleen, peripheral blood, lung, liver, and peritoneal cavity. These macrophages exert migration and phagocytosis functions, as well as response to LPS stimulation. Since M-CSF-differentiated macrophages have been proposed as pro-tumor M2 macrophages and humanized M-CSF macrophages are present in multiple tissues, a humanized M-CSF mouse model may be an appropriate experimental melanoma model for studying the roles of macrophages in melanoma development.

1.3.7   Targeting Macrophages for Melanoma Therapy

Because of the multifunctions of macrophages on promoting tumor progression and metastasis, many approaches have been developed to target macrophages for studying the mechanisms of macrophages on tumor development and to treat tumor patients.

Liposome-Based Assay A liposome is an artificially prepared vesicle structure composed of a bilayer of phospholipid. Drugs loaded in liposome can be recognized and phagocytosed by macrophages. Therefore, loading drugs into liposomes provides an efficient means of targeting macrophages. In addition, the structure of liposomes can avoid rapid degradation of chemotherapy agents in the serum and have less toxicity than regular chemotherapy reagents [96]. Liposome-encapsulated clodronate (LIP-CLOD) sulfate induces macrophage apoptosis and is a commonly used agent to deplete macrophages in animal models. Experimentally, deletion of macrophages with the LIP-CLOD significantly inhibits angiogenesis and melanoma growth in a human melanoma xenograft model [90]. In agreement with this, Banciu et al. showed that the antitumor growth effect of liposomal prednisolone phosphate is dependent on the deletion of TAMs in a mouse B16 melanoma model [97]. Clinical trials have shown that liposomal-based chemotherapeutic agents have better clinical efficacy. A combination of liposome-encapsulated doxorubicin (LD)

Table 1.2 Summary of drugs that target macrophages

Name	Pathways	Clinical indication	Therapy combination	ClinicalTrials.gov identifier	Phase
PLX3397	M-CSFR	Metastatic breast cancer	Eribulin	NCT01596751	I/II
		Advanced solid tumors	Paclitaxel	NCT01525602	I
		Advanced castration-resistant prostate cancer		NCT01499043	II
		Unresectable or metastatic melanoma	Vemurafenib	NCT01826448	I
		Glioblastoma	Temozolomide and radiation	NCT01790503	I/II
		Recurrent glioblastoma		NCT01349036	II
		Solid tumors		NCT01004861	I
AMG 820	M-CSFR	Advanced solid tumors	No	NCT01444404	I
ARRY-382	M-CSFR	Advanced solid tumors	No	NCT01316822	I

with docetaxel and trastuzumab has been used in a phase II clinical trial for treating stages II and IIIA human HER2-overexpressing breast cancer patients. The combination therapy has better patient responses and fewer cardiotoxicity. However, whether the combination efficacy is dependent on the targeting macrophages or the improvement of delivery system remains unknown.

CCL-2 Inhibitor CCL-2 is the most potent chemoattractant for monocytes/macrophages and plays critical roles in macrophage differentiation and survival. Several studies indicated that targeting CCL-2 in combination with other anticancer therapies might be used for melanoma therapy. Bindarit, a small molecule that inhibits the LPS-induced MCP-1 expression and blocks CCL-2-induced inflammation, significantly inhibits melanoma progression in preclinical model [90]. A recent study also indicated that the antitumor activity of BRAF inhibitors is associated with their ability to decrease the expression of CCL-2, and combination therapy with BRAFi and an anti-CCL-2 antibody has a synergistic effect on reducing tumor growth in mouse melanoma xenograft and de novo tumorigenesis models [98].

M-CSF Receptor Inhibitor M-CSF is highly expressed in melanoma cell lines, as well as melanoma-associated macrophages. M-CSF is the most potent growth factor that activates multiple survival signaling pathways for macrophages through binding M-CSF receptor (M-CSFR). Several M-CSFR inhibitors are now in the clinical trials for advanced or metastatic solid cancers, including melanomas. M-CSFR inhibitor ARRY-382 is now in phase I clinical trial for treating solid tumors (ClinicalTrials.gov Identifier: NCT01316822). Anti-M-CSFR antibody, IMC-CS4 from Lilly (NCT01346358), and AMG 820 from Amgen (NCT01444404) are also in clinical trials for advanced solid tumors. A study from our lab demonstrated that macrophages confer melanoma resistance to BRAF inhibitors, and targeting macrophages with an M-CSF receptor, GW2580, significantly increases the antitumor activity of BRAFi in a mouse xenograft model. Accordingly, an M-CSFRi, PLX3397 developed by Plexxikon Inc., increases the antitumor activity of BRAF inhibitor in a BRAF-mutant colon cancer xenograft model. Based on this finding, a phase I clinical trial with the combination of vemurafenib with PLX3397 in BRAF-mutant melanoma patients is under way. In addition, combination therapy with chemotherapy and PLX3397 is now also in the clinical trial for breast cancer and other types of solid cancers. These clinical trials (summarized in Table 1.2), if successful, will switch the current focus of cancer therapy from tumor cells to both cancer cells and tumor microenvironment.

1.3.8   Myeloid-Derived Suppressor Cells

Of note, another population of myeloid cells, myeloid-derived suppressor cells (MDSCs), is phenotypically and functionally similar to TAMs. MDSCs are composed of a mixed heterogeneous population of early myeloid progenitors, immature granulocytes, macrophages, and dendritic cells at different stages of differentiation. MDSCs express many similar markers with TAMs. The major difference is human macrophages express CD11c, and MHC-II, but MDSCs do not express these molecules. Interested readers can further learn about this topic in some excellent reviews.

1.3.9   Cross Talk Between MAFs and Macrophages

In addition, the cross talk between tumor cells and stromal cells and interaction between stromal cells occur in the tumor microenvironment, which in turn affects tumor development. Erez et al. demonstrated that tumor cells educate fibroblast to produce pro-inflammatory cytokines and chemokines, which promote macrophage recruitment, angiogenesis, and tumor growth in an NF-κB-dependent manner [99]. Accordingly, melanoma cells also induce fibroblasts to produce multiple chemokines, such as CCL2, IL-8, CXCL1, and CXCL3 [25, 100]. All of these factors increase the infiltration of immune cells, including macrophages. These factors also have direct roles on melanoma growth. For example, IL-8 can increase melanoma cell tumor growth and metastasis. A recent study from Samaniego indicated that CD90-positive fibroblasts surrounding peri-tumoral vessels secrete CCL-2 to recruit

CCR2-positive leukocytes at the tumor periphery in a preclinical melanoma model [101]. The interaction between macrophages and CAFs is reciprocal. In prostate cancer, macrophages increase the effect of epithelial-mesenchymal transition of fibroblasts, leading to their enhanced reactivity. Conversely, CAFs increase monocyte recruitment toward tumor site and promote monocyte differentiation into TAMs. Therefore, CAFs and TAMs synergize to promote tumor progression [102]. However, whether these phenotypic changes occur in melanomas remains unknown.

1.4 Hypoxic Tumor Microenvironment

In vivo oxygen levels range from roughly 2–3 % in the brain, liver, and myocardium, 9–10 % in the spleen, up to 13–14 % in the alveoli of the lung. In the skin, normal oxygen levels range from 1.5 to 5 % O_2. Such oxygen concentration in the skin is sufficient for the stabilization of HIF-1α [103]. Under normal conditions, melanocytes in the dermal-epidermal junction are physiologically hypoxic, and hypoxia is crucial for melanocyte transformation [103]. Malignant tumors rapidly outgrow their blood supplies, resulting in uneven distribution of vasculature [4]. Hypoxia is invariably present in solid tumors when malignant tumor size is more than 1 mm in diameter. As a result, pockets of hypoxic regions can be visualized by immunohistochemistry with either antibodies to pimonidazole [5] or CAIX [104]. Under normoxic conditions, prolyl hydroxylase domain protein 2 (PHD2) constitutively prolyl hydroxylates HIF-α in a site-specific manner. This allows for binding of the von Hippel-Lindau (VHL) protein, a component of an E3 ubiquitin ligase complex that targets HIF-α for degradation. Under hypoxia, this modification, which is inherently oxygen-dependent, is attenuated, thereby allowing HIF-α to escape degradation and activate genes involved in cellular, local, and systemic adaptation to hypoxia. There are two main isoforms of HIF-α, HIF-1α and HIF-2α. HIF-1α and HIF-2α are transcription factors that have common transcriptional targets, including genes involved in angiogenesis, invasion, and metastasis [105]. However, they also regulate distinct subsets of genes during hypoxia. For example, genes activated by HIF-1α alone are involved in glycolysis and apoptosis [106–108], whereas genes activated by HIF-2α alone include the SCF Oct4 [109] and ABCG2 [110]. The observation that nuclear HIF-1α is detected in the normal skin suggests that HIF-1α is activated in melanocytes, which is consistent with the finding that HIF-1α is an MITF transcriptional target in melanocytes [111].

1.4.1 Hypoxia and Melanoma Initiation and Progression

Hypoxia has broad effects on tumor cells, and it is known to induce tumor resistance to both chemo- and radiation therapies [6]. Hypoxia promotes genetic instability [112], favors growth of hypoxia-tolerant tumor cell clones [113], encourages growth of cells with attenuated function of the TP53 tumor suppressor [114], and reduces drug-induced apoptosis [115].

There have been increasing numbers of studies about the role of HIFs in melanoma progression, metastasis, and chemotherapy resistance. Melanocytes are more prone to oncogenic transformation when grown in a hypoxic microenvironment, and this is in part due to stabilization of HIF-1α, because HIF-1α-deficient melanocytes grown in hypoxic conditions show a diminished transformation capacity and delayed tumor growth in vivo. On the other hand, the expression of a nondegradable form of HIF-1α protein leads to transformation of cells in normoxic conditions and to the growth of very aggressive melanomas [41]. These observations suggest that the low oxygen microenvironment in the skin, by enabling HIF-1α stabilization, provides a permissive environment in which HIF-1α acts as tumor promoter in cells that are genetically unstable and have acquired oncogenic mutations.

Erythropoietin, a potent cytoprotective cytokine increasing cell survival under hypoxic conditions, promotes melanoma cell survival by activating AKT-dependent signaling pathway [116]. HIF-1α is necessary for the AKT-mediated transformation of melanocytes [117]. Widmer et al. found that hypoxia influences driving metastatic progression by promoting a switch from a proliferative to an invasive phenotype in melanoma cells [118]. The exposure of proliferative melanoma cells to hypoxic microenvironment downregulates melanocytic marker expression and increases their invasive potential in an HIF-1α-dependent manner [118]. HIF-1α and HIF-2α are also found to drive melanoma invasion and invadopodium formation through PDGFRα and focal adhesion kinase-mediated activation of SRC and by coordinating ECM degradation in *Pten*-deficient, *Braf*-mutant mouse model [119]. These studies suggest that hypoxia induces invasiveness and metastasis in melanoma cells.

Furthermore, we found that oncogenic BRAF^{V600E} mutation increases HIF-1α expression and melanoma survival under hypoxic conditions, which suggests that effects of the oncogenic BRAF^{V600E} mutation may be partially mediated through HIF-1α pathway [120]. Also, we found that hypoxia increased melanoma cells migration and drug resistance, accompanied by increased Snail and decreased E-cadherin expression [121]. Hypoxia upregulates *Snail* expression via HIF-2α and leads to increased metastatic capacity and drug resistance in melanoma cells. Solid tumors, including melanoma, with hypoxic regions have a poorer prognosis than their well-oxygenated counterparts, independent of treatment [122, 123]. Both HIF-1α and HIF-2α are overexpressed in melanoma [124]. In conclusion, hypoxia in tumor microenvironments plays important roles in melanoma progression and treatment resistance.

1.4.2 Targeting Hypoxic Tumor Cells for Treatment

The increased resistance of *hypoxic* cells to all forms of cancer therapy presents a major barrier to the successful treatment of most solid tumors. Despite early promise in cancer treatment, antiangiogenic therapies have only provided modest benefits in delaying tumor progression and have not translated into prolongation of overall survival time. Recent evidences demonstrate that VEGF inhibitors have the paradoxical enhancement of tumor progression by generating a more aggressive tumor phenotype [7, 125, 126]. Among the observed mechanisms demonstrated to abrogate sensitivity to antiangiogenic therapy is the observation that VEGF inhibitor therapy induces hypoxia-dependent alterations in gene expression resulting in an *increase* in the invasive and/or metastatic capabilities of different tumor types [8, 126–128]. These findings argue that hypoxia triggers an adaptive response by which tumor cells that culminates in their capacity to evade unfavorable environments and metastasize to other sites. These observations further underscore the significance of targeting hypoxic tumor cells to inhibit tumor progression.

Hypoxia-activated prodrugs (HAPs) target regions of tumor hypoxia within tumor cells. HAPs may offer the potential, alone and in combination with conventional chemotherapy, of improving cancer therapy. There are several companies developing HAPs: Novacea, Inc., Proacta Inc., and Threshold Pharmaceuticals, Inc. These companies are developing the following drug candidates: AQ4N (Novacea), PR-104 (Proacta), and TH-302 (Threshold Pharmaceuticals).

TH-302 is a 2-nitroimidazole-triggered HAP. Under hypoxic conditions, TH-302 releases bromo-isophosphoramide mustard (Br-IPM), which induces DNA cross-linking [129]. Preclinical models demonstrate that TH-302 exhibits hypoxia-dependent activation and a broad spectrum of hypoxia-dependent cytotoxicity across many different human cancer cell lines [130]. Phase I clinical trials have determined the safety and tolerability of TH-302 in different human cancers and even demonstrated a partial response in a patient with metastatic melanoma [131, 132]. It is recently shown that TH-302-induced DNA damage as measured by γH2AX was initially only present in the hypoxic regions and then radiated to the entire tumor in a time-dependent manner, consistent with TH-302 having a "bystander effect" [133]. The study also showed a strong correlation between the magnitude of tumor hypoxia as measured by pimonidazole staining and TH-302 efficacy, suggesting that pimonidazole staining patient biopsies may be useful as a biomarker to select patients for TH-302 treatment. In summary, HAPs may represent a novel class of drug to eliminate hypoxic treatment-resistant tumor cells.

1.5 Summary and Future Outlook

Recently, a shift has been put in motion from conventional chemotherapy to targeted therapies, spurred by our advanced understanding of cancer genetics. Understanding the biology of tumor microenvironment will contribute extensively to this shift and is thus an exciting avenue of cancer research in the coming years. Already, clinical trials targeting tumor microenvironment are under way. If successful, the results have the potential to change the current paradigm of cancer therapy, changing the focus from specific alteration in protein-coding oncogenes or tumor suppressor genes—which may be difficult to treat—to therapies focused on tumor-stromal cells.

The combinations of these two treatments are more likely to induce sustained and complete clinical responses.

Acknowledgement The work is supported by NIH grants (AR054593, CA25874, CA114046)

References

1. Li G, Satyamoorthy K, Meier F, Berking C, Bogenrieder T, Herlyn M (2003) Function and regulation of melanoma-stromal fibroblast interactions: when seeds meet soil. Oncogene 22:3162–3171
2. Kondo T, Hearing VJ (2011) Update on the regulation of mammalian melanocyte function and skin pigmentation. Expert Rev Dermatol 6:97–108
3. Hockel M, Schlenger K, Aral B, Mitze M, Schaffer U, Vaupel P (1996) Association between tumor hypoxia and malignant progression in advanced cancer of the uterine cervix. Cancer Res 56:4509–4515
4. Wachsberger P, Burd R, Dicker AP (2003) Tumor response to ionizing radiation combined with antiangiogenesis or vascular targeting agents: exploring mechanisms of interaction. Clin Cancer Res 9:1957–1971
5. Post DE, Devi NS, Li Z et al (2004) Cancer therapy with a replicating oncolytic adenovirus targeting the hypoxic microenvironment of tumors. Clin Cancer Res 10:8603–8612
6. Harrison L, Blackwell K (2004) Hypoxia and anemia: factors in decreased sensitivity to radiation therapy and chemotherapy? Oncologist 9(Suppl 5):31–40
7. Bikfalvi A, Moenner M, Javerzat S, North S, Hagedorn M (2011) Inhibition of angiogenesis and the angiogenesis/invasion shift. Biochem Soc Trans 39:1560–1564
8. Paez-Ribes M, Allen E, Hudock J et al (2009) Antiangiogenic therapy elicits malignant progression of tumors to increased local invasion and distant metastasis. Cancer Cell 15:220–231
9. Yamaguchi Y, Brenner M, Hearing VJ (2007) The regulation of skin pigmentation. J Biol Chem 282:27557–27561
10. Andersen K, Nesland JM, Holm R, Florenes VA, Fodstad O, Maelandsmo GM (2004) Expression of S100A4 combined with reduced E-cadherin expression predicts patient outcome in malignant melanoma. Mod Pathol 17:990–997
11. Huber MA, Kraut N, Park JE et al (2003) Fibroblast activation protein: differential expression and serine protease activity in reactive stromal fibroblasts of melanocytic skin tumors. J Invest Dermatol 120:182–188
12. Faraone D, Aguzzi MS, Toietta G et al (2009) Platelet-derived growth factor-receptor alpha strongly inhibits melanoma growth in vitro and in vivo. Neoplasia 11:732–742
13. Okamoto-Inoue M, Nakayama J, Hori Y, Taniguchi S (2000) Human malignant melanoma cells release a factor that inhibits the expression of smooth muscle alpha-actin. J Dermatol Sci 23:170–177
14. Tsukamoto H, Mishima Y, Hayashibe K, Sasase A (1992) Alpha-smooth muscle actin expression in tumor and stromal cells of benign and malignant human pigment cell tumors. J Invest Dermatol 98:116–120
15. Anderberg C, Pietras K (2009) On the origin of cancer-associated fibroblasts. Cell Cycle 8:1461–1462
16. Kalluri R, Zeisberg M (2006) Fibroblasts in cancer. Nat Rev Cancer 6:392–401
17. Xing F, Saidou J, Watabe K (2010) Cancer associated fibroblasts (CAFs) in tumor microenvironment. Front Biosci 15:166–179
18. Wandel E, Grasshoff A, Mittag M, Haustein UF, Saalbach A (2000) Fibroblasts surrounding melanoma express elevated levels of matrix metalloproteinase-1 (MMP-1) and intercellular adhesion molecule-1 (ICAM-1) in vitro. Exp Dermatol 9:34–41

19. Wandel E, Raschke A, Hildebrandt G et al (2002) Fibroblasts enhance the invasive capacity of melanoma cells in vitro. Arch Dermatol Res 293:601–608

20. Loffek S, Zigrino P, Angel P, Anwald B, Krieg T, Mauch C (2005) High invasive melanoma cells induce matrix metalloproteinase-1 synthesis in fibroblasts by interleukin-1alpha and basic fibroblast growth factor-mediated mechanisms. J Invest Dermatol 124:638–643

21. Kanekura T, Chen X, Kanzaki T (2002) Basigin (CD147) is expressed on melanoma cells and induces tumor cell invasion by stimulating production of matrix metalloproteinases by fibroblasts. Int J Cancer 99:520–528

22. Adam B, Toth L, Pasti G, Balazs M, Adany R (2006) Contact stimulation of fibroblasts for tenascin production by melanoma cells. Melanoma Res 16:385–391

23. Anderberg C, Li H, Fredriksson L et al (2009) Paracrine signaling by platelet-derived growth factor-CC promotes tumor growth by recruitment of cancer-associated fibroblasts. Cancer Res 69:369–378

24. Guan S, Fan J, Han A, Chen M, Woodley DT, Li W (2009) Non-compensating roles between Nckalpha and Nckbeta in PDGF-BB signaling to promote human dermal fibroblast migration. J Invest Dermatol 129:1909–1920

25. Li L, Dragulev B, Zigrino P, Mauch C, Fox JW (2009) The invasive potential of human melanoma cell lines correlates with their ability to alter fibroblast gene expression in vitro and the stromal microenvironment in vivo. Int J Cancer 125:1796–1804

26. Gartner MF, Wilson EL, Dowdle EB (1992) Fibroblast-dependent tumorigenicity of melanoma xenografts in athymic mice. Int J Cancer 51:788–791

27. Cornil I, Theodorescu D, Man S, Herlyn M, Jambrosic J, Kerbel RS (1991) Fibroblast cell interactions with human melanoma cells affect tumor cell growth as a function of tumor progression. Proc Natl Acad Sci USA 88:6028–6032

28. Satyamoorthy K, Li G, Vaidya B, Patel D, Herlyn M (2001) Insulin-like growth factor-1 induces survival and growth of biologically early melanoma cells through both the mitogen-activated protein kinase and beta-catenin pathways. Cancer Res 61:7318–7324

29. Otsuka T, Takayama H, Sharp R et al (1998) c-Met autocrine activation induces development of malignant melanoma and acquisition of the metastatic phenotype. Cancer Res 58:5157–5167

30. Willenberg A, Saalbach A, Simon JC, Anderegg U (2012) Melanoma cells control HA synthesis in peritumoral fibroblasts via PDGF-AA and PDGF-CC: impact on melanoma cell proliferation. J Invest Dermatol 132:385–393

31. Pasonen-Seppanen S, Takabe P, Edward M et al (2012) Melanoma cell-derived factors stimulate hyaluronan synthesis in dermal fibroblasts by upregulating HAS2 through PDGFR-PI3K-AKT and p38 signaling. Histochem Cell Biol 138:895–911

32. Abety AN, Fox JW, Schonefuss A et al (2012) Stromal fibroblast-specific expression of ADAM-9 modulates proliferation and apoptosis in melanoma cells in vitro and in vivo. J Invest Dermatol 132:2451–2458

33. Guaiquil V, Swendeman S, Yoshida T, Chavala S, Campochiaro PA, Blobel CP (2009) ADAM9 is involved in pathological retinal neovascularization. Mol Cell Biol 29:2694–2703

34. John JK, Paraiso KH, Rebecca VW et al (2012) GSK3beta inhibition blocks melanoma cell/host interactions by downregulating N-cadherin expression and decreasing FAK phosphorylation. J Invest Dermatol 132:2818–2827

35. Bar J, Feniger-Barish R, Lukashchuk N et al (2009) Cancer cells suppress p53 in adjacent fibroblasts. Oncogene 28:933–936

36. Addadi Y, Moskovits N, Granot D et al (2010) p53 status in stromal fibroblasts modulates tumor growth in an SDF1-dependent manner. Cancer Res 70:9650–9658

37. Lujambio A, Akkari L, Simon J et al (2013) Non-cell-autonomous tumor suppression by p53. Cell 153:449–460

38. Box NF, Terzian T (2008) The role of p53 in pigmentation, tanning and melanoma. Pigment Cell Melanoma Res 21:525–533

39. Nguyen DX, Bos PD, Massague J (2009) Metastasis: from dissemination to organ-specific colonization. Nat Rev Cancer 9:274–284

40. Orgaz JL, Sanz-Moreno V (2013) Emerging molecular targets in melanoma invasion and metastasis. Pigment Cell Melanoma Res 26:39–57
41. Bedogni B, Powell MB (2009) Hypoxia, melanocytes and melanoma – survival and tumor development in the permissive microenvironment of the skin. Pigment Cell Melanoma Res 22:166–174
42. Ntayi C, Hornebeck W, Bernard P (2003) Influence of cultured dermal fibroblasts on human melanoma cell proliferation, matrix metalloproteinase-2 (MMP-2) expression and invasion in vitro. Arch Dermatol Res 295:236–241
43. Zigrino P, Kuhn I, Bauerle T et al (2009) Stromal expression of MMP-13 is required for melanoma invasion and metastasis. J Invest Dermatol 129:2686–2693
44. Ulmer A, Korber V, Schmid H, Fierlbeck G (1998) Increased activity of cathepsin B in fibroblasts isolated from primary melanoma in comparison to fibroblasts from normal skin. Exp Dermatol 7:14–17
45. Yin M, Soikkeli J, Jahkola T, Virolainen S, Saksela O, Holtta E (2012) TGF-beta signaling, activated stromal fibroblasts, and cysteine cathepsins B and L drive the invasive growth of human melanoma cells. Am J Pathol 181:2202–2216
46. Goldstein LJ, Chen H, Bauer RJ, Bauer SM, Velazquez OC (2005) Normal human fibroblasts enable melanoma cells to induce angiogenesis in type I collagen. Surgery 138:439–449
47. Tsunoda S, Nakamura T, Sakurai H, Saiki I (2007) Fibroblast growth factor-2-induced host stroma reaction during initial tumor growth promotes progression of mouse melanoma via vascular endothelial growth factor A-dependent neovascularization. Cancer Sci 98:541–548
48. Balsamo M, Scordamaglia F, Pietra G et al (2009) Melanoma-associated fibroblasts modulate NK cell phenotype and anti-tumor cytotoxicity. Proc Natl Acad Sci USA 106:20847–20852
49. Khalili JS, Liu S, Rodriguez-Cruz TG et al (2012) Oncogenic BRAF(V600E) promotes stromal cell-mediated immunosuppression via induction of interleukin-1 in melanoma. Clin Cancer Res 18:5329–5340
50. Edward M, Quinn JA, Pasonen-Seppanen SM, McCann BA, Tammi RH (2010) 4-Methylumbelliferone inhibits tumour cell growth and the activation of stromal hyaluronan synthesis by melanoma cell-derived factors. Br J Dermatol 162:1224–1232
51. Alemany R (2012) Design of improved oncolytic adenoviruses. Adv Cancer Res 115:93–114
52. Chai L, Liu S, Mao Q, Wang D, Li X, Zheng X et al (2012) A novel conditionally replicating adenoviral vector with dual expression of IL-24 and arresten inserted in E1 and the region between E4 and fiber for improved melanoma therapy. Cancer Gene Ther 19:247–254
53. Viale DL, Cafferata EG, Gould D et al (2013) Therapeutic improvement of a stroma-targeted CRAd by incorporating motives responsive to the melanoma microenvironment. J Invest Dermatol 133(11):2576–2584
54. Kraman M, Bambrough PJ, Arnold JN et al (2010) Suppression of anti-tumor immunity by stromal cells expressing fibroblast activation protein-alpha. Science 330:827–830
55. Lee J, Fassnacht M, Nair S, Boczkowski D, Gilboa E (2005) Tumor immunotherapy targeting fibroblast activation protein, a product expressed in tumor-associated fibroblasts. Cancer Res 65:11156–11163
56. Loeffler M, Kruger JA, Niethammer AG, Reisfeld RA (2006) Targeting tumor-associated fibroblasts improves cancer chemotherapy by increasing intratumoral drug uptake. J Clin Invest 116:1955–1962
57. Tran E, Chinnasamy D, Yu Z et al (2013) Immune targeting of fibroblast activation protein triggers recognition of multipotent bone marrow stromal cells and cachexia. J Exp Med 210:1125–1135
58. Hofheinz RD, Al-Batran SE, Hartmann F et al (2003) Stromal antigen targeting by a humanised monoclonal antibody: an early phase II trial of sibrotuzumab in patients with metastatic colorectal cancer. Onkologie 26:44–48
59. Eager RM, Cunningham CC, Senzer N et al (2009) Phase II trial of talabostat and docetaxel in advanced non-small cell lung cancer. Clin Oncol (R Coll Radiol) 21:464–472

60. Narra K, Mullins SR, Lee HO et al (2007) Phase II trial of single agent Val-boroPro (Talabostat) inhibiting fibroblast activation protein in patients with metastatic colorectal cancer. Cancer Biol Ther 6:1691–1699

61. Mantovani A, Sica A (2010) Macrophages, innate immunity and cancer: balance, tolerance, and diversity. Curr Opin Immunol 22:231–237

62. Porta C, Subhra Kumar B, Larghi P, Rubino L, Mancino A, Sica A (2007) Tumor promotion by tumor-associated macrophages. Adv Exp Med Biol 604:67–86

63. Qian BZ, Pollard JW (2010) Macrophage diversity enhances tumor progression and metastasis. Cell 141:39–51

64. Solinas G, Germano G, Mantovani A, Allavena P (2009) Tumor-associated macrophages (TAM) as major players of the cancer-related inflammation. J Leukoc Biol 86:1065–1073

65. Torisu H, Ono M, Kiryu H et al (2000) Macrophage infiltration correlates with tumor stage and angiogenesis in human malignant melanoma: possible involvement of TNFalpha and IL-1alpha. Int J Cancer 85:182–188

66. Duluc D, Delneste Y, Tan F et al (2007) Tumor-associated leukemia inhibitory factor and IL-6 skew monocyte differentiation into tumor-associated macrophage-like cells. Blood 110:4319–4330

67. Pixley FJ, Stanley ER (2004) M-CSF regulation of the wandering macrophage: complexity in action. Trends Cell Biol 14:628–638

68. Roca H, Varsos ZS, Sud S, Craig MJ, Ying C, Pienta KJ (2009) CCL2 and interleukin-6 promote survival of human CD11b+ peripheral blood mononuclear cells and induce M2-type macrophage polarization. J Biol Chem 284:34342–34354

69. Solinas G, Schiarea S, Liguori M et al (2010) Tumor-conditioned macrophages secrete migration-stimulating factor: a new marker for M2-polarization, influencing tumor cell motility. J Immunol 185:642–652

70. Bennicelli JL, Guerry D (1993) Production of multiple cytokines by cultured human melanomas. Exp Dermatol 2:186–190

71. Lazar-Molnar E, Hegyesi H, Toth S, Falus A (2000) Autocrine and paracrine regulation by cytokines and growth factors in melanoma. Cytokine 12:547–554

72. Paglia D, Oran A, Lu C, Kerbel RS, Sauder DN, McKenzie RC (1995) Expression of leukemia inhibitory factor and interleukin-11 by human melanoma cell lines: LIF, IL-6, and IL-11 are not coregulated. J Interferon Cytokine Res 15:455–460

73. Richmond A, Yang J, Su Y (2009) The good and the bad of chemokines/chemokine receptors in melanoma. Pigment Cell Melanoma Res 22:175–186

74. Umemura N, Saio M, Suwa T et al (2008) Tumor-infiltrating myeloid-derived suppressor cells are pleiotropic-inflamed monocytes/macrophages that bear M1- and M2-type characteristics. J Leukoc Biol 83:1136–1144

75. Wang T, Ge Y, Xiao M et al (2012) Melanoma-derived conditioned media efficiently induce the differentiation of monocytes to macrophages that display a highly invasive gene signature. Pigment Cell Melanoma Res 25:493–505

76. Brocker EB, Zwadlo G, Holzmann B, Macher E, Sorg C (1988) Inflammatory cell infiltrates in human melanoma at different stages of tumor progression. Int J Cancer 41:562–567

77. Bernengo MG, Quaglino P, Cappello N, Lisa F, Osella-Abate S, Fierro MT (2000) Macrophage-mediated immunostimulation modulates therapeutic efficacy of interleukin-2 based chemoimmunotherapy in advanced metastatic melanoma patients. Melanoma Res 10:55–65

78. Brocker EB, Zwadlo G, Suter L, Brune M, Sorg C (1987) Infiltration of primary and metastatic melanomas with macrophages of the 25F9-positive phenotype. Cancer Immunol Immunother 25:81–86

79. Makitie T, Summanen P, Tarkkanen A, Kivela T (2001) Tumor-infiltrating macrophages (CD68(+) cells) and prognosis in malignant uveal melanoma. Invest Ophthalmol Vis Sci 42:1414–1421

80. Varney ML, Johansson SL, Singh RK (2005) Tumour-associated macrophage infiltration, neovascularization and aggressiveness in malignant melanoma: role of monocyte chemotactic protein-1 and vascular endothelial growth factor-A. Melanoma Res 15:417–425

81. Jensen TO, Schmidt H, Moller HJ et al (2009) Macrophage markers in serum and tumor have prognostic impact in American Joint Committee on Cancer stage I/II melanoma. J Clin Oncol 27:3330–3337

82. Storr SJ, Safuan S, Mitra A et al (2012) Objective assessment of blood and lymphatic vessel invasion and association with macrophage infiltration in cutaneous melanoma. Mod Pathol 25:493–504

83. Emri E, Egervari K, Varvolgyi T et al (2012) Correlation among metallothionein expression, intratumoural macrophage infiltration and the risk of metastasis in human cutaneous malignant melanoma. J Eur Acad Dermatol Venereol 27(3):e320–327

84. Bianchini F, Massi D, Marconi C et al (2007) Expression of cyclo-oxygenase-2 in macrophages associated with cutaneous melanoma at different stages of progression. Prostaglandins Other Lipid Mediat 83:320–328

85. Zaidi MR, Davis S, Noonan FP et al (2011) Interferon-gamma links ultraviolet radiation to melanomagenesis in mice. Nature 469:548–553

86. Handoko HY, Rodero MP, Boyle GM et al (2013) UVB-induced melanocyte proliferation in neonatal mice driven by CCR2-independent recruitment of Ly6c(low)MHCII(hi) macrophages. J Invest Dermatol 133:1803–1812

87. Kang K, Hammerberg C, Meunier L, Cooper KD (1994) CD11b+ macrophages that infiltrate human epidermis after in vivo ultraviolet exposure potently produce IL-10 and represent the major secretory source of epidermal IL-10 protein. J Immunol 153:5256–5264

88. Wang T, Herlyn M (2013) The macrophage: a new factor in UVR-induced melanomagenesis. J Invest Dermatol 133:1711–1713

89. Marconi C, Bianchini F, Mannini A, Mugnai G, Ruggieri S, Calorini L (2008) Tumoral and macrophage uPAR and MMP-9 contribute to the invasiveness of B16 murine melanoma cells. Clin Exp Metastasis 25:225–231

90. Gazzaniga S, Bravo AI, Guglielmotti A et al (2007) Targeting tumor-associated macrophages and inhibition of MCP-1 reduce angiogenesis and tumor growth in a human melanoma xenograft. J Invest Dermatol 127:2031–2041

91. Hansen BD, Schmidt H, von der Maase H, Sjoegren P, Agger R, Hokland M (2006) Tumour-associated macrophages are related to progression in patients with metastatic melanoma following interleukin-2 based immunotherapy. Acta Oncol 45:400–405

92. Kono K, Salazar-Onfray F, Petersson M et al (1996) Hydrogen peroxide secreted by tumor-derived macrophages down-modulates signal-transducing zeta molecules and inhibits tumor-specific T cell-and natural killer cell-mediated cytotoxicity. Eur J Immunol 26:1308–1313

93. Zou W (2006) Regulatory T cells, tumour immunity and immunotherapy. Nat Rev Immunol 6:295–307

94. Landsberg J, Kohlmeyer J, Renn M et al (2012) Melanomas resist T-cell therapy through inflammation-induced reversible dedifferentiation. Nature 490:412–416

95. Schneemann M, Schoeden G (2007) Macrophage biology and immunology: man is not a mouse. J Leukoc Biol 81:579 (discussion 80)

96. Kelly C, Jefferies C, Cryan SA (2011) Targeted liposomal drug delivery to monocytes and macrophages. J Drug Delivery 2011:727241

97. Banciu M, Metselaar JM, Schiffelers RM, Storm G (2008) Anti-tumor activity of liposomal prednisolone phosphate depends on the presence of functional tumor-associated macrophages in tumor tissue. Neoplasia 10:108–117

98. Knight DA, Ngiow SF, Li M et al (2013) Host immunity contributes to the anti-melanoma activity of BRAF inhibitors. J Clin Invest 123:1371–1381

99. Erez N, Truitt M, Olson P, Arron ST, Hanahan D (2010) Cancer-associated fibroblasts are activated in incipient neoplasia to orchestrate tumor-promoting inflammation in an NF-kappaB-dependent manner. Cancer Cell 17:135–147

100. Gallagher PG, Bao Y, Prorock A et al (2005) Gene expression profiling reveals cross-talk between melanoma and fibroblasts: implications for host-tumor interactions in metastasis. Cancer Res 65:4134–4146

101. Samaniego R, Estecha A, Relloso M et al (2013) Mesenchymal contribution to recruitment, infiltration, and positioning of leukocytes in human melanoma tissues. J Invest Dermatol 133(9):2255–2264

102. Comito G, Giannoni E, Segura CP et al (2013) Cancer-associated fibroblasts and M2-polarized macrophages synergize during prostate carcinoma progression. Oncogene 33(19): 2423–2431

103. Bedogni B, Powell MB (2006) Skin hypoxia: a promoting environmental factor in melanomagenesis. Cell Cycle 5:1258–1261

104. Pires IM, Bencokova Z, Milani M et al (2010) Effects of acute versus chronic hypoxia on DNA damage responses and genomic instability. Cancer Res 70:925–935

105. Keith B, Simon MC (2007) Hypoxia-inducible factors, stem cells, and cancer. Cell 129:465–472

106. Patel SA, Simon MC (2008) Biology of hypoxia-inducible factor-2alpha in development and disease. Cell Death Differ 15:628–634

107. Rankin EB, Giaccia AJ (2008) The role of hypoxia-inducible factors in tumorigenesis. Cell Death Differ 15:678–685

108. Rankin EB, Rha J, Unger TL et al (2008) Hypoxia-inducible factor-2 regulates vascular tumorigenesis in mice. Oncogene 27:5354–5358

109. Covello KL, Kehler J, Yu H et al (2006) HIF-2alpha regulates Oct-4: effects of hypoxia on stem cell function, embryonic development, and tumor growth. Genes Dev 20:557–570

110. Martin CM, Ferdous A, Gallardo T et al (2008) Hypoxia-inducible factor-2alpha transactivates Abcg2 and promotes cytoprotection in cardiac side population cells. Circ Res 102:1075–1081

111. Busca R, Berra E, Gaggioli C et al (2005) Hypoxia-inducible factor 1{alpha} is a new target of microphthalmia-associated transcription factor (MITF) in melanoma cells. J Cell Biol 170:49–59

112. Bristow RG, Hill RP (2008) Hypoxia and metabolism. Hypoxia, DNA repair and genetic instability. Nat Rev Cancer 8:180–192

113. Brahimi-Horn MC, Chiche J, Pouyssegur J (2007) Hypoxia and cancer. J Mol Med 85:1301–1307

114. Lee SJ, No YR, Dang DT et al (2013) Regulation of hypoxia-inducible factor 1alpha (HIF-1alpha) by lysophosphatidic acid is dependent on interplay between p53 and Kruppel-like factor 5. J Biol Chem 288:25244–25253

115. Schnitzer SE, Schmid T, Zhou J, Brune B (2006) Hypoxia and HIF-1alpha protect A549 cells from drug-induced apoptosis. Cell Death Differ 13:1611–1613

116. Kumar SM, Yu H, Fong D, Acs G, Xu X (2006) Erythropoietin activates the phosphoinositide 3-kinase/Akt pathway in human melanoma cells. Melanoma Res 16:275–283

117. Bedogni B, Welford SM, Cassarino DS, Nickoloff BJ, Giaccia AJ, Powell MB (2005) The hypoxic microenvironment of the skin contributes to Akt-mediated melanocyte transformation. Cancer Cell 8:443–454

118. Widmer DS, Hoek KS, Cheng PF et al (2013) Hypoxia contributes to melanoma heterogeneity by triggering HIF1alpha-dependent phenotype switching. J Invest Dermatol 133:2436–2443

119. Hanna SC, Krishnan B, Bailey ST et al (2013) HIF1alpha and HIF2alpha independently activate SRC to promote melanoma metastases. J Clin Invest 123:2078–2093

120. Kumar SM, Yu H, Edwards R et al (2007) Mutant V600E BRAF increases hypoxia inducible factor-1alpha expression in melanoma. Cancer Res 67:3177–3184

121. Liu S, Kumar SM, Martin JS, Yang R, Xu X (2011) Snail1 mediates hypoxia-induced melanoma progression. Am J Pathol 179:3020–3031

122. Bachmann IM, Ladstein RG, Straume O, Naumov GN, Akslen LA (2008) Tumor necrosis is associated with increased alphavbeta3 integrin expression and poor prognosis in nodular cutaneous melanomas. BMC Cancer 8:362

123. Chang SH, Worley LA, Onken MD, Harbour JW (2008) Prognostic biomarkers in uveal melanoma: evidence for a stem cell-like phenotype associated with metastasis. Melanoma Res 18:191–200

124. Giatromanolaki A, Sivridis E, Kouskoukis C, Gatter KC, Harris AL, Koukourakis MI (2003) Hypoxia-inducible factors 1alpha and 2alpha are related to vascular endothelial growth factor expression and a poorer prognosis in nodular malignant melanomas of the skin. Melanoma Res 13:493–501

125. Bergers G, Hanahan D (2008) Modes of resistance to anti-angiogenic therapy. Nat Rev Cancer 8:592–603

126. Ebos JM, Kerbel RS (2011) Antiangiogenic therapy: impact on invasion, disease progression, and metastasis. Nat Rev Clin Oncol 8:210–221

127. Ebos JM, Lee CR, Kerbel RS (2009) Tumor and host-mediated pathways of resistance and disease progression in response to antiangiogenic therapy. Clin Cancer Res 15:5020–5025

128. Pennacchietti S, Michieli P, Galluzzo M, Mazzone M, Giordano S, Comoglio PM (2003) Hypoxia promotes invasive growth by transcriptional activation of the met protooncogene. Cancer Cell 3:347–361

129. Duan JX, Jiao H, Kaizerman J et al (2008) Potent and highly selective hypoxia-activated achiral phosphoramidate mustards as anticancer drugs. J Med Chem 51:2412–2420

130. Meng F, Evans JW, Bhupathi D et al (2012) Molecular and cellular pharmacology of the hypoxia-activated prodrug TH-302. Mol Cancer Ther 11:740–751

131. Ganjoo KN, Cranmer LD, Butrynski JE et al (2011) A phase I study of the safety and pharmacokinetics of the hypoxia-activated prodrug TH-302 in combination with doxorubicin in patients with advanced soft tissue sarcoma. Oncology 80:50–56

132. Weiss GJ, Infante JR, Chiorean EG et al (2011) Phase 1 study of the safety, tolerability, and pharmacokinetics of TH-302, a hypoxia-activated prodrug, in patients with advanced solid malignancies. Clin Cancer Res 17:2997–3004

133. Sun JD, Liu Q, Wang J et al (2012) Selective tumor hypoxia targeting by hypoxia-activated prodrug TH-302 inhibits tumor growth in preclinical models of cancer. Clin Cancer Res 18:758–770

Chapter 2
The Role of the Immune System and Immunoregulatory Mechanisms Relevant to Melanoma

Cara Haymaker, Geok Choo Sim, Marie-Andree Forget, Jie Qing Chen, Chantale Bernatchez, and Laszlo Radvanyi

Abstract A hallmark of melanoma is its inherent immunogenicity through both innate and adaptive immune mechanisms. However, a number of factors inhibit these immune responses through intrinsic mechanisms in tumor cells or adaptive resistance triggered by the immune response via negative feedback. Understanding how these processes are balanced in context of pathways regulating T-cell activation, migration, and differentiation, and T-cell dysfunction in tumors has become a critical area of research. This chapter describes the immunoregulatory mechanisms in the melanoma tumor microenvironment and how positive and negative signaling elements can be harnessed to facilitate enhanced anti-tumor immune responses through immunotherapy.

Keywords Melanoma • Immune cells • Immunotherapy • Anti-tumor immunity • Cytokines

C. Haymaker, PhD • M.-A. Forget, PhD • C. Bernatchez, PhD
Department of Melanoma Medical Oncology, The University of Texas,
MD Anderson Cancer Center, Houston, TX, USA
e-mail: chaymaker@mdanderson.org; mforget@mdanderson.org;
cbernatchez@mdanderson.org

G.C. Sim, PhD
Department of Melanoma Medical Oncology, The University of Texas,
MD Anderson Cancer Center, Houston, TX, USA

Moffit Cancer Center, Tampa, FL, USA
e-mail: gcsim1@yahoo.co.uk

J.Q. Chen
Department of Melanoma Medical Oncology, The University of Texas,
MD Anderson Cancer Center, Houston, TX, USA

Lion Biotechnologies, Tampa, FL, USA

L. Radvanyi (✉)
Department of Melanoma Medical Oncology, The University of Texas,
MD Anderson Cancer Center, Houston, TX, USA

EMD Serono Research and Development Institute, Billerica, MA, USA

© Springer Science+Business Media New York 2016
C.A. Torres-Cabala, J.L. Curry (eds.), *Genetics of Melanoma*, Cancer Genetics,
DOI 10.1007/978-1-4939-3554-3_2

2.1 Introduction

One of the key starting points in a discussion of anti-melanoma immunity is whether the immune system evolved to recognize tumor antigens and mount an adaptive (T-cell-mediated) antitumor immune response together with key components of innate immunity operating either in a facilitative or inhibitory role. This fundamental question needs to frame any detailed discussion of the mechanisms of antitumor immunity and the development of cancer immunotherapies relevant to melanoma. The adaptive immune system has a remarkable capacity to recognize foreign pathogens, such as bacteria, viruses, and fungal infections as one of the most primordial life-preserving functions throughout evolution. This powerful response against foreign invaders however is also counterbalanced by equally powerful immunoregulatory mechanisms designed to limit damage to normal tissues (autoimmunity) and prevent runaway immune responses (immunopathology) that can ultimately kill the host. Both of these fundamental immunological processes also intersect during wound healing due to the need to curtail any opportunistic infections in wounds or due to tissue damage that may be caused by infection while at the same time limiting inflammation in resolving parts of the wound to initiate tissue repair. From an evolutionary biology perspective, both these two contrasting functions of the immune system evolved over millions of years culminating in mammals and humans as a mechanism of protection against infectious disease while preventing immunopathology mainly as a protective mechanism during reproductive years, thus perpetuating the species. In addition, these processes evolved to their present forms in context with the development of an adaptive immune system consisting of highly specific antigen receptor-expressing lymphocytes [T-cell receptor (TCR)-expressing T cells mediating cell-mediated immunity and immunoglobulin receptor-expressing B cells mediating antibody-dependent immunity through opsonization] together with a more primordial innate immune system that developed cross-circuiting or cross-communication with adaptive immunity as a critical initiator of T- and B-cell responses as well as suppressive lymphocyte responses.

Thus, with these biological realities in mind, a fundamental question that emerges is whether the immune system also "evolved" to fight cancer (abnormal growth and differentiation of self-tissues that threaten life) as an intrinsic process during evolution to preserve the species or is the anticancer immune response an evolutionary "fluke of nature" based on how the immune system evolved to distinguish self from non-self (foreign antigens). Cancer can be viewed as an "altered non-self" that the immune system by default evolved some capacity to recognize, but rather inefficiently due to the suppressive counterbalances (e.g., central T-cell tolerance during T-cell differentiation in the thymus gland, immunosuppressive cytokines such as TGF-β, Foxp3$^+$ T-regulatory cells, myeloid cells during wound healing) that exist that protect us from autoimmunity and immunopathology. Aging is another parameter that now enters this discussion. In this context, cancer (including melanoma) is really a disease of aging where cumulative genetic and tissue damage (e.g., from cumulative UV radiation) together with chronic inflammation leads to abnormal cellular proliferation, immortalization, invasiveness, and then ultimately metastatic spread that kills the host. As human aging has become a reality with lifespan increasing beyond original evolutionary constraints, the immune system is now faced with a new and unexpected selective pressure to somehow modify its essential evolutionary function away from simply fighting infection to maintain life only through the reproductive years. However, both the innate and adaptive arms of the immune system significantly weaken during aging, as manifested in thymic involution reducing naive T cells, reduced NK cell function, suppressed dendritic cell activation, chronic inflammation mediated by abnormally activated macrophages, and oligoclonal expansions of T-cell clones (e.g., CMV-specific CD8$^+$ T cells) together with senescence (caused by telomere shortening and terminal T-cell differentiation). Ultimately, all these evolutionary processes and consequences are shaping how the immune system is "learning" to cope with melanoma and other forms of cancer.

Due to the damage to local tissues caused by primary tumors and metastatic growth, all tumors, including melanoma, are intrinsically "immunogenic" and drive a wound healing response attracting innate myeloid and granulocytic cells. The inflammation and damage to both normal stromal tissue and cancer cells in this process releases tumor antigens presented on class I and class II major histocompatibility complex (MHC) molecules activating CD8$^+$ and CD4$^+$ αβ TCR$^+$ T cells. Tumors can induce an immune response both systemically and at the tumor site against tumor antigens inducing T-cell responses and other stress-induced molecules that are recognized by innate lymphocytes (NK cells and γδ T cells) and antigen-presenting cells (dendritic cells). However, unlike a successfully resolved infection by a foreign pathogen or a normal wound healing response, it has become readily apparent that immunosuppressive mechanisms both systemically and in the tumor microenvironment are triggered during cancer progression and advanced cancer (manifested as metastases from seeded circulating tumor cells), limiting the effectiveness of an antitumor immune response. However, despite these processes, de novo adaptive immune responses against both primary and metastatic melanoma occur in almost all patients and, thus, questions arise as to what role these responses play in the overall course of the disease and patient survival, why some patients with melanoma mount more effective adaptive immune responses against both local and disseminated tumors manifested by higher lymphocyte infiltration into the tumor bed that can be boosted by immunotherapy, and what biomarkers are associated with this enhanced level of "immunocompetence."

It is in this conceptual framework that we will discuss the key processes regulating immune responses against melanoma both at the tumor site and systemically, the cellular components of the immune infiltrates in the melanoma tumor microenvironment, and how tumors can regulate immune responses in the host systemically in uninvolved secondary lymphatic tissues (tumor-draining lymph nodes and uninvolved nodes, as well as the spleen). We will introduce the concept of how and why melanoma is considered an "immunogenic" tumor regulated by inflammation and how critical inflammatory molecules can either be drivers of cancer cell survival and growth or act as initiators of adaptive cytotoxic T-cell responses that can eradicate tumor cells by recognition of tumors antigens presented on MHC molecules. In some cases, tumor-associated stromal cells, such as tumor-associated fibroblasts (TAFs) and endothelial cells (from tumor angiogenic processes), can also be targeted. We will also discuss how the normal checks and balances that evolved in the immune system during evolution to prevent runaway inflammation and autoimmunity, manifested as negative feedback mechanisms at different stages of the immune responses or during normal T-cell differentiation, can inhibit adaptive immune responses against these "wounds" and some of the key molecules and signaling pathways involved in this process such as the T-cell "checkpoint" molecules (e.g., CTLA-4 and PD-1) that have emerged to be exciting new cancer immunotherapy targets. Lastly, we attempt to bring together the concepts discussed into a unifying set of principles that can be used to drive immune biomarker research and how these immune system biomarkers can be used as prognostic tools or as tools to determine which patients are more apt to respond to immune intervention (immunotherapy) against their melanoma, especially at the advanced stages. Our hope is that these biomarkers can be eventually used to select patients for specific types of immunotherapies or combination therapies with targeted drugs or chemotherapies. A minimal knowledge of basic immunology is assumed, including the major components of the innate and adaptive immune response and knowledge of T-cell antigen recognition and activation processes involving positive costimulatory molecules and negative costimulatory molecules or checkpoints, the major types of T-cell responses, as well as the major cytokines involved. There are some excellent textbooks and overviews on basic immunology that the reader can consult if needed [1, 2].

2.2 Melanoma as an "Immunogenic" Tumor: Lymphocytes and the Tumor Microenvironment

2.2.1 Melanoma Is a Heterogeneous Entity of Tumor Cells, Hematopoietic Cells, and Resident and Nonresident Stromal Cells Regulating the Melanoma "Wound"

Melanoma is a heterogeneous entity of cells comprised of distinct clones of cancer cells, with different proliferative and invasiveness capacities, and stromal cells. In the tumor microenvironment, constant interaction between cancer cells and different stromal cells could either promote tumor rejection or tumor progression. In many cases, melanoma cells appear to "manipulate" the stromal cells within or surrounding the tumor to drive their growth, survival, and evasion from attack by immune cells. The stromal compartment in the tumor microenvironment itself is complex and comprised of numerous cell types that are categorized as resident and nonresident stromal cells [3]. Resident stromal cells including tumor-associated fibroblasts (TAFs), tumor-associated endothelial cells (TECs), and mesenchymal cells are cell populations that reside within stroma. Melanoma cells and resident stromal cells are a good source of a broad array of growth factors, proinflammatory cytokines (IL-6, IL-8, TNF-α) [4, 5], and chemokines (CXCL12, CCL5) [6–8]. Acting in either an autocrine or paracrine manner, tumor-derived cytokines and

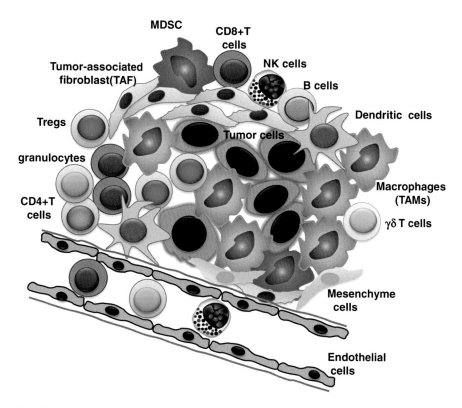

Fig. 2.1 Tumor microenvironment in melanoma. The tumor microenvironment is composed of many cell types that are recruited through the production of cytokines and chemokines. These include nonresident stromal cells such as tumor-associated fibroblasts (TAFs) and mesenchymal cells as well as various innate and adaptive immune cells [dendritic cells, tumor-associated macrophages (TAMs), myeloid-derived suppressor cells (MDSC), CD4+ and CD8+ T cells, γδ T cells, granulocytes, B cells, and NK cells]. Immune cells can be found within the tumor (intratumoral) as well as surrounding the tumor (peritumoral)

chemokines support tumor growth while recruiting nonresident stromal cells, comprised of various innate and adaptive immune cells (such as dendritic cells, tumor-associated macrophages (TAMs), myeloid-derived suppressor cells (MDSCs), T cells, γδ T cells, granulocytes, B cells, and NK cells) to the tumor site (Fig. 2.1).

In many melanoma tumors, lymphocytes, especially CD8+ T cells that recognize melanoma antigens (such as Melan-A/MART-1, gp100) and NK cells, can be found to differing degrees [9, 10]. These cells can produce high amounts of IFN-γ and express high levels of cytotoxic molecules such as granzyme B and perforin and play a positive role in limiting rising malignancies and in facilitating tumor rejection. The presence of CD8+ T cells has been correlated with better clinical response and survival in patients with melanoma and with other cancer types [11–13]. The infiltration of other cell types, such as IFN-γ-secreting-γδ T cells and NK/T cells, within the tumor tissue has also shown a favorable clinical outcome [14, 15]. However, in parallel to the infiltration of antitumor immune cells, negative immune regulators with immunosuppressive function such as TAMs, suppressive T-regulatory cells (Tregs), and MDSCs also accumulated in melanoma tumors [16–19]. These cells contribute to cancer progression by limiting the efficacy of CD8- and NK cell-mediated antitumor responses via various immunosuppressive mechanisms such as secretion of TGF-β, IL-10, IL-6, and IL-1, IDO expression in the tumor microenvironment reducing tryptophan, sequestration of growth factors such as IL-2 from T cells, and the release of factors mediating oxidative stress [20–22]. In this regard, the accumulation of Tregs in the tumor microenvironment significantly contributes to a decline in antitumor CD8$^+$ and Th1 CD4$^+$ T-cell responses and decreased overall survival and relapse-free survival [23, 24]. In addition, the presence of immunosuppressive TAMs exhibiting M2 phenotype was associated with poor survival in patients with melanoma [16, 17].

Furthermore, close interactions between positive and negative immune regulators with cancer cells in the tumor microenvironment could result in the polarization of "good" immune cells to "bad" immune cells that turn from mediating "antitumor" to "pro-tumor" effects. For instance, the presence of the immunosuppressive cytokine TGF-β, together with a low antigen signal in the tumor microenvironment, facilitates the conversion of conventional CD4$^+$ T cells to induced regulatory T cells (iTregs) that can suppress antitumor responses mediated by CD8$^+$ cytotoxic T cells and NK cells. In addition, many of the infiltrated-CD8$^+$ T cells in melanoma tumors were found to be dysfunctional [25–27] or incompletely differentiated in a TGF-β-dependent manner [28], thereby lacking the capability to mediate tumor rejection. Thus, the diverse communication of immune cells with cancer cells and within the tumor microenvironment dictates the final outcome of anti- or pro-tumor responses.

Moreover, the extent of infiltration by various antitumor and immunosuppressive immune cells, together with pro- and anti-inflammatory cytokines and chemokines that are present in the tumor microenvironment, contributes to different inflammation states of tumors: non-inflamed, over-inflamed, and well-balanced inflammation. The overall inflammatory nature of a tumor, either being non-inflamed, over-inflamed, or having well-balanced inflammation, would rely on how cancer cells and stromal cells interact and on their activation state. In a well-balanced inflammation tumor, both positive and negative immune regulators are present in the tumor microenvironment and operating to promote "good inflammation" that could lead to tumor rejection. However, some melanoma tumors are non-inflamed and lack T-cell accumulation in the tumor microenvironment, whereas some tumors are over-inflamed and contain massive accumulation of innate immune cells that promote a "bad" inflammation state and facilitate tumorigenesis [9]. This concept will also be discussed in context of tumor-related biomarkers later. Recently, specific gene expression patterns that were associated with different states of inflammation and immune cell infiltration of melanoma tumors have been identified. In this regard, CD8$^+$ T-cell-infiltrated but not non-inflamed tumors have showed a type I IFN transcriptional profile as well as the expression of key chemokines, and these gene signatures may implicate an association with the activation of innate immune responses [29, 30]. Melanoma patients having T-cell-inflamed tumors showed expression of a chemokine signature for T-cell recruitment (CCL2, CCL3, CCL4, CCL5, CXCL9, and CXCL10) had a more favorable clinical outcome [9, 30].

Paradoxically, the activation of antitumor-related cytokine secretion, for example, IFN-γ, which is traditionally considered to be important in mediating tumor-specific responses, has been shown to participate in immunosuppressive mechanisms. For example, the presence of Th1 producing IFN-γ cells was linked to the promotion of MDSC accumulation and the lack of efficient antitumor responses [31]. Recently, Spranger et al. have showed that infiltrating-CD8+ T cells were responsible for the recruitment of Tregs and for an increase of IDO and PD-L1 expression in the melanoma tumor microenvironment [20]. These data suggest that strong inflammation mediated by IFN-γ could activate a negative feedback immune response by recruiting immunosuppressors (e.g., Tregs and MDSC) to counteract the local inflammation and to suppress the tumor-specific responses. Taken together, it is crucial to understand how the interaction between stromal cells and cancer cells contributes to the different state of inflammation and outcome of immune responses to further improve current immunotherapy against melanoma.

2.2.2 The Concept of Melanoma Tumor Antigens Recognized by T Lymphocytes of the Adaptive Immune System

Just like the majority of cells that compose the human body, melanoma tumor cells express class I major MHC molecules. Although the expression level may vary from tumor to tumor, these MHC class I molecules are a way for the immune system to identify a tumor cell and engender its destruction. Each MHC class I molecule expressed at the cell surface forms a complex with an 8–12-amino acid long peptide. Peptides are usually the degradation product of an intracellular protein or from the extracellular compartment if the protein was internalized by a professional antigen-presenting cell (APC) like dendritic cells (DCs) or macrophages (Fig. 2.2). The complex formed by the MHC class I molecule and the peptide at the surface of the cell can be recognized specifically by the TCR of a CD8+ T lymphocyte (CD8+ T cell) and trigger different activation signals leading to proliferation and/or cytotoxic functions. A similar process exists for CD4+ T-helper cells, but in this case, longer 10–15-amino acid length peptides (usually derived from extracellular and secreted proteins) are presented on MHC class II molecules.

During development, CD8+ T cells have been selected in the thymus to recognize MHC class I in a process called positive selection. A second step called negative selection aimed to eliminate T cells recognizing self-peptide to prevent autoimmune responses. Mature CD8+ T cells spared from that "negative selection" are believed to be able to eliminate only cells presenting peptides from foreign proteins such as a virus. A protein from which a derived peptide triggers the recognition and action of a T cell is called an antigen. This definition extends further than viral, bacterial, fungal, and other "foreign" proteins to also overexpressed self-proteins or antigens

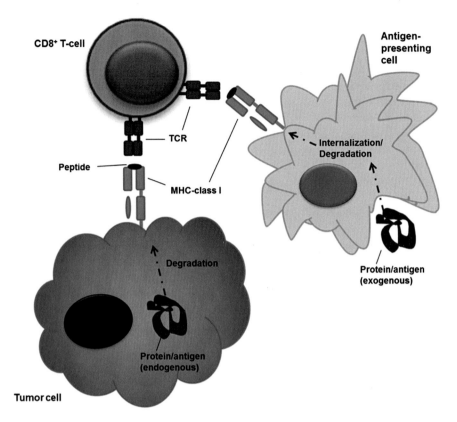

Fig. 2.2 MHC class I peptide presentation. The T-cell receptor (TCR) of a CD8[+] T lymphocyte (CD8[+] T cell) can specifically recognize peptides presented at the cell surface as a complex with MHC class I molecules. These peptides are the result of protein degradation. Intracellular proteins, for example, in tumor cells, can be degraded into small peptides which, if they possess strong affinity to bound the intracellular MHC-I molecule, will then migrate to the surface of the cell to be presented to a CD8[+] T cell. If MHC-I-peptide complex is recognized by the T cell, this will trigger different activation signals leading to proliferation and/or cytotoxic functions of the T cell. Peptides can also originate from degradation of extracellular proteins. These proteins are internalized by a professional antigen-presenting cell (APC) like dendritic cells (DCs) or macrophages before being degraded and loaded on MHC-I to be presented, as a complex, to the CD8[+] T cell

induced under conditions of stress and cancer, as we will further demonstrate in this section. These overexpressed self-proteins normally ignored by the immune system, together with protein products from mutated genes, constitute what are termed tumor-associated antigens (TAAs).

TAAs are generally defined as proteins expressed by tumor cells with a weak or nonexistent expression in normal tissues, especially vital tissues such as the brain, lungs, and heart. TAA immunogenicity, which is defined as its capacity to be presented on MHC (i.e., a peptide-bound MHC class I or class II molecules on the cell surface) and recognized by the immune system (i.e., peptide-MHC complex recognized by a TCR), has to be proven before being designated as a TAA. The field has actually attributed four qualities that would constitute the ideal TAA [32]. In addition from being absent from normal tissues, it is preferable that TAA are involved in tumor progression so it is more beneficial when targeted. The ideal TAA also has known peptides that can be recognized by T cells and presented naturally, complexed with MHC class I and class II at the surface of tumor cells [32].

The TAA can be classified into four families: shared cancer/testis antigens, differentiation antigens, antigens overexpressed in cancer cells, and antigens derived from somatic mutations of tumor cells [33]. It is in the cancer/testis family that we find the first TAA to have been identified, MAGE-1 [34]. These TAA were expressed during development but are now silenced in mature, normal cells with the exception of spermatozoids, which makes these antigens great targets with very few off-target effects (side effects) for the patient. However, unsuspected low levels of expression of these proteins in normal indispensable tissues can lead to high toxicity like it was observed when the TAA MAGE-A3 was targeted with an engineered MAGE-A3-specific T cell, resulting in neurologic problems and even death [35]. NY-ESO-1, which is found in melanoma tumor cells as well as other cancers, is part of this family [36]. The TAAs in the melanocyte differentiation family are often expressed at lower levels in normal cells from which the tumor has arisen. The most common TAAs in this family are the proteins gp100, tyrosinase, tyrosinase-related protein 1 and 2 (TRP1 and TRP1), and MART-1, which are expressed in melanocytes through their role in melanin biosynthesis but also found highly expressed in melanoma cancer cells [37]. Targeting these TAA in immunotherapy can usually give rise to non-life-threatening side effects like skin depigmentation. The difference between the overexpressed antigen family and the differentiation antigens is that the expression of the overexpressed antigens is not restricted to the tissue where the tumor emerged but is also found in other normal tissues [33].

The last category, the mutated Ag, has been a subject of great interest lately with the use of exomic sequencing methods to rapidly identify mutations generating mutated proteins/peptides that can be recognized by T cells that have infiltrated the tumor [38, 39]. It was recently demonstrated using a murine model of chemically induced tumors that some protein mutations generated highly immunogenic peptides sufficient to mediate the tumor eradication by T cells recognizing the specific mutation [38]. This represents a major advantage when targeting TAA for therapy given the absence of expression of this type of mutation in normal tissues. The T cells that are specific against this mutated protein either do not recognize or have a weak recognition for the wild-type version of the protein or the wild-type version is simply not expressed. Conversely, when some of the resident tumor cells lack expression of such an immunogenic peptide, the cancer immunoediting phenomenon occurs, which will be subsequently discussed, and gives the tumor cells the capacity to overpower the action of the immune system [38]. In humans, it is a well-known fact that cancers caused by mutations such as in smoke (MCA) for lung cancer or UV for melanoma are themselves enriched with mutations. It was recently demonstrated that a mutated antigen isolated from a melanoma tumor cell line that was recognized by autologous tumor-infiltrating lymphocytes (TILs) was responsible for tumor regression when these TILs were massively expanded in vitro and adoptively transferred to the patient (discussed in a later section) [39].

There is another category of TAA which the literature does not include in the four families: the viral TAA. Some solid tumors like nasopharyngeal cancer originates from a viral infection which gives rise to immunogenic peptides coming from that virus and also expressed by tumor cells [40]. For melanoma, viruses are not considered a primary cause of tumor genesis; however sequences of the K-type human endogenous retrovirus (HERV-K) were found in melanoma tumor cells but not in normal melanoma [41]. UV radiation has been reported to induce HERV-K activation which could in turn participate in the malignant transformation of melanoma cells [42, 43]. A peptide from the HERV-K-MEL found in melanoma was able to bind MHC class I and to be recognized by CD8$^+$ T cells taken from the blood of melanoma patients [44]. Even though HERV-K-MEL was not initially classified as a TAA in the four families of TAA because of is endogenous genomic origin, the fact that it is expressed in cancer cells and not normal cells, and that it is immunogenic and may participate in driving tumor progression, qualifies it has a TAA for melanoma.

2.3   The Immune System Can Be "Two-Faced" Either Inhibiting or Facilitating Early Melanoma Progression

The immune system can be a "two-edged sword" in regulating tumor development or tumor control. Research is now just beginning to understand the factors that play a role in the immune system helping drive cancer versus those playing a role later in eradicating cancer cells through innate and adaptive mechanisms both at the earliest stages of cancer initiation (called "tumor immunosurveillance") or at more advanced stages through immunotherapeutic interventions. The line between these two processes is still "fuzzy" and is still being defined. Moreover, the immune system can be a driver of cancer in two scenarios: (1) early cancer formation and (2) generating immune-resistant tumor cell subsets in more advanced disease through immunoselecting antigen-loss variants, variants that lose key ligands (e.g., MHC class I) sensed by the adaptive and innate immune systems, and through triggering epithelial-to-mesenchymal transition in tumor cells that are more metastatic and have tumor stem cell-like properties.

2.3.1   Immune System as a Driver of Melanoma Initiation

It has long been known that chronic inflammation through innate immune system mediators regulating wound healing can drive cancer development and initial progression. Cytokines such as TNF-α, IL-1α, IL-1β, and IL-17 and its associated cytokine IL-23, as well as IFN-γ, are key players regulating both CD8$^+$ CTL and CD4$^+$ T-helper responses that can drive tumor initiation [45–48]. These cytokines (TNF-α, IFN-γ, IL-1α/β) are not only products of adaptive immune responses but can also be produced by innate immune system cells such as macrophages, granulocytes, and NK cells homing to damaged or stressed tissues [45].

Building on our theme of cancer as a "wound that never heals," growing data in melanoma indicates that UV radiation-damaged melanocytes and keratinocytes in the skin can trigger a stress response that activates an innate inflammatory response through the influx of innate immune cells but at the same time triggers the release of mediators, such as IL-10, that inhibit DC activation and initiation of an adaptive immune response [49]. This may also be a protective mechanism to prevent immunopathology at the stressed site, but, in terms of cancer initiation, this protective pathway "does not know" that a cancerous situation is causing the initial stress. For example, in a recent study by Zaidi et al., IFN-γ was found to be a key mediator in cutaneous melanoma initiation after UVB irradiation in a new hepatocyte growth factor/scatter factor transgenic mouse model [50]. UVB, but not UVA irradiation of neonatal pups, led to melanocytic tumors reminiscent of human melanoma that was prevented by blocking IFN-γ, but not type I IFN [50]. The source of IFN-γ facilitating tumor formation was found to be from activated CCR2 chemokine receptor-positive macrophages infiltrating into the damaged skin area via localized production of CCR2 ligands [50]. IFN-γ-positive macrophages were also found in >70 % of human melanoma examined [50]. IFN-γ and IL-12 as innate immune system drivers can also lead to the activation of other "bystander" macrophages and myeloid cells to express inducible nitric oxide synthase (iNOS) releasing nitric oxide (NO) that together with reactive oxygen species (ROS) can cause a highly reactive compound, peroxynitrite, that causes DNA damage and protein tyrosine nitration [51–55]. This together with other mutations in melanocytes induced by UVB-induced DNA damage can set off a chain reaction of events that leads to more genetic damage, more inflammation, and then cancer formation. Activated macrophages also produce IL-6, IL-1, and TNF-α, which activates NF-κB in transformed cells protecting cells from apoptosis. In fact, activated macrophages (that also increase with aging in humans) are drivers of many types of cancer initiation not just melanoma; underscoring how chronic inflammation during aging (also called "inflammaging") is a major driver of cancer [56–58]. For further information and concepts of the role of inflammation and cancer, an excellent review on the role of inflammation as a driver of cancer initiation has recently been published by Trinchieri and colleagues [45, 59].

2.3.2 Cancer Immunosurveillance

The notion that the immune system can detect transformed cells in early subclinical cancerous lesions has been suggested for over 100 years and was first formulated into a working hypothesis by Macfarlane Burnet in the 1950s as the "cancer immunosurveillance hypothesis" [60]. Cellular transformation induces cell stress and it was postulated that ligands appear on the surface of transformed cells that are recognized by innate immune cells such as NK cells and macrophages for removal of these cells by cytotoxic killing and phagocytosis. With the discovery of adaptive immunity and the model of clonal selection in the 1950s, Burnet proposed that antigen-specific T cells recognize mutated antigens or altered self-antigens in these early transformed cells and killed these cells off in most cases before tumor arises and that only under conditions of immunosuppression or compromised antigen-specific lymphocyte function would cancer arise [60, 61]. Thus, the notion of the cancer mutanome (of huge interest currently in tumor immunology) is not new, but back then the molecular tools, including knowledge of the TCR and MHC restriction, was not yet discovered. It was during this time in the 1960s that Jacques Miller (also at the Walter and Eliza Hall Institute with Burnet) discovered that T lymphocytes differentiated in the thymus gland and that athymic animals or early thymus removal obliterated T-cell development [62]. The cancer immunosurveillance hypothesis was debated and a number of indirect sources of evidence were used to support it, such as the increased incidence of cancer with aging due to the successive loss of immunocompetence, the development of cancer under other immuno-compromised situations such as after organ transplantation and the development of secondary cancers in individuals treated with high-dose chemotherapy for a previous cancer, and autopsy data that found that many women and men have latent, preinvasive ductal breast carcinomas and in situ prostate carcinomas that seemed to have remained dormant. Fast forwarding to the 1970s, a problem emerged with the introduction of athymic nude mice that were thought to completely lack any T cells (the first immunodeficient mouse model available as a result of a random mutation during inbreeding) that set the field back unfortunately for more than a decade due to unsubstantiated dogma that arises in the scientific community. Here, in a number of careful longitudinal studies in nude mouse strains, Stutman and colleagues found that the incidence or rates of spontaneous cancers, including leukemias, lymphomas, and virally induced sarcomas and sarcomas induced by methylcholanthrene (MCA), were not increased relative to non-immunocompromised mice, including those syngeneic with nude mouse strains [63–65]. This seemed to cast the death knoll for the immune system as being a sentinel against cancer until further research on nude mouse strains in the 1990s after the discovery of NK cells (MHC nonrestricted effector cells) found that NK cells exist in relatively normal numbers and activity in nude mice [66–68]. Moreover, a considerable amount of extrathymic T-cell differentiation (e.g., gut-associated lymphoid system) was found to occur in aged nude mice indicating that the nude mouse was a bad model to address the cancer immunosurveillance hypothesis [66–68]. Actually, this was already hinted at by a paper by Stutman himself in 1975 showing delayed tumor appearance in older nude mice in comparison with younger nude mice after murine sarcoma virus infection that was mediated by transfer of splenocytes from the older nude mice into the younger ones [64].

The development of gene knockout mouse strains in the 1990s allowed researchers to determine whether specific cell types and cytokines play a role in the antitumor immune response and whether immunosurveillance of early preneoplastic and neoplastic lesions occurs. In addition, monoclonal antibodies specific for cytokines and cell surface proteins became available that could either block the effects of specific cytokines or deplete specific lymphocyte subsets in vivo through complement-mediated or antibody-dependent cellular cytotoxicity (ADCC)-mediated pathways. Using these approaches, the group of Rob Schreiber began to elegantly resurrect Burnet's original idea using a spontaneous sarcoma tumor model arising in mice after carcinogen treatment with the carcinogen MCA [69, 70]. Using this model they showed an increased MCA sarcoma incidence in mice lacking type II IFN (IFN-γ) as well as STAT1 the key transcriptional factor activated downstream of IFN-γ and type I IFN signaling. Similar results were found by injecting blocking IFN-γ antibodies. Later, a more immunodeficient mouse model lacking the recombinase-activating gene (RAG) preventing all T- and B-lymphocyte development was also found to have increased incidence of both MCA-induced sarcoma and another spontaneous tumors. Similar results were obtained with mice lacking NK T cells [71–75].

Another important concept emanating from these studies was "immunoediting": the notion that the adaptive immune response can control tumor growth, especially early on, but also selects for tumor cell variants in the primary tumor that are resistant to the T-cell response as a result of antigen loss or other immunosuppressive mechanisms. Thus, the immune system "immunoedits" or "immunoselects" resistant tumor variants that can grow faster and evade further adaptive T-cell responses [71–74]. Work showing that tumors developing after MCA treatment in RAG knockout mice grow slower and many times can even be rejected when transplanted into wild-type syngeneic mice while those originating in wild-type mice grew faster when transplanted into other naive wild-type mice and were almost never rejected elegantly gave proof to this concept [71–74]. Since then, many groups are now studying the molecular mechanisms of this immunoediting process. As discussed below, this concept is also emerging to be critical at all stages of cancer where the immune system is constantly engaging tumors throughout the body and placing constant "immune pressure" on tumors leading to selective survival of resistant tumor stem-like cells either as a result of acquired or in intrinsic mechanisms.

2.3.3   Immunoselection of Resistant Tumor Subtypes by the Innate and Adaptive Immune Response

A number of studies in animal tumor models of melanoma using the B16 tumor cell line as well as spontaneous animal tumor models employing the *BRAF^{V600E}* oncogene together with PTEN knockdown specifically in melanocytes [using a tyrosinase or dopachrome tautomerase (DCT) promoters] have shown that the adaptive immune response leads to tumor antigen escape variants and preferential survival melanoma tumor cells with cancer stem cell properties. For example, in a recent study using the B16 model, adoptive cell therapy with melanoma-specific T cells was found to elicit a down-modulation of melanoma tumor antigen expression (MART-1, tyrosinase, and gp100) mediated through a mechanism involving tumor-localized TNF-α [76]. This led to renewed tumor growth. However, the loss of melanoma tumor antigen expression was transient and not permanent such that cessation of the immune response or neutralization of TNF-α resulted in tumor antigen re-expression [76]. Thus, proinflammatory cytokines like TNF-α released during an antitumor adaptive immune response can directly down-modulate antigen expression. The mechanism behind the transient nature of this process will need to be worked out but may be associated with an inflammation-induced dedifferentiation phenomenon or the selective survival of tumor cells with stem-like properties that lack tumor antigen expression.

This latter scenario is now gaining traction in the field in recent studies using an anti-melanoma vaccine model in which an incomplete antitumor immune response led to the preferential survival of melanoma stem-like cells that have lost antigen expression as well as other cell adhesion molecules (e.g., E-cadherin and claudin family tight junction protein) in a process that is beginning to be called "pseudo-epithelial-mesenchymal transition" (pseudo-EMT) after the well-documented EMT events that occur in epithelial malignancies [77–80]. These concepts have been elegantly studied by Vile and colleagues who used a B16 melanoma cDNA library-based vaccine approach using the vesicular stomatitis virus (VSV) vector [81]. When this melanoma VSV-cDNA vaccine was given in a suboptimal way so that an incomplete tumor eradication is ensued by limiting the number of booster inoculations of the vaccine, established tumors shrank, but then regrew after a while. Analysis of these early regrowing tumors revealed that they were composed of these pseudo-EMT melanoma cells that could be cultured as nonadherent, suspended cells in much the same way as tumor stem cells from epithelial cancers like breast, lung, and prostate cancer. These stem-like melanoma cells grew as nonadherent spheres (so-called melanospheres) and were tumorigenic when transplanted into naive mice [81]. However, as found in the study mentioned above, the phenotype of these stem-like cells were not stable; after 1–2 weeks in culture, they became adherent again and could be treated again with a new VSV-cDNA vaccine [81]. This underscores an interesting concept that the immune system may place a transient, but not permanent, selective pressure on melanoma tumors inducing phenotypic alteration that evades the immune response, but not a permanent genetic change. This is good news for immunotherapy, but also suggests that we need to be highly cautious. Immunotherapies, such as vaccines and adoptive cell therapy that do not induce a strong enough response eradicating the tumor completely or invoking an irreversible dormant state, may actually select for this pseudo-EMT phenomenon in melanoma manifested by the survival of melanoma stem-like cells that can migrate to other areas of the body or eventually regrow at the original tumor sites. These stem-like cells have also been found to be slowly dividing (so-called slow cycling cells exhibiting high levels of mitochondrial respiration and are resistant to chemotherapy or targeted drugs (e.g., MAPK pathway inhibitors) aimed at inhibiting rapidly cycling tumor cells [82].

The exact molecular mechanisms of this induction of this resistant transient melanoma stem-like cells and what cytokines or other signaling pathways are involved will need to be investigated. Nevertheless, it emphasizes the dynamic nature of the immune system-tumor interaction and how the immune system, via proinflammatory signaling pathways, can lead to an "adaptive resistance" of the tumor against further immune attack. Recently, this has been elegantly demonstrated by the role of adaptive immune cytokines, such as IFN-γ, at the tumor site inducing the expression of immunosuppressive molecules by tumor cells (e.g., PD-1 ligand) that then feedback inhibits the local effector T-cell response [20].

2.4   Evolution at Play: Counterbalancing Immune Regulatory Factors in Melanoma Through "Adaptive Resistance"

As part of the different strategies to escape the immune system, the melanoma tumor microenvironment has evolved to suppress its action both locally and systemically (see Fig. 2.3 for a summary of the major mechanism discussed in this section). This includes utilizing suppressive cells within the immune system as well as directly through the tumor interaction with local T cells. Suppressive immune cells that are found within and around the tumor include MDSCs, T-regulatory cells

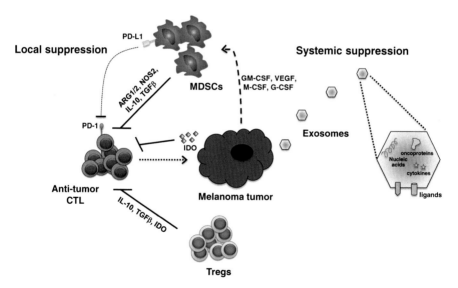

Fig. 2.3 Mechanisms of tumor-induced immunosuppression and adaptive resistance. Suppression exerted on the immune system by the tumor can be both local and systemic in nature. Locally, tumors can directly suppress invading antitumor CTL through the production of factors such as IDO (indoleamine 2,3-dioxygenase) or indirectly via the recruitment of suppressive immune cells such as Tregs and MDSCs. These cells, in turn, can mediate suppression through the production of cytokines such as IL-10 and TGF-β as well as through the production of arginase 1/2 (ARG1/2) and nitric oxide synthase 2 (NOS2). Direct suppression can also be mediated by the expression of inhibitory ligands such as programmed death ligand 1 (PD-L1) whose receptor, programmed death 1 (PD-1), is expressed on activated T cells. Tumors can induce systemic suppression via the production of exosomes expressing inhibitory ligands and containing suppressive cytokines, oncoproteins, and nucleic acids. Exosomes are able to help generate a "tumor-friendly" environment allowing for metastasis and promoting tumor growth

(Tregs), and type II CD4+ T-helper cells (Th2 cells). Some major mechanisms of T-cell suppression by MDSCs involve their production of arginases 1 and 2 (ARG1 and ARG2) and nitric oxide synthase 2 (NOS2) as well as nitric oxide (NO) and ROS and peroxynitrite. Both ARG1 and ARG2 as well as NOS2 synthesize L-arginine and block translation of a component of the TCR-signaling complex (the CD3ζ chain), inhibiting T-cell proliferation and inducing T-cell apoptosis [83, 84]. Peroxynitrite is the product of nitric oxide and superoxide anion. Increased levels of peroxynitrite have been correlated with a bad prognosis in multiple types of solid tumors including melanoma [55]. Peroxynitrate production by MDSCs within the immediate environment of the T cells has been shown to induce nitration of the TCR and CD8 molecules, thereby affecting their specific peptide-binding ability, resulting in the T-cell failure to respond to antigenic stimulation [85]. MDSCs can also suppress activated CTL, macrophages, and NK cells within the tumor microenvironment through secretion of suppressive cytokines such as IL-10 and the expression of membrane-bound TGF-β [86, 87]. Immature myeloid cells (IMCs) undergo differentiation into MDSCs in response to cytokines and other host factors that are released during cancer and some infections. MDSCs are induced by the tumor microenvironment due to the inflammatory nature of the tumor site. Tumor cells have been shown to produce the cytokines GM-CSF, G-CSF, M-CSF, and VEGF which all favor MDSC development [88]. In addition, stromal cells, activated T cells, and macrophages within and around the tumor produce other cytokines such as IL-1β, IL-4, IL-13, IL-6, IL-10, IFN-γ, and PGE that all aid in the generation of MDSCs from normal circulating IMCs [88].

As mentioned above, Tregs can be found within the melanoma tumor microenvironment and are a major factor mediating immunosuppression. Tumor production of the chemokines CCL2 and CCL22 has been shown to recruit Tregs to the tumor site, driven by mediated expression of the chemokine receptor CCR4 by the Tregs [89, 90]. At the tumor site, Tregs are able to suppress activation and proliferation of T cells indirectly through their secretion of IL-10 and TGF-β. Some studies have shown that Tregs are able to mediate direct suppression of activated T cells via cell-to-cell contact. Recently, the Whiteside group demonstrated that Tregs are in fact able to kill CD8+ T cells through Fas-mediated apoptosis in cancer patients [91]. The different subsets of Tregs within the tumor microenvironment may also be important to different degrees. For example, it has been demonstrated in melanoma that expression of ICOS marks a subset of highly activated Tregs found at the tumor site but not in the blood that are able to mediate stronger suppression than their ICOS[lo] counterparts [92]. Tregs are also able to inhibit activated effector cells through their generation of adenosine via CD39 and CD73. CD39 converts adenosine triphosphate (ATP) and adenosine diphosphate (ADP) into adenosine monophosphate (AMP). CD73, in turn, degrades AMP into adenosine. ATP is released by damaged or dying cells and has a proinflammatory effect on the innate immune system [93]. Conversely, the presence of adenosine induces the expression of adenosine receptors on local cells including activated effector T cells and induces anergy [94].

Not only does the tumor induce inactivation of antitumor CTLs by the body's own immune system, the tumor cell itself utilizes inhibitory molecules expressed by the CTL to induce further suppression/inactivation. Two major pathways that have been extensively studied are the CTLA-4/CD80/CD86 and the PD-1/PD-L1/PD-L2 inhibitory pathways. Cytotoxic T-lymphocyte antigen-4 (CTLA-4) is upregulated on T cells following activation and is also expressed on Tregs. CTLA-4 provides a natural break for immune activation as it displays a high affinity for the costimulatory ligands CD80 and CD86 (expressed on APCs) effectively blocking the ability of the T cells to receive stimulation through CD28. In fact, a recent study has shown that CTLA-4 actively pulls CD86 from the surface of an APC and internalizes it, removing the ability of the APC to costimulate reactive T cells [95]. However, the expression of CD80 or CD86 on the tumor cells has not been shown to be induced in response to the presence of T cells in or around the tumor.

Conversely, another inhibitory molecule that is upregulated on T cells following activation, programmed death receptor 1 (PD-1), is found to be highly expressed in T cells within melanoma tumors. PD-1 has two known ligands, PD-L1 and PD-L2. Expression of PD-L1 is induced on the tumor cells due to the presence of the inflammatory cytokine, interferon-gamma (IFN-γ). Ligation of PD-1 by PD-L1 or PD-L2 results in a strong brake on the T cell in terms of cytokine secretion, proliferation, and killing potential. Recently, it was found that expression of PD-L1 by the tumor occurs after tumor invasion by T cells in direct response to IFN-γ production by T cells [20]. Thus, the tumor is able to respond to the presence of activated T cells producing inflammatory cytokines and mediate their suppression. Other immune modulatory molecules are expressed by the melanoma tumor and tumor-associated antigen-presenting cells including herpes virus entry mediator (HVEM). HVEM interaction with B and T-lymphocyte attenuator (BTLA) on T cells results in suppression of cytokine production and proliferation. Melanoma cell expression of HVEM has been shown to mediate direct suppression of activated CD8$^+$ T cells [96]. While HVEM is not expressed on normal melanocytes, it remains unclear what factor induces its expression by melanoma tumor cells.

Another major mechanism of tumor-driven immunosuppression is the secretion of indoleamine 2,3-dioxygenase (IDO) by the tumor cells. IDO is an enzyme that catalyzes tryptophan degradation. T cells undergo cell cycle arrest in the absence of tryptophan. This mechanism for local immunosuppression was first described in mouse models and human xenograft models. This study showed that most human tumors express IDO and that T cells fail to proliferate and reject such tumors in mouse [97]. More recent work has shown that the presence of IDO in the tumor is a direct result of IFN-γ production by CD8$^+$ T cells [20]. Furthermore, the presence of IDO in melanoma lymph node metastases has been shown to correlate with a high level of Treg infiltration and decreased survival [98]. Thus the tumor is responding directly to the attack by the immune system by producing factors and expressing ligands that in turn aid in immunosuppression.

Melanoma tumors are also able to suppress the immune system systemically through the release of exosomes carrying proteins, miRNAs, and mRNA that circulate through the blood [99–101]. Exosomes are small vesicles naturally released by the tumor. Initially this was considered a random process but recent data has suggested that, instead, this provides a way for the tumor cells to communicate with each other as well as educate niches to be permissive to the development of metastases [102, 103]. In fact, exosomes have been shown to carry oncoproteins such as the MET protein, which in turn induces secretion of VEGF and prepares the environment for metastatic development [103]. Exosomes are able to influence a permissive immune niche for tumor growth through a skewing of the development of myeloid cells toward the MDSC state through delivery of cytokines and other key factors involved in their development to distant hematopoietic sites in the body [104].

Although the tumor microenvironment has evolved to aid its own growth and development through taking advantage of features of the immune system, many emerging therapies are counterbalancing the immune response against the tumor. Adoptive T-cell therapy, blockade of inhibitory signaling pathways through the use of blocking antibodies, and the addition of cytokines to aid the growth and survival of tumor reactive T cells will all be discussed in a later section.

2.4.1 Immunotherapy: Enhancing De Novo Antitumor Immunity

Until recently, treatment options for solid tumors such as melanoma were surgery, chemotherapy, and radiotherapy. Although these treatments can be very effective, some patients affected by aggressive cancers such as metastatic stage IV melanoma often have to face the failure of treatment. In the past three decades, a new type of treatment using biological resources has come to the forefront of cancer therapy, immunotherapy. Immunotherapy capitalizes on the use of different components of the immune system such as antibodies and immune cells to eradicate the tumor cells. This concept is based around the fact that the tumor expresses TAA, as previously discussed, and so it is seen by the immune system as a foreign object that needs to be eliminated. Immunotherapy is also about providing tools to activate the immune cells and/or protecting them against suppression generated by the tumor and/or its environment. Immunotherapy of cancer can be divided into four categories: cytokines, vaccines, antibodies, and cell based. This section will generally address these different categories specifically regarding melanoma treatment.

Melanoma has been considered the pioneer cancer regarding development of immunotherapy due to the richness of TAA-specific CD8+ T cells found in melanoma patients' tumors and blood [105, 106]. One of the first types of immunotherapy to be applied was the use of cytokines as sole agents. The immune response is a complex sequence of events that requires communication between the immune cells and the surrounding environment. Cytokines are small proteins that play an important mediator role in the communication network. There are over 200 known cytokines involved, both locally and systemically, in different spheres of the immune response. The specificity of the cytokine response is ensured by the expression of the corresponding receptor(s) on the surface of the target cell. At the site of secretion, the gradient created and the short half-life of cytokines also dictates the response. Capitalizing on the importance of cytokines in the mediation of the immune response, IL-2 was the first to be used as a systemic treatment in melanoma. An antitumor response was observed in these patients but only 3–5 % achieved a complete and durable response [107, 108]. Aside from activation of antitumor T cells, administration of systemic IL-2 can also lead to the activation of Tregs, which express a receptor that is highly specific for that cytokine [109]. Activation of these Tregs can block the antitumor response, diminishing the effect of the therapy. Another side effect of IL-2 therapy that is encountered, especially when using high doses, is the vascular leak syndrome that occurs with a massive release of cytokines such as IL-1, IFN-γ, and tumor necrosis factor alpha (TNF-α). These cytokines interfere with vascular permeability, which can result in serious complications for the patient such as pulmonary edema [110]. Renal, gastric, and neurologic toxicities have also been reported in patients treated with high doses of IL-2 [111]. In an effort to avoid such side effects, different groups have been working toward developing synthetic or chimeric versions of this cytokine, which represents a promising avenue for immunotherapy, especially if used in combination with the other types of immunotherapy subsequently described here [112–115]. Aside from IL-2, which has so far been the most popular cytokine to be used as a front line treatment, other cytokines such as IFN-α, IL-12, IFN-γ, TNF-α, GM-CSF, IL-15, and IL-21 have either been tested or are currently being used in ongoing clinical trials [116, 117] and www.clinicaltrials.gov. These cytokines have been used either in a recombinant form, as a fusion protein, or in a gene vector.

Another type of immunotherapy that has been widely tested in metastatic stage IV melanoma is the peptide vaccine. Capitalizing on the innate presence of T cells with directed specificity against defined MHC class 1 peptides derived from TAA such as MART-1, tyrosinase, and gp100, clinical trials have been carried out with vaccines containing these peptides with the addition of Montanide ISA (*incomplete Freund's adjuvant*) and cytokines such as IL-2 to boost the patient's endogenous antitumor response. Aside from reports of higher levels of antigen-specific T cells in the blood post-vaccination, no significant clinical response was obtained. However, one study using a gp100 peptide reported a higher clinical response when compared to IL-2 alone and brought hope for this cost-effective strategy [118]. However, questions have been raised regarding the use of other types of peptide such as those generated from mutations and identified by exome sequencing of the tumor. It is believed that these peptide could be able to raise a more potent and durable endogenous antitumor response [38, 119]. In addition, questions have also been raised around the use of Montanide as an adjuvant as it may not be optimal to generate potent immune responses at the tumor site [120]. Research efforts are now being pushed toward the development of new strategies to enhance immunogenicity of peptides with the use of new adjuvants such as crystals or viral plant particles. APC subsets, such as DC, have also been used in combination with peptides or the whole protein to help boost the endogenous antitumor response by delivering the antigen to the tumor site and providing additional costimulation to T cells. Our group is currently conducting a clinical trial combining MART-1 peptide-loaded DC, high-dose IL-2, and adoptive transfer of TIL which will be discussed later in this section. Other trials using peptide-pulsed DC or engineered DC-expressing TAA are also currently ongoing (www.clinicaltrials.gov). Although promising, there is still much debate about the optimal type of DC to be used in this vaccine setting [121].

Tumor cells have also been used in vaccination. Whole cell lysates, generated by multiple rounds of freeze/thaw to generate tumor necrosis or irradiation to induce apoptosis, have been given as a sole agent or combined with the administration of preloaded or fused DC (www.clinicaltrials.gov). Although this approach provides access to a myriad of different known and unknown TAAs to be included in the vaccine, no major benefit was reported for melanoma. Interestingly, other cancer cell components, such as exosomes [122–124], are also being explored for use in a vaccine. Melanoma tumor cells have the capacity to secrete microvesicules called exosomes, which may contain TAA such as gp100, MART-1, and tyrosinase [125]. These exosomes can be used as components of an antitumor vaccine to boost the immune response. However, one must be careful with the use of naturally derived exosomes for it has been shown that these microvesicules can contain immunosuppressive factors and even receptors, which could suppress the immune response [122–124, 126]. They can also contain oncoproteins such as MET which is an oncogenic tyrosine kinase receptor, which can favor metastasis and induce vascular leakage [102, 103].

As described in previous sections, the tumor microenvironment takes advantage of the presence of inhibitory molecules on both immune and cancer cells to suppress the antitumor immune response. Conversely, this also provides a target to block these immune checkpoints. Current methods use antibodies directed against inhibitory molecules found on the invading T cells such as cytotoxic T-lymphocyte antigen 4 (CTLA-4) and programmed death receptor 1 (PD-1). Another method is designed to block the inhibitory ligands found on the tumor cells and the MDSCs within the tumor microenvironment such as programmed death ligand 1 (PD-L1). Anti-CTLA-4 (drug name ipilimumab, marketed by Bristol-Myers Squibb as Yervoy) was the first checkpoint inhibitor to gain FDA approval for the treatment of melanoma. In a recent melanoma phase III clinical trial, patients who received anti-CTLA-4 showed an improved overall survival of 10 months had an overall response rate of 10.9 with 60 % maintaining an objective response rate for 2 years post treatment [127]. While anti-CTLA-4 has been proven effective in some patients, the side effects can be severe. The use of this antibody causes the breakdown of immune tolerance to normal body tissues resulting in an increased risk of autoimmunity as well as gastrointestinal toxicities, hepatitis, and dermatitis.

Antibodies directed against PD-1 (nivolumab and MK3475) have also shown considerable efficacy in clinical trials in melanoma as well as in other types of cancer. The Bristol-Myers Squibb anti-PD-1 antibody (nivolumab), which blocks the binding of PD-1 to both PD-L1 and PD-L2, showed significant effectiveness in late-stage melanoma with a 31 % response rate and median response duration of 24 months [128]. Blockade of PD-1, using another antibody generated at Merck (lambrolizumab), resulted in a 38 % overall response rate with 81 % durable response at 11 months after initiation of treatment of stage III/IV melanoma [129]. Interestingly, the adverse side effects of anti-PD-1 therapies are not as severe as those using anti-CTLA-4. Although the risk of autoimmunity is still present in anti-PD-1 therapy, most patients experienced rash, diarrhea, and fatigue.

The use of antibodies directed against PD-L1 has been less utilized in the treatment of melanoma than the anti-PD-1 therapy but still shows therapeutic efficacy. Cellular inhibition through PD-1 can be due to its binding either PD-L1 or PD-L2. Thus blocking PD-1 in fact blocks both these pathways, while PD-L1 blockade only blocks the one. However, 2 independent phase I/II dose escalation trials have demonstrated that treatment of melanoma with anti-PD-L1 results in 17 % (BMS-936559) and 38 % (MPDL3280A) response rate [130]. Such positive results have increased the interest in the use of antibodies as therapeutic agents in melanoma.

Alternatively, antibodies directed against important T-cell costimulatory molecules such as OX40 and 4-1BB are regaining ground in the treatment of melanoma. In this case, however, the antibodies are agonistic in nature and so induce a positive feedback signal to the T cells. The combination of anti-OX40 and IL-2 has been shown to be effective in mouse models [131]. The combination of anti-OX40 and anti-CTLA-4 therapy in metastatic melanoma is also being examined in a current phase I/II clinical trial. In addition, different strategies targeting 4-1BB are emerging to be potentially effective.

While the methods described above are able to induce tumor regression in some patients, currently some of the most effective treatments for late-stage melanoma are cell based and referred to as adoptive cell therapy (ACT). This involves the isolation of TAA-specific T cells from the patients' blood or tumor. As a number of melanoma TAA are characterized (e.g., MART-1, gp100), these cells can be isolated from the blood and expanded in vitro in an antigen-specific matter and then infused back into the patient. This method has been tested using CD8$^+$ T-cell clones (homogenous population) directed against MART-1 and gp100 MHC class 1 peptides. One study from 2002 reported tumor regression in 2 out of the 10 patients infused with the TAA-specific clones [132]. Subsequent work revealed that persistence of the transferred cells and gain of a memory phenotype after infusion were important to achieve clinical response [133]. The use of selected CD4$^+$ T-cell clones directed against the NY-ESO1 antigen in melanoma has also been tested but with little reported success [134]. In addition, the identification of other epitopes to generate CD4$^+$ T-cell clones is challenging and so does not play in favor of the use of that subset in ACT [135].

Expanding TAA-specific T cells of known reactivity is limited by the number of known epitopes and only provides for reactivity against those epitopes for a defined MCH-class I type, the most popular being HLA-A0201. Another cell-based approach is based on the concept that the T cells found at the tumor site will be enriched for reactivity against multiple known and unknown TAAs. This involves the surgical resection of a tumor and expansion of the tumor-infiltrating lymphocytes (TILs) followed by infusion into the patient. Adoptive transfer of TIL for the treatment of metastatic melanoma was first performed at the National Cancer

Institute [136]. In this study, TIL ACT was followed by IL-2 therapy to aid T cell growth in vivo. By 1994, TIL ACT in metastatic melanoma had a response rate of 34 % [107]. In the years that followed, it was found that non-myeloablative chemotherapy prior to TIL ACT improved the response rate to around 50 % at three independent institutions [137–139]. Lymphodepletion prior to TIL transfer aids in the removal of suppressive immune cells such as Tregs and provides access to endogenous cell survival cytokines such as IL-7 and IL-15. Interestingly, while the presence of a high percentage of CD8+ T cells in the infusion product was found to significantly correlate with clinical response [138, 139], infusion of CD8+ T cells alone did not improve clinical efficacy above the transfer of bulk TIL [140]. However, the use of total body irradiation prior to TIL infusion was successful in increasing the response rate up to 72 % [137].

Given the success of TIL in the treatment of melanoma, some researchers have attempted to manipulate the TIL to enhance their antitumor functions and persistence after treatment through the secretion of cytokines (e.g., IL-12) [141]. Current clinical trials at MD Anderson are exploring whether inducing expression of a chemokine receptor (CXCR2) might aid in the migration of TIL to the tumor site or make the TIL unable to be suppressed by secreted factors (DN TGF-βR).

TCR gene therapy is another way to induce an antitumor response that has been tested using PBMCs virally manipulated to express a foreign TCR to induce recognition of known TAAs such as MART-1 [142]. In early clinical trials, only two patients showed regression of tumor metastases and had persistence of the infused, genetically engineered T cells at 1 year after infusion. The possibility of engineered TCR signaling not being powerful enough to generate an antitumor response and persistence was suggested and so a new TCR was generated against MART-1. This new TCR demonstrated a higher affinity for the MART-1 peptide and was used to treat an additional 20 patients followed by IL-2 with prior lymphodepletion. While a 30 % objective clinical response was observed, some patients experienced a strong autoimmune response such as hearing loss due to the destruction of normal melanocytes in the ear as well as in the skin and eye [143]. A recent study using anti-MAGE-A3-engineered T cells showed clinical effectiveness but also generated severe neurologic toxicities resulting in the death of two patients [35]. Overall, these studies highlight the powerful responses generated by the use of the engineered TCRs showing a strong affinity for a specific peptide and are making the field aware of the importance of selecting the right TAA to target to avoid dramatic off-target consequences.

Chimeric antigen receptors (CARs) represent another mechanism by which PBMCs and potentially TIL can be manipulated to express selected anti-TAAs. CAR T cells are generated to express a monoclonal antibody as a receptor to recognize a given TAA. This allows the T cell to have reactivity against tumor antigens that does not require processing and presentation of the antigen, hence no MHC restrictions. CARs have been very popular in treatment of some hematologic cancers with the last couple of years demonstrating very promising results [144–146]. CAR-engineered T cells are a powerful tool by which it is possible to generate a strong immune response; however, studies in solid tumors other than melanoma using an anti-erbb2 CAR have also shown that there is great risk associated with such a high potent response [147]. Again, precaution has to be taken in the selection of the target and its expression in normal cells. Mechanisms for quick destruction of the CAR-expressing cells are also being developed to eradicate the cells if needed. Still, clinical trials using anti-VEGFR-engineered CAR T cells are currently recruiting patients with stage IV melanoma (www.clinicaltrial.com). Additionally, based on preclinical data showing anti-melanoma tumor responses and increased survival in mouse xenograft models, other clinical trials are recruiting patients for treatment using anti-GD2 and anti-GD3 CAR T cells in solid cancer [148, 149].

The cellular-based immunotherapies are a great example of how the combination of treatments can be used to obtain clinical success. Transfer of TAA-specific cells combined with cytokines and sometimes booster vaccines has been achieving better results in clinical trials than cell product transfer alone. Antibodies like anti-CTLA-4 and anti-PD-1 are now being added to the treatments to improve therapy. As single-therapy agents, the new compounds do not always show the expected results; however, their use is setting the stage for the combination of multiple targeted agents as well as a combination of cell-based and antibody-based immunotherapy. Many questions remain regarding when and which immunotherapy should be applied for the treatment of melanoma. The use of biomarkers to aid in this decision-making process is attractive but remains unclear. For example, in an anti-PD-1 study, the presence of PD-L1 in the tumor emerged as a biomarker for response to therapy [128]. However, this has not yet been confirmed in other studies. Another example is the presence of TIL in the tumor as a biomarker for ACT. If it was possible to know prior to resection if the tumor is infiltrated with lymphocytes and their functional quality, we could know whether TIL ACT is appropriate and if not which other treatment to use [150]. One thing is clear; immunoselection is one of the worst enemies of immunotherapy. This is why it is vital to target multiple tumor antigens and combine cell-based and antibody-based therapy to maximize antitumor responses and persistence of TAA-specific cells.

2.5 Biomarkers of Active and Suppressive Immune Regulatory Mechanisms in Melanoma Patients: Is the Presence of Immunosuppressive Factors in the Tumor Microenvironment Bad or Good?

More and more evidences emerged and showed that the classification of cancer related to estimating the clinical outcome should base on the tumor microenvironment, considering the effects of the host immune response. The immunological status of the microenvironment among different immunotherapies could explain the difference between response and resistance of melanoma patients or predict patient prognosis. Currently, there are several approaches to study or measure the role of the immune system in melanoma. As shown in the model in Fig. 2.4, key biomarkers can be measured in an interaction between tumor- and host-derived factors regulating the degree of T cell infiltration into tumors and the phenotype and antitumor

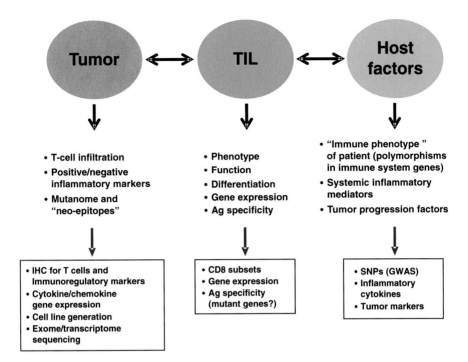

Fig. 2.4 Systems biology approach to biomarker discovery for melanoma immunotherapy. Biomarkers can be used to measure the interaction between tumor- and host-derived factors and the regulation of T-cell infiltration into tumors and the phenotype and antitumor activity of the TIL. This approach may allow physicians to delineate patients who may respond to immunotherapy prior to therapy

activity of these TILs. It can delineate patients who are responding to immunotherapy as well as predicting who may respond before therapy.

Gene expression profiling using Nanostring nCounter™ analysis system could accurate quantify the RNA levels from fresh-frozen and FFPE samples in small amounts of total RNA [151]. This new technology could identify different genes panels, such as immunology panel, inflammatory panel, and cancer-related gene panel, as potential immunotherapy targets for melanoma [152] or as biomarkers to predict melanoma patient prognosis, and therefore identify the patients who would benefit from immunotherapy. Messina et al. found that 12-chemokine (CCL18, CCL19, CCL2, CCL21, CCL3, CCL4, CCL5, CCL8, CXCL10, CXCL11, CXCL13, and CXCL9) gene expression signature (GES) score was associated with better overall survival in metastatic melanoma [30]. Same results were shown by Tanese et al. when they compared the gene expression profile between iNOS-positive and iNOS-negative tumor samples and found CXCL10 expression was upregulated in iNOS-negative groups and had the most favorable prognosis [153], while inducible nitric oxide synthase (iNOS) and nitrotyrosine (NT) expression in patients with stage III melanoma strongly corrected with poor survival [55]. Although *BRAF V600E, KIT, and NRAS* mutations are the most important drivers of melanoma development and could predict the poor outcome of melanoma patients [154], epigenetic analysis found the DNA methylation is associated with melanoma progression [155, 156].

Patients with a high ratio of T-cell infiltration have clinical responses to melanoma vaccines and anti-CTLA-4 monoclonal antibody (ipilimumab) therapies [157, 158]. Steven A. Rosenberg's group also found an overall increase of total number of CD8$^+$ T-cell infiltration in metastatic melanoma between the responders to TIL therapy and the nonresponders; however, there was no significant difference [159]. One possible reason may be that the infiltrations of inflammatory and lymphocytic cells were not randomly distributed in the tumor. For example, they found a significant increase of FoxP3$^+$ CD4 Treg cells in the intratumoral areas compared with peritumoral areas [159] and illustrated the selective accumulation of T cells in tumor. Galen et al. set up an immunoscore approach by immunohistochemical technology to analyze the location, density, and function of different immune cell types. It is important and useful for routine clinical use for classification of cancer, identification of the prognostic factors for disease-free survival (DFS) and overall survival (OS), and the potential targets for immunotherapy [160–162].

Recent studies suggested the immunosuppressive mechanisms in tumor microenvironment that inhibit T-cell activation [163] might also explain the reason for resistance of tumor immunotherapies. Gajewski's group found that the inhibitory pathways might have a negative feedback loop. Their results show that CD8$^+$ T-cell-infiltrated metastatic melanomas had higher expression of inhibitory factors, indoleamine-2,3-dioeygenase (IDO), PD-L1/B7-H1, and FoxP3$^+$ regulatory T cells (Tregs), and therefore are candidates for T-cell function inhibitors at the tumor site [20].

2.6 Conclusions: Where Is It All Heading?

The immune system has a remarkable capacity to recognize and control cancer growth and eradicate cancer cells through a variety of innate and adaptive effector mechanisms both at early stages and later stages either through de novo mechanisms or by clinical interventions that enhance immune responses through immunotherapy, as described in this chapter.

Much progress has occurred in our molecular understanding of cancer and how it interacts with the immune system and what key immune system drivers or blockers in melanoma can be harnessed to treat early- and late-stage disease. A key concept that has become apparent is that we need to view each tumor differently as an independent entity and that the tumor microenvironment needs to be viewed in context of the whole organism (cancer patient) where it forms a new ecosystem within the host as a "wound that never heals" or as "wounds in different parts of the body that have great trouble healing." It has become apparent that tumors can regulate the immune response in the host both at short and long distances (e.g., exosomes can travel long distances through the circulation as can some dislodged tumor cells). For example, metastatic melanoma cells can induce the differentiation of suppressive MDSCs from monocytes through prostaglandins and COX-2 as well as through the release of

TGF-β. These MDSCs can express chemokine receptors (e.g., CCR7) that promote their homing not only to local but also in some cases distal lymphoid organs (lymph nodes and spleen) that do not harbor any tumor cells at all. At these sites, these MDSCs can set up an environment of systemic immunosuppression, especially in context of tumor-derived antigens that can be carried to these sites by these suppressive myeloid cells or, as recently demonstrated, through the uptake of tumor-derived exosomes that can traffic to these sites [122–124]. Tumor-derived exosomes can not only contain tumor biomarkers and tumor antigens but also contain factors, such as micro-RNA and other non-coding RNA, and immunosuppressive proteins that can be internalized by MDSCs at these local and distal lymphoid organ sites inducing T-cell tolerance, T-regulatory cell activation, and the inhibition of effector T-cell responses through the uptake of exosome-derived mediators directly into responding T cells [122–124]. Thus, tumors can elicit long-distance control over immune responses. This necessitates us to study the cancer patient as a whole ecosystem linking biomarkers of the immune response and tumor progression and metastasis and control in a systems biology approach looking at both systemic and tumor-localized proteomic and genomic factors regulating these processes.

Another area in which key concepts are rapidly changing is how we view the presence or detection of immunosuppressive pathways, especially at the tumor site. In the Introduction, we introduced the concept that the immune system is just beginning to recognize cancer as a problem, especially now in this new human age where life spans are increasing in length. Up until recently human evolution is needed to deal with the "enemy" of infectious disease to ensure survival through reproductive age. This protective process also needed coevolution of a counteractive process to limit or balance highly activated or powerful immune responses by invoking negative feedback processes that inhibit adaptive inflammatory responses to prevent immunopathology and autoimmunity. We are now also beginning that in fact this negative feedback or suppression of overly strong immune responses is also the key problem preventing effective tumor control during de novo immune responses or during responses elicited during immunotherapy. Thus, the focus of immunotherapy has shifted recently into both activating stronger antitumor responses (e.g., through cancer vaccines and proinflammatory cytokines like IL-2) and preventing this feedback inhibition through immunomodulators that inhibit signaling pathways, such as CTLA-4, PD-1, amino acid deprivation, and suppressive cytokines (e.g., TGF-β). The latter has been collectively called immune "checkpoints," with "checkpoint blockade" using drugs and antibodies used to overcome these negative factors or checkpoints. Thus, an effective immune response against cancer must balance these two processes and future work will need to identify the situations (specific types of cancer and cancer stages and locations in the body) and how we fine-tune this balance between regulating these two processes. In addition, immune-based biomarkers in different patients will be critical to determine when and how we should use immune-activating or checkpoint blockade or both in specific circumstances. These biomarkers will identify patients with an active de novo antitumor response, using antitumor immune response measurements both in the blood and the tumor microenvironment (e.g., tumor biopsies) or those where a de novo response is weak or missing. Therapies will need to manipulate the immune response based on these biomarkers, where in the former case, more activation and/or checkpoint blockade may be applied and, in the latter case, a stronger immune-activating regimen (both against the tumor and enhancing overall "immunocompetence") may be needed. This new reality has also beginning to transform the way we interpret the detection of immunosuppressive biomarkers especially at the tumor site. Recent biomarker data now suggests that it is not the tumor cells that intrinsically turn on immunosuppressive pathways at the tumor site, but rather the immune system itself is orchestrating this. Thus, biomarkers of immunosuppression are being reinterpreted as being positive markers and not negative markers indicative of a stronger innate and adaptive immune response rather than a suppressed response. This contrasting view to our previously held beliefs will rewrite how we study antitumor immunity and how we apply immunotherapy. As shown in Fig. 2.5, this new conceptual framework can allow us to stratify patients toward different types or groups of thera-

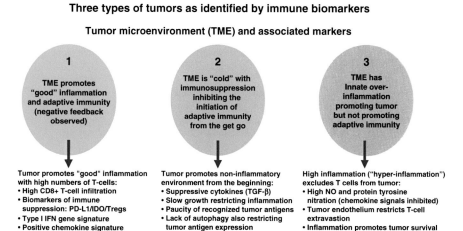

Three types of tumors as identified by immune biomarkers

Tumor microenvironment (TME) and associated markers

1
TME promotes "good" inflammation and adaptive immunity (negative feedback observed)

Tumor promotes "good" inflammation with high numbers of T-cells:
• High CD8+ T-cell infiltration
• Biomarkers of immune suppression: PD-L1/IDO/Tregs
• Type I IFN gene signature
• Positive chemokine signature
• Permissive tumor endothelium

2
TME is "cold" with immunosuppression inhibiting the initiation of adaptive immunity from the get go

Tumor promotes non-inflammatory environment from the beginning:
• Suppressive cytokines (TGF-β)
• Slow growth restricting inflammation
• Paucity of recognized tumor antigens
• Lack of autophagy also restricting tumor antigen expression

3
TME has Innate over-inflammation promoting tumor but not promoting adaptive immunity

High inflammation ("hyper-inflammation") excludes T cells from tumor:
• High NO and protein tyrosine nitration (chemokine signals inhibited)
• Tumor endothelium restricts T-cell extravastion
• Inflammation promotes tumor survival over adaptive immune response

Fig. 2.5 New conceptual framework can allow us to stratify patients toward different types or groups of therapies based on the characteristics of their tumor-localized immune response. The goldilocks principle of tumors based on immune biomarkers: (1) "good" inflammation where a balanced set of innate immune factors and adaptive immune factors coupled with chemokine expression and DC activation leads to a high degree of T-cell infiltration versus too much infiltration by other myeloid cells such as macrophages and MDSCs; (2) non-inflammatory or "cold" tumor microenvironment that limits inflammation and infiltration by adaptive immune cells through cancer cell-derived powerful, intrinsic immunosuppression, such as high TGF-β release; and (3) "hyper-inflammation" in which the local inflammatory response is directed away from a more balance set of factors facilitating the migration of T cells and other adaptive immune cells into the tumor microenvironment and their survival and effector function toward an *over-production* of innate cytokines such as IL-1α and IL-1β, TNF-α, IL-6, IL-12, VEGF, endothelins, and Toll-like receptor agonists that not only feedback inhibit T cells but also drive strong NFκB activation in tumor cells and tumor cell survival and further secretion of these "negative" factors in a positive feedback loop. This latter tumor microenvironment may be exemplified by high peroxynitrite and protein nitration that can inhibit the function of key proteins such as chemokines and chemokine receptors or the activation of endothelial cells needed to drive T cells into the tumor

pies based on the characteristics of their tumor-localized immune response or markers in context to their systemic immune system or state of their overall immune system or "immune health" that will have another set of measured values. This will be the new reality for cancer care.

References

1. Frank SA (2002) Immunology and evolution of infectious disease. Princeton University Press, Princeton, NJ
2. Janeway CAJ, Travers P, Walport M, Shlomchik MJ (2001) Immunobiology: the immune system in health and disease, 5th edn. Garland Science, New York, NY
3. Schiavoni G, Gabriele L, Mattei F (2013) The tumor microenvironment: a pitch for multiple players. Front Oncol 3:90
4. Lu C, Kerbel RS (1994) Cytokines, growth factors and the loss of negative growth controls in the progression of human cutaneous malignant melanoma. Curr Opin Oncol 6:212–220
5. Bar-Eli M (1999) Role of interleukin-8 in tumor growth and metastasis of human melanoma. Pathobiology 67:12–18
6. Di Cesare S, Marshall JC, Fernandes BF, Logan P, Antecka E, Filho VB, Burnier MN Jr (2007) In vitro characterization and inhibition of the CXCR4/CXCL12 chemokine axis in human uveal melanoma cell lines. Cancer Cell Int 7:17
7. Mrowietz U, Schwenk U, Maune S et al (1999) The chemokine RANTES is secreted by human melanoma cells and is associated with enhanced tumour formation in nude mice. Br J Cancer 79:1025–1031
8. Bergenwald C, Westermark G, Sander B (1997) Variable expression of tumor necrosis factor alpha in human malignant melanoma localized by in situ hybridization for mRNA. Cancer Immunol Immunother 44:335–340
9. Harlin H, Meng Y, Peterson AC et al (2009) Chemokine expression in melanoma metastases associated with CD8+ T-cell recruitment. Cancer Res 69:3077–3085
10. Balsamo M, Scordamaglia F, Pietra G et al (2009) Melanoma-associated fibroblasts modulate NK cell phenotype and antitumor cytotoxicity. Proc Natl Acad Sci USA 106:20847–20852
11. Azimi F, Scolyer RA, Rumcheva P et al (2012) Tumor-infiltrating lymphocyte grade is an independent predictor of sentinel lymph node status and survival in patients with cutaneous melanoma. J Clin Oncol 30:2678–2683
12. Fridman WH, Pages F, Sautes-Fridman C, Galon J (2012) The immune contexture in human tumours: impact on clinical outcome. Nat Rev Cancer 12:298–306
13. Senovilla L, Vacchelli E, Galon J et al (2012) Trial watch: prognostic and predictive value of the immune infiltrate in cancer. Oncoimmunology 1:1323–1343
14. Cordova A, Toia F, La Mendola C et al (2012) Characterization of human gammadelta T lymphocytes infiltrating primary malignant melanomas. PLoS One 7:e49878
15. Metelitsa LS, Wu HW, Wang H et al (2004) Natural killer T cells infiltrate neuroblastomas expressing the chemokine CCL2. J Exp Med 199:1213–1221
16. Makitie T, Summanen P, Tarkkanen A, Kivela T (2001) Tumor-infiltrating macrophages (CD68(+) cells) and prognosis in malignant uveal melanoma. Invest Ophthalmol Vis Sci 42:1414–1421
17. Bronkhorst IH, Ly LV, Jordanova ES, Vrolijk J, Versluis M, Luyten GP, Jager MJ (2011) Detection of M2-macrophages in uveal melanoma and relation with survival. Invest Ophthalmol Vis Sci 52:643–650
18. Martin-Orozco N, Li Y, Wang Y et al (2010) Melanoma cells express ICOS ligand to promote the activation and expansion of T-regulatory cells. Cancer Res 70:9581–9590

19. Gros A, Turcotte S, Wunderlich JR, Ahmadzadeh M, Dudley ME, Rosenberg SA (2012) Myeloid cells obtained from the blood but not from the tumor can suppress T-cell proliferation in patients with melanoma. Clin Cancer Res 18:5212–5223

20. Spranger S, Spaapen RM, Zha Y, Williams J, Meng Y, Ha TT, Gajewski TF (2013) Up-regulation of PD-L1, IDO, and T(regs) in the melanoma tumor microenvironment is driven by CD8(+) T cells. Sci Transl Med 5:200ra116

21. Kerkar SP, Restifo NP (2012) Cellular constituents of immune escape within the tumor microenvironment. Cancer Res 72:3125–3130

22. Gabrilovich DI, Ostrand-Rosenberg S, Bronte V (2012) Coordinated regulation of myeloid cells by tumours. Nat Rev Immunol 12:253–268

23. Siddiqui SA, Frigola X, Bonne-Annee S et al (2007) Tumor-infiltrating Foxp3-CD4+CD25+ T cells predict poor survival in renal cell carcinoma. Clin Cancer Res 13:2075–2081

24. Curiel TJ, Coukos G, Zou L et al (2004) Specific recruitment of regulatory T cells in ovarian carcinoma fosters immune privilege and predicts reduced survival. Nat Med 10:942–949

25. Harlin H, Kuna TV, Peterson AC, Meng Y, Gajewski TF (2006) Tumor progression despite massive influx of activated CD8(+) T cells in a patient with malignant melanoma ascites. Cancer Immunol Immunother 55:1185–1197

26. Appay V, Jandus C, Voelter V et al (2006) New generation vaccine induces effective melanoma-specific CD8+ T cells in the circulation but not in the tumor site. J Immunol 177:1670–1678

27. Zippelius A, Batard P, Rubio-Godoy V et al (2004) Effector function of human tumor-specific CD8 T cells in melanoma lesions: a state of local functional tolerance. Cancer Res 64:2865–2873

28. Wu RC, Liu S, Chacon JA et al (2012) Detection and characterization of a novel subset of CD8(+)CD57(+) T cells in metastatic melanoma with an incompletely differentiated phenotype. Clin Cancer Res 18:2465–2477

29. Gajewski TF, Woo SR, Zha Y, Spaapen R, Zheng Y, Corrales L, Spranger S (2013) Cancer immunotherapy strategies based on overcoming barriers within the tumor microenvironment. Curr Opin Immunol 25:268–276

30. Messina JL, Fenstermacher DA, Eschrich S et al (2012) 12-Chemokine gene signature identifies lymph node-like structures in melanoma: potential for patient selection for immunotherapy? Sci Rep 2:765

31. Cripps JG, Wang J, Maria A, Blumenthal I, Gorham JD (2010) Type 1 T helper cells induce the accumulation of myeloid-derived suppressor cells in the inflamed Tgfb1 knockout mouse liver. Hepatology 52:1350–1359

32. Romero P, Cerottini JC, Speiser DE (2004) Monitoring tumor antigen specific T-cell responses in cancer patients and phase I clinical trials of peptide-based vaccination. Cancer Immunol Immunother 53:249–255

33. Pilla L, Rivoltini L, Patuzzo R, Marrari A, Valdagni R, Parmiani G (2009) Multipeptide vaccination in cancer patients. Expert Opin Biol Ther 9:1043–1055

34. van der Bruggen P, Traversari C, Chomez P et al (1991) A gene encoding an antigen recognized by cytolytic T lymphocytes on a human melanoma. Science 254:1643–1647

35. Morgan RA, Chinnasamy N, Abate-Daga D et al (2013) Cancer regression and neurological toxicity following anti-MAGE-A3 TCR gene therapy. J Immunother 36:133–151

36. Jager E, Chen YT, Drijfhout JW et al (1998) Simultaneous humoral and cellular immune response against cancer-testis antigen NY-ESO-1: definition of human histocompatibility leukocyte antigen (HLA)-A2-binding peptide epitopes. J Exp Med 187:265–270

37. Anichini A, Maccalli C, Mortarini R et al (1993) Melanoma cells and normal melanocytes share antigens recognized by HLA-A2-restricted cytotoxic T cell clones from melanoma patients. J Exp Med 177:989–998

38. Matsushita H, Vesely MD, Koboldt DC et al (2012) Cancer exome analysis reveals a T-cell-dependent mechanism of cancer immunoediting. Nature 482:400–404

39. Robbins PF, Lu YC, El-Gamil M et al (2013) Mining exomic sequencing data to identify mutated antigens recognized by adoptively transferred tumor-reactive T cells. Nat Med 19:747–752
40. Niedobitek G (2000) Epstein-Barr virus infection in the pathogenesis of nasopharyngeal carcinoma. Mol Pathol 53:248–254
41. Muster T, Waltenberger A, Grassauer A et al (2003) An endogenous retrovirus derived from human melanoma cells. Cancer Res 63:8735–8741
42. Schanab O, Humer J, Gleiss A et al (2011) Expression of human endogenous retrovirus K is stimulated by ultraviolet radiation in melanoma. Pigment Cell Melanoma Res 24:656–665
43. Serafino A, Balestrieri E, Pierimarchi P et al (2009) The activation of human endogenous retrovirus K (HERV-K) is implicated in melanoma cell malignant transformation. Exp Cell Res 315:849–862
44. Schiavetti F, Thonnard J, Colau D, Boon T, Coulie PG (2002) A human endogenous retroviral sequence encoding an antigen recognized on melanoma by cytolytic T lymphocytes. Cancer Res 62:5510–5516
45. Trinchieri G (2012) Cancer and inflammation: an old intuition with rapidly evolving new concepts. Annu Rev Immunol 30:677–706
46. Dunn JH, Ellis LZ, Fujita M (2012) Inflammasomes as molecular mediators of inflammation and cancer: potential role in melanoma. Cancer Lett 314:24–33
47. Melnikova VO, Bar-Eli M (2009) Inflammation and melanoma metastasis. Pigment Cell Melanoma Res 22:257–267
48. Richmond A, Yang J, Su Y (2009) The good and the bad of chemokines/chemokine receptors in melanoma. Pigment Cell Melanoma Res 22:175–186
49. Dore JF, Pedeux R, Boniol M, Chignol MC, Autier P (2001) Intermediate-effect biomarkers in prevention of skin cancer. IARC Sci Publ 154:81–91
50. Zaidi MR, Davis S, Noonan FP et al (2011) Interferon-gamma links ultraviolet radiation to melanomagenesis in mice. Nature 469:548–553
51. Ahmed B, Van Den Oord JJ (2000) Expression of the inducible isoform of nitric oxide synthase in pigment cell lesions of the skin. Br J Dermatol 142:432–440
52. Kuchel JM, Barnetson RS, Halliday GM (2003) Nitric oxide appears to be a mediator of solar-simulated ultraviolet radiation-induced immunosuppression in humans. J Invest Dermatol 121:587–593
53. Grimm EA, Sikora AG, Ekmekcioglu S (2013) Molecular pathways: inflammation-associated nitric-oxide production as a cancer-supporting redox mechanism and a potential therapeutic target. Clin Cancer Res 19:5557–5563
54. Grimm EA, Ellerhorst J, Tang CH, Ekmekcioglu S (2008) Constitutive intracellular production of iNOS and NO in human melanoma: possible role in regulation of growth and resistance to apoptosis. Nitric Oxide 19:133–137
55. Ekmekcioglu S, Ellerhorst J, Smid CM, Prieto VG, Munsell M, Buzaid AC, Grimm EA (2000) Inducible nitric oxide synthase and nitrotyrosine in human metastatic melanoma tumors correlate with poor survival. Clin Cancer Res 6:4768–4775
56. Bonafe M, Storci G, Franceschi C (2012) Inflamm-aging of the stem cell niche: breast cancer as a paradigmatic example: breakdown of the multi-shell cytokine network fuels cancer in aged people. Bioessays 34:40–49
57. Shaw AC, Joshi S, Greenwood H, Panda A, Lord JM (2010) Aging of the innate immune system. Curr Opin Immunol 22:507–513
58. Franceschi C, Bonafe M, Valensin S, Olivieri F, De Luca M, Ottaviani E, De Benedictis G (2000) Inflamm-aging. An evolutionary perspective on immunosenescence. Ann NY Acad Sci 908:244–254
59. Goldszmid RS, Trinchieri G (2012) The price of immunity. Nat Immunol 13:932–938
60. Burnet M (1957) Cancer; a biological approach. I. The processes of control. Br Med J 1:779–786
61. Burnet M (1957) Cancer: a biological approach. III. Viruses associated with neoplastic conditions. IV. Practical applications. Br Med J 1:841–847

62. Miller JF (1961) Immunological function of the thymus. Lancet 2:748–749
63. Stutman O (1974) Tumor development after 3-methylcholanthrene in immunologically deficient athymic-nude mice. Science 183:534–536
64. Stutman O (1975) Delayed tumour appearance and absence of regression in nude mice infected with murine sarcoma virus. Nature 253:142–144
65. Stutman O (1979) Chemical carcinogenesis in nude mice: comparison between nude mice from homozygous matings and heterozygous matings and effect of age and carcinogen dose. J Natl Cancer Inst 62:353–358
66. Seki S, Takeda K, Abo T (1995) The function and role of extrathymic T cells. Nihon Rinsho 53:2846–2857
67. Budzynski W, Radzikowski C (1994) Cytotoxic cells in immunodeficient athymic mice. Immunopharmacol Immunotoxicol 16:319–346
68. Pawelec G (1994) MHC-unrestricted immune surveillance of leukemia. Cancer Biother 9:265–288
69. Kaplan DH, Shankaran V, Dighe AS, Stockert E, Aguet M, Old LJ, Schreiber RD (1998) Demonstration of an interferon gamma-dependent tumor surveillance system in immunocompetent mice. Proc Natl Acad Sci USA 95:7556–7561
70. Shankaran V, Ikeda H, Bruce AT, White JM, Swanson PE, Old LJ, Schreiber RD (2001) IFNgamma and lymphocytes prevent primary tumour development and shape tumour immunogenicity. Nature 410:1107–1111
71. Vesely MD, Schreiber RD (2013) Cancer immunoediting: antigens, mechanisms, and implications to cancer immunotherapy. Ann NY Acad Sci 1284:1–5
72. Schreiber RD, Old LJ, Smyth MJ (2011) Cancer immunoediting: integrating immunity's roles in cancer suppression and promotion. Science 331:1565–1570
73. Dunn GP, Bruce AT, Sheehan KC et al (2005) A critical function for type I interferons in cancer immunoediting. Nat Immunol 6:722–729
74. Dunn GP, Bruce AT, Ikeda H, Old LJ, Schreiber RD (2002) Cancer immunoediting: from immunosurveillance to tumor escape. Nat Immunol 3:991–998
75. Smyth MJ, Crowe NY, Godfrey DI (2001) NK cells and NKT cells collaborate in host protection from methylcholanthrene-induced fibrosarcoma. Int Immunol 13:459–463
76. Landsberg J, Kohlmeyer J, Renn M et al (2012) Melanomas resist T-cell therapy through inflammation-induced reversible dedifferentiation. Nature 490:412–416
77. Caramel J, Papadogeorgakis E, Hill L et al (2013) A switch in the expression of embryonic EMT-inducers drives the development of malignant melanoma. Cancer Cell 24:466–480
78. Garrido MC, Requena L, Kutzner H, Ortiz P, Perez-Gomez B, Rodriguez-Peralto JL (2014) Desmoplastic melanoma: expression of epithelial-mesenchymal transition-related proteins. Am J Dermatopathol 36:238–242
79. Taddei ML, Giannoni E, Morandi A et al (2014) Mesenchymal to amoeboid transition is associated with stem-like features of melanoma cells. Cell Commun Signal 12:24
80. Dou J, He X, Liu Y et al (2014) Effect of downregulation of ZEB1 on vimentin expression, tumour migration and tumourigenicity of melanoma B16F10 cells and CSCs. Cell Biol Int 38:452–461
81. Pulido J, Kottke T, Thompson J et al (2012) Using virally expressed melanoma cDNA libraries to identify tumor-associated antigens that cure melanoma. Nat Biotechnol 30:337–343
82. Roesch A, Fukunaga-Kalabis M, Schmidt EC et al (2010) A temporarily distinct subpopulation of slow-cycling melanoma cells is required for continuous tumor growth. Cell 141:583–594
83. Rodriguez PC, Zea AH, Culotta KS, Zabaleta J, Ochoa JB, Ochoa AC (2002) Regulation of T cell receptor CD3zeta chain expression by L-arginine. J Biol Chem 277:21123–21129
84. Rodriguez PC, Quiceno DG, Ochoa AC (2007) L-arginine availability regulates T-lymphocyte cell-cycle progression. Blood 109:1568–1573
85. Nagaraj S, Gupta K, Pisarev V et al (2007) Altered recognition of antigen is a mechanism of CD8+ T cell tolerance in cancer. Nat Med 13:828–835

86. Sinha P, Clements VK, Bunt SK, Albelda SM, Ostrand-Rosenberg S (2007) Cross-talk between myeloid-derived suppressor cells and macrophages subverts tumor immunity toward a type 2 response. J Immunol 179:977–983

87. Li H, Han Y, Guo Q, Zhang M, Cao X (2009) Cancer-expanded myeloid-derived suppressor cells induce anergy of NK cells through membrane-bound TGF-beta 1. J Immunol 182:240–249

88. Gabrilovich DI, Nagaraj S (2009) Myeloid-derived suppressor cells as regulators of the immune system. Nat Rev Immunol 9:162–174

89. Ishida T, Ueda R (2006) CCR4 as a novel molecular target for immunotherapy of cancer. Cancer Sci 97:1139–1146

90. Kimpfler S, Sevko A, Ring S et al (2009) Skin melanoma development in ret transgenic mice despite the depletion of CD25+Foxp3+ regulatory T cells in lymphoid organs. J Immunol 183:6330–6337

91. Strauss L, Bergmann C, Whiteside TL (2009) Human circulating CD4+CD25highFoxp3+ regulatory T cells kill autologous CD8+ but not CD4+ responder cells by Fas-mediated apoptosis. J Immunol 182:1469–1480

92. Strauss L, Bergmann C, Szczepanski MJ, Lang S, Kirkwood JM, Whiteside TL (2008) Expression of ICOS on human melanoma-infiltrating CD4+CD25highFoxp3+ T regulatory cells: implications and impact on tumor-mediated immune suppression. J Immunol 180:2967–2980

93. Zitvogel L, Kepp O, Galluzzi L, Kroemer G (2012) Inflammasomes in carcinogenesis and anticancer immune responses. Nat Immunol 13:343–351

94. Zarek PE, Huang CT, Lutz ER et al (2008) A2A receptor signaling promotes peripheral tolerance by inducing T-cell anergy and the generation of adaptive regulatory T cells. Blood 111:251–259

95. Qureshi OS, Zheng Y, Nakamura K et al (2011) Trans-endocytosis of CD80 and CD86: a molecular basis for the cell-extrinsic function of CTLA-4. Science 332:600–603

96. Derre L, Rivals JP, Jandus C et al (2010) BTLA mediates inhibition of human tumor-specific CD8+ T cells that can be partially reversed by vaccination. J Clin Invest 120:157–167

97. Uyttenhove C, Pilotte L, Theate I et al (2003) Evidence for a tumoral immune resistance mechanism based on tryptophan degradation by indoleamine 2,3-dioxygenase. Nat Med 9:1269–1274

98. Brody JR, Costantino CL, Berger AC et al (2009) Expression of indoleamine 2,3-dioxygenase in metastatic malignant melanoma recruits regulatory T cells to avoid immune detection and affects survival. Cell Cycle 8:1930–1934

99. Simpson RJ, Jensen SS, Lim JW (2008) Proteomic profiling of exosomes: current perspectives. Proteomics 8:4083–4099

100. Lasser C, Eldh M, Lotvall J (2012) Isolation and characterization of RNA-containing exosomes. J Vis Exp 59:e3037

101. Valadi H, Ekstrom K, Bossios A, Sjostrand M, Lee JJ, Lotvall JO (2007) Exosome-mediated transfer of mRNAs and microRNAs is a novel mechanism of genetic exchange between cells. Nat Cell Biol 9:654–659

102. Hood JL, San RS, Wickline SA (2011) Exosomes released by melanoma cells prepare sentinel lymph nodes for tumor metastasis. Cancer Res 71:3792–3801

103. Peinado H, Aleckovic M, Lavotshkin S et al (2012) Melanoma exosomes educate bone marrow progenitor cells toward a pro-metastatic phenotype through MET. Nat Med 18:883–891

104. Bunt SK, Sinha P, Clements VK, Leips J, Ostrand-Rosenberg S (2006) Inflammation induces myeloid-derived suppressor cells that facilitate tumor progression. J Immunol 176:284–290

105. Rosenberg SA (1999) A new era for cancer immunotherapy based on the genes that encode cancer antigens. Immunity 10:281–287

106. Kvistborg P, Shu CJ, Heemskerk B et al (2012) TIL therapy broadens the tumor-reactive CD8(+) T cell compartment in melanoma patients. Oncoimmunology 1:409–418

107. Rosenberg SA, Yannelli JR, Yang JC et al (1994) Treatment of patients with metastatic melanoma with autologous tumor-infiltrating lymphocytes and interleukin 2. J Natl Cancer Inst 86:1159–1166
108. Rosenberg SA, Yang JC, Topalian SL et al (1994) Treatment of 283 consecutive patients with metastatic melanoma or renal cell cancer using high-dose bolus interleukin 2. JAMA 271:907–913
109. Zhang H, Chua KS, Guimond M et al (2005) Lymphopenia and interleukin-2 therapy alter homeostasis of CD4+CD25+ regulatory T cells. Nat Med 11:1238–1243
110. Parmiani G, Rivoltini L, Andreola G, Carrabba M (2000) Cytokines in cancer therapy. Immunol Lett 74:41–44
111. Poust JC, Woolery JE, Green MR (2013) Management of toxicities associated with high-dose interleukin-2 and biochemotherapy. Anticancer Drugs 24:1–13
112. Levin AM, Bates DL, Ring AM et al (2012) Exploiting a natural conformational switch to engineer an interleukin-2 'superkine'. Nature 484:529–533
113. Carmenate T, Pacios A, Enamorado M, Moreno E, Garcia-Martinez K, Fuente D, Leon K (2013) Human IL-2 mutein with higher antitumor efficacy than wild type IL-2. J Immunol 190:6230–6238
114. Heaton KM, Ju G, Grimm EA (1993) Human interleukin 2 analogues that preferentially bind the intermediate-affinity interleukin 2 receptor lead to reduced secondary cytokine secretion: implications for the use of these interleukin 2 analogues in cancer immunotherapy. Cancer Res 53:2597–2602
115. Heaton KM, Rippon MB, El-Naggar A, Tucker SL, Ross MI, Balch CM (1993) Prognostic implications of DNA index in patients with stage III cutaneous melanoma. Am J Surg 166:648–652 (discussion 652–643)
116. Dranoff G (2004) Cytokines in cancer pathogenesis and cancer therapy. Nat Rev Cancer 4:11–22
117. Tarhini AA, Gogas H, Kirkwood JM (2012) IFN-alpha in the treatment of melanoma. J Immunol 189:3789–3793
118. Schwartzentruber DJ, Lawson DH, Richards JM et al (2011) gp100 peptide vaccine and interleukin-2 in patients with advanced melanoma. N Engl J Med 364:2119–2127
119. Lu YC, Yao X, Li YF et al (2013) Mutated PPP1R3B is recognized by T cells used to treat a melanoma patient who experienced a durable complete tumor regression. J Immunol 190:6034–6042
120. Hailemichael Y, Dai Z, Jaffarzad N et al (2013) Persistent antigen at vaccination sites induces tumor-specific CD8(+) T cell sequestration, dysfunction and deletion. Nat Med 19:465–472
121. Klechevsky E, Banchereau J (2013) Human dendritic cells subsets as targets and vectors for therapy. Ann NY Acad Sci 1284:24–30
122. Taylor DD, Gercel-Taylor C (2011) Exosomes/microvesicles: mediators of cancer-associated immunosuppressive microenvironments. Semin Immunopathol 33:441–454
123. Roberson CD, Atay S, Gercel-Taylor C, Taylor DD (2010) Tumor-derived exosomes as mediators of disease and potential diagnostic biomarkers. Cancer Biomark 8:281–291
124. Taylor DD, Gercel-Taylor C (2005) Tumour-derived exosomes and their role in cancer-associated T-cell signalling defects. Br J Cancer 92:305–311
125. Mears R, Craven RA, Hanrahan S et al (2004) Proteomic analysis of melanoma-derived exosomes by two-dimensional polyacrylamide gel electrophoresis and mass spectrometry. Proteomics 4:4019–4031
126. Yang C, Kim SH, Bianco NR, Robbins PD (2011) Tumor-derived exosomes confer antigen-specific immunosuppression in a murine delayed-type hypersensitivity model. PLoS One 6:e22517
127. Hodi FS, O'Day SJ, McDermott DF et al (2010) Improved survival with ipilimumab in patients with metastatic melanoma. N Engl J Med 363:711–723
128. Topalian SL, Hodi FS, Brahmer JR et al (2012) Safety, activity, and immune correlates of anti-PD-1 antibody in cancer. N Engl J Med 366:2443–2454

129. Hamid O, Robert C, Daud A et al (2013) Safety and tumor responses with lambrolizumab (anti-PD-1) in melanoma. N Engl J Med 369:134–144
130. Brahmer JR, Tykodi SS, Chow LQ et al (2012) Safety and activity of anti-PD-L1 antibody in patients with advanced cancer. N Engl J Med 366:2455–2465
131. Redmond WL, Triplett T, Floyd K, Weinberg AD (2012) Dual anti-OX40/IL-2 therapy augments tumor immunotherapy via IL-2R-mediated regulation of OX40 expression. PLoS One 7:e34467
132. Yee C, Thompson JA, Byrd D, Riddell SR, Roche P, Celis E, Greenberg PD (2002) Adoptive T cell therapy using antigen-specific CD8+ T cell clones for the treatment of patients with metastatic melanoma: in vivo persistence, migration, and antitumor effect of transferred T cells. Proc Natl Acad Sci USA 99:16168–16173
133. Chapuis AG, Thompson JA, Margolin KA et al (2012) Transferred melanoma-specific CD8+ T cells persist, mediate tumor regression, and acquire central memory phenotype. Proc Natl Acad Sci USA 109:4592–4597
134. Hunder NN, Wallen H, Cao J et al (2008) Treatment of metastatic melanoma with autologous CD4+ T cells against NY-ESO-1. N Engl J Med 358:2698–2703
135. Muranski P, Restifo NP (2009) Adoptive immunotherapy of cancer using CD4(+) T cells. Curr Opin Immunol 21:200–208
136. Rosenberg SA, Packard BS, Aebersold PM et al (1988) Use of tumor-infiltrating lymphocytes and interleukin-2 in the immunotherapy of patients with metastatic melanoma. A preliminary report. N Engl J Med 319:1676–1680
137. Dudley ME, Yang JC, Sherry R et al (2008) Adoptive cell therapy for patients with metastatic melanoma: evaluation of intensive myeloablative chemoradiation preparative regimens. J Clin Oncol 26:5233–5239
138. Besser MJ, Shapira-Frommer R, Treves AJ et al (2010) Clinical responses in a phase II study using adoptive transfer of short-term cultured tumor infiltration lymphocytes in metastatic melanoma patients. Clin Cancer Res 16:2646–2655
139. Radvanyi LG, Bernatchez C, Zhang M et al (2012) Specific lymphocyte subsets predict response to adoptive cell therapy using expanded autologous tumor-infiltrating lymphocytes in metastatic melanoma patients. Clin Cancer Res 18:6758–6770
140. Dudley ME, Gross CA, Somerville RP et al (2013) Randomized selection design trial evaluating CD8+-enriched versus unselected tumor-infiltrating lymphocytes for adoptive cell therapy for patients with melanoma. J Clin Oncol 31:2152–2159
141. Zhang L, Feldman SA, Zheng Z et al (2012) Evaluation of gamma-retroviral vectors that mediate the inducible expression of IL-12 for clinical application. J Immunother 35:430–439
142. Morgan RA, Dudley ME, Wunderlich JR et al (2006) Cancer regression in patients after transfer of genetically engineered lymphocytes. Science 314:126–129
143. Johnson LA, Morgan RA, Dudley ME et al (2009) Gene therapy with human and mouse T-cell receptors mediates cancer regression and targets normal tissues expressing cognate antigen. Blood 114:535–546
144. Kalos M, Levine BL, Porter DL, Katz S, Grupp SA, Bagg A, June CH (2011) T cells with chimeric antigen receptors have potent antitumor effects and can establish memory in patients with advanced leukemia. Sci Transl Med 3:95ra73
145. Grupp SA, Kalos M, Barrett D et al (2013) Chimeric antigen receptor-modified T cells for acute lymphoid leukemia. N Engl J Med 368:1509–1518
146. Kochenderfer JN, Dudley ME, Feldman SA et al (2012) B-cell depletion and remissions of malignancy along with cytokine-associated toxicity in a clinical trial of anti-CD19 chimeric-antigen-receptor-transduced T cells. Blood 119:2709–2720
147. Morgan RA, Yang JC, Kitano M, Dudley ME, Laurencot CM, Rosenberg SA (2010) Case report of a serious adverse event following the administration of T cells transduced with a chimeric antigen receptor recognizing ERBB2. Mol Ther 18:843–851
148. Yvon E, Del Vecchio M, Savoldo B et al (2009) Immunotherapy of metastatic melanoma using genetically engineered GD2-specific T cells. Clin Cancer Res 15:5852–5860

149. Lo AS, Ma Q, Liu DL, Junghans RP (2010) Anti-GD3 chimeric sFv-CD28/T-cell receptor zeta designer T cells for treatment of metastatic melanoma and other neuroectodermal tumors. Clin Cancer Res 16:2769–2780

150. Angell H, Galon J (2013) From the immune contexture to the Immunoscore: the role of prognostic and predictive immune markers in cancer. Curr Opin Immunol 25:261–267

151. Reis PP, Waldron L, Goswami RS et al (2011) mRNA transcript quantification in archival samples using multiplexed, color-coded probes. BMC Biotechnol 11:46

152. Beard RE, Abate-Daga D, Rosati SF, Zheng Z, Wunderlich JR, Rosenberg SA, Morgan RA (2013) Gene expression profiling using nanostring digital RNA counting to identify potential target antigens for melanoma immunotherapy. Clin Cancer Res 19:4941–4950

153. Tanese K, Grimm EA, Ekmekcioglu S (2012) The role of melanoma tumor-derived nitric oxide in the tumor inflammatory microenvironment: its impact on the chemokine expression profile, including suppression of CXCL10. Int J Cancer 131:891–901

154. Mann GJ, Pupo GM, Campain AE et al (2013) BRAF mutation, NRAS mutation, and the absence of an immune-related expressed gene profile predict poor outcome in patients with stage III melanoma. J Invest Dermatol 133:509–517

155. Marzese DM, Scolyer RA, Huynh JL et al (2014) Epigenome-wide DNA methylation landscape of melanoma progression to brain metastasis reveals aberrations on homeobox D cluster associated with prognosis. Hum Mol Genet. 1;23(1):226–38

156. Griewank KG, Ugurel S, Schadendorf D, Paschen A (2013) New developments in biomarkers for melanoma. Curr Opin Oncol 25:145–151

157. Gajewski TF, Louahed J, Brichard VG (2010) Gene signature in melanoma associated with clinical activity: a potential clue to unlock cancer immunotherapy. Cancer J 16:399–403

158. Ji RR, Chasalow SD, Wang L et al (2012) An immune-active tumor microenvironment favors clinical response to ipilimumab. Cancer Immunol Immunother 61:1019–1031

159. Ahmadzadeh M, Felipe-Silva A, Heemskerk B, Powell DJ Jr, Wunderlich JR, Merino MJ, Rosenberg SA (2008) FOXP3 expression accurately defines the population of intratumoral regulatory T cells that selectively accumulate in metastatic melanoma lesions. Blood 112:4953–4960

160. Galon J, Pages F, Marincola FM et al (2012) Cancer classification using the immunoscore: a worldwide task force. J Transl Med 10:205

161. Galon J, Pages F, Marincola FM et al (2012) The immune score as a new possible approach for the classification of cancer. J Transl Med 10:1

162. Fridman WH, Galon J, Pages F, Tartour E, Sautes-Fridman C, Kroemer G (2011) Prognostic and predictive impact of intra- and peritumoral immune infiltrates. Cancer Res 71: 5601–5605

163. Gajewski TF, Meng Y, Harlin H (2006) Immune suppression in the tumor microenvironment. J Immunother 29:233–240

Part II
Clinical and Pathological Aspects of Melanoma

Chapter 3
Epidemiology and Clinical Characteristics of Melanoma

Ana Ciurea

Abstract Melanoma represents a significant and growing health problem throughout the world. Global incidence is approximately 160,000 new cases per year, with 48,000 deaths. According to the Centers for Disease Control and Prevention, the rates of melanoma have doubled in the United States in the past 30 years. Melanoma is now the fifth most common cancer among men and the sixth most common cancer in women in the United States. Among people under age 50, women are about 30 % more likely than men to develop the disease. By contrast, among people aged 50 and older, men are nearly twice as likely as women to develop melanoma, and by age 60, men are nearly three times more likely to develop melanoma. The annual incidence of melanoma among whites has increased by more than 70 % over the past two decades. Increases have been most rapid among whites aged 60 and older.

Melanoma is completely curable if detected and resected early in its evolution. There is general consensus that early detection offers the greatest opportunity for reducing melanoma mortality in the short term. Education, coupled with regular complete physical examination and self-skin examination, is vitally an important method in reducing deaths from melanoma.

In order for the healthcare professional to make a clinical diagnosis of a possible melanoma as early in its course as possible, he/she must have a high index of suspicion for melanoma and thorough knowledge of the clinical features of early melanomas, common pigmented lesions which must be differentiated from melanoma, and the characteristics of variants of atypical melanocytic nevi which are commonly seen in association with a higher risk for melanoma.

Keywords Melanoma • Epidemiology • Incidence • Ultraviolet radiation • Classification • Clinical characteristics • Diagnosis • Early recognition

A. Ciurea, MD (✉)
Department of Dermatology, The University of Texas, MD Anderson Cancer Center,
1400, Pressler St., Unit 1452, Houston, TX 77030, USA
e-mail: amciurea@mdanderson.org

© Springer Science+Business Media New York 2016
C.A. Torres-Cabala, J.L. Curry (eds.), *Genetics of Melanoma*, Cancer Genetics,
DOI 10.1007/978-1-4939-3554-3_3

3.1 Epidemiology of Melanoma

The incidence of the most dangerous skin cancer has considerably increased in recent decades in most countries. The steepest rise in incidence rates have been in men >60 years of age and in lower socioeconomic areas [1–3]. For any given stage and all ages, men have poorer melanoma survival than women. The rising incidence rates of melanoma for older men has worsened for the 25-year period from 1983 to 2007, during which men aged 60–64 years experienced a twofold increase in incidence, whereas men aged 75–79 years had a fourfold increase [4]. Between 1992 and 2004, the incidence of melanoma increased for tumors of all histologic subtypes and thicknesses. While this increase may be attributed to higher rates of melanoma screening, the sharpest increase in incidence was evident among low socioeconomic status (SES) areas, where individuals are least likely to undergo screening, suggesting that increasing incidence rates are not simply an artifact of screening [5].

The most common body sites for melanoma historically have included the trunk, head, and neck in men and extremities in women [6]. Caini et al. [7] found that the nevus count >25 was associated with melanoma on usually nonexposed sites, such as the legs or trunk. In addition, skin and hair color correlate with the body site for melanoma, which may be attributed to genetic variability [7, 8].

Recent studies have found a left-sided predominance for skin cancers, including melanoma, possibly related to poor ultraviolet A (UVA)–filtering side windows in automobiles [9].

While melanoma is much more common in whites than in darker skinned populations, the incidence among US Hispanics and non-Hispanic blacks is rising in certain regions of the country. Based on data from the California Cancer Registry between 1988 and 2001, there was a 1.8 % per year increase in incidence of invasive melanomas in Hispanic patients, and a disproportionate increase in the number of tumors thicker than 1.5 mm. Hispanic patients of lower SES had a higher risk of thick tumors (>2 mm) and higher rates of the nodular melanoma subtype [10]. In addition, several studies have shown that both Hispanics and non-Hispanics blacks tend to present with later stage disease and carry a poorer prognosis than non-Hispanic whites [10–12].

Black patients have a lower incidence of melanoma than whites; however, the 5-year relative survival rate for blacks is 74.1 % compared with 92 % for whites [12]. The majority of melanomas in dark-skinned patients occur on sun protected areas, such as lower extremity, trunk, and hip [12, 13]. These atypical locations may contribute to lower survival for black patients.

In terms of histologic subtypes of melanoma, the nodular subtype accounts for only 14 % of all melanomas but comprises a high percentage (37 %) of fatal cases [14]. Based on the US Surveillance Epidemiology and End Result (SEER) data from 1992 to 2004, T4 (>4 mm) melanoma increased by 3.86 % annually, with individuals in the lowest SES groups and those ≥65 years of age having the largest percent increases in these thick tumors. However, this increase in thick tumors was not associated with a disproportionate increase in nodular melanomas, which are characterized by rapid growth that tends to preclude early detection [3, 5].

3.1.1 Risk Factors

The main environmental risk factor is excessive exposure of fair-skinned individuals to ultraviolet radiation (UV). Both UVA and ultraviolet B (UVB) radiation from the sun have been proven to cause skin cancer in humans, including melanoma. It has been suggested that intermittent sun exposure resulted in sunburns in unacclimatized fair skin is a greater risk factor for melanoma than chronic lifetime sun exposure [15, 16].

The patients with an increased number of benign melanocytic lesions have an increased risk for the development of melanoma. More than five atypical (dysplastic) nevi that are larger than 5 mm in diameter and are asymmetric in shape and color with irregular edges is also a risk factor for melanoma, especially if they occur in families as a manifestation of the dysplastic nevus syndrome [17, 18]. There is a correlation between CDKN2A mutations in family members with dysplastic nevus syndrome in about 20 % of the patients, and CDK4 mutations have been described [19]. High-risk alleles with high penetrance are often expressed in familial clusters in an autosomal-dominant pattern, and approximately a third of melanoma families have a germline mutation in CDKN2A.

Large congenital nevi (>20 cm in diameter) have an estimated lifetime risk between 5 and 20 % for malignant transformation [20].

Further risk factors include phenotypic factors (pale skin, light eyes and hair, presence of freckles, inability to tan, burns easily), personal history of melanoma (3–5 % risk of developing a second melanoma in the absence of atypical nevi), immunosuppression, DNA repair defects (e.g., xeroderma pigmentosum), and equatorial latitudes [21, 22].

In the past few years, research has also confirmed that indoor ultraviolet (UV) tanning is at least as dangerous as solar UV, and possibly more dangerous. Close to 90 % of melanomas can be attributed to ultraviolet radiation emitted by the sun and tanning beds.

Nearly 30 million people tan indoors in the United States every year; 2.3 million of them are teens. Frequent tanners using new high-pressure sunlamps may receive as much as 12 times the annual UVA dose compared to the dose they receive from sun exposure. Indoor ultraviolet tanning bed users are 74 % more likely to develop melanoma than those who have never tanned indoors [22]. Additionally, the more time a person has spent tanning indoors, the higher the risk. One tanning bed session raises melanoma risk by 20 %, according to Boniol et. al. [23].

It has been suggested that the incidence of melanoma in children and adolescents is also increasing [24]. The absolute numbers remain small, yet melanoma incidence increased 50 % among patients younger than 20 years of age during a 20-year study period recently reported by Cormier at al. The overall average melanoma incidence was 5.4 per one million children and adolescents; there was a 2.5 % relative yearly incidence increase between 1998 and 2007.

A history of cancer in childhood is a risk factor for subsequent malignancy, primary basal cell carcinoma [25]. An analysis of childhood cancer survivors for subsequent melanoma risk revealed a standardized incidence ration (SIR) of 2.42 (95 % confidence interval, 1.77–3.23). The childhood cancer cases were generally those treated with radiation [26, 27].

The reasons for the increase in melanoma detection is children and adolescents remain unclear and are likely multifactorial. Most children with melanoma have no family history of disease and no history of predisposing factors including congenital and atypical nevi. The increased incidence may be attributable to changes in sun-related behavior and/or geographic changes leading to increased UV exposure.

3.1.2 Novel Risk Factors

Melanoma screening and educational efforts are generally targeted to individuals with established and identifiable risk factors. While the following novel risk factors are not as common, they represent a growing burden that may require innovative educational and behavioral interventions.

3.1.2.1 Melanocortin-1 Receptor

The melanocortin-1 receptor (MC1R) is one of the key genes that regulates skin color. Variants in MC1R commonly seen in individuals with red hair and exquisite sun sensitivity typical for Fitzpatrick skin phototype I. The contribution of MC1R gene variants to the development of early onset melanoma is unknown. Reduced photo protection secondary to MC1R dysfunction involves pigmentary and non-pigmentary mechanisms (reduced DNA repair, effects on cell proliferation and possibly immunological reaction) [28]. In an Australian population-based, case–control family study, MC1R sequencing of 565 young (18–39 years) patients with invasive cutaneous melanoma, 409 unrelated controls, and 518 sibling controls revealed that some MC1R variants were important determinants of early onset melanoma, with strong associations in men and those with none or few nevi or with high childhood sun exposure [29, 37].

3.1.2.2 Immunosuppression

Organ transplant recipients are at greatly increased risk of developing a wide variety of skin cancers, particularly epithelial skin cancers. While transplant patients are at far greater risk of squamous cell carcinomas, they also develop more melanomas compared to the general population [30]. The age-adjusted incidence rate of melanoma among renal transplantation recipients was 55.9 diagnoses per 100,000 populations, representing a 3.6-fold greater risk in age-adjusted, standardized risk from the SEER population [31, 32].

HIV infection has also been linked with melanoma risk [30]. Comparing HIV-infected individuals with demographically similar individuals who were not infected with HIV, Silverberg et al. [33] found elevated risks of melanoma [relative risk (RR) = 1.8 (95 % CI, 1.3–2.6)].

Melanoma-related mortality is significantly elevated in HIV-infected compared with HIV-uninfected patients, independent of the melanoma stage or receipt of cancer treatment (HR 1.72; CI, 1.09–2.70).

3.1.2.3 Parkinson's Disease

An association between Parkinson's disease (PD) and melanoma has long been suspected, but whether the association is with the dopaminergic treatments or with the disease itself remains a question. Emerging epidemiologic evidence suggests links between Parkinson's disease (PD) and cancer, especially lower risk of smoking-related cancer and higher risk of melanoma, although the interpretation of the current clinical studies pose limitations, and well-conducted prospective studies are needed for improved understanding of a potential biologic PD and melanoma association [34, 35].

3.1.3 International Trends

There has been a global trend of increasing melanoma incidence in people of European descent [22]. Interestingly, Croatia has one of the highest increases in melanoma incidence. Melanoma mortality remains the highest in Australia and New Zealand, where the incidence is 40–60 cases per 100,000 inhabitants [22, 36].

3.1.4 Melanoma Mortality

According to data from the Connecticut Tumor Registry between 1950 and 2007, mortality rates more than tripled in men (1.6–4.9 per 100,000) and doubled in women (1.3–2.6 per 100,000) [4]. For any given stage and across all ages, men have had poorer melanoma survival than women, and more than 50 % of all melanoma deaths are in white men 50 years of age and older [4, 5]. Lower education level and SES are also associated with decreased survival. The total number of melanoma in the United States in 2015 is estimated at 73,870 which is responsible for 9940 deaths.

3.1.5   Clinical Strategies for Earlier Recognition and Identification

Early detection is crucial in reducing melanoma morbidity and mortality. Potential interventions include screening, risk factors education, self-skin examinations, increasing total body skin screenings by physicians, creating specialized skin cancer clinics, and developing diagnostic tools through advances in technology. Recent advances in imaging technologies including examining dermatoscopy, total body photography (TBP), confocal microscopy, and other new diagnostic aides could potentially lead to improved, more accurate diagnosis of melanoma.

3.2   Clinical Characteristics: Types of Primary Melanomas

The traditional clinicopathologic types of melanoma include superficial spreading melanoma, nodular melanoma, lentigo maligna melanoma (LMM), and acral lentiginous melanoma. A number of less common melanoma variants (desmoplastic melanoma, ocular melanoma, mucosal melanoma, clear cell sarcoma, animal-type melanoma, and malignant melanoma in association with blue nevus) may present with unusual manifestations defined by clinical and histologic findings. Recently, mutually exclusive oncogenic mutations in melanomas involving NRAS (15–20 %), BRAF (50 %), CKIT (2 %), and GNAQ/GNA11 (50 % of uveal melanomas) have been identified. This might herald the beginning of a new molecular classification of melanoma in which the biologically distinct subsets share a common oncogenic mechanism, behave clinically in a similar fashion, and require similar clinical management.

3.2.1   Superficial Spreading Melanoma

Superficial spreading melanoma is the most common histologic subtype in the United States and represents the highest proportion of fatal melanomas.

It affects fair-skinned adults of all ages, with the median age in the fifth decade. The upper back in both sexes and legs in women are the most common sites. Superficially spreading melanoma typically involves intermittently sun-exposed anatomical sites such as the trunk and extremities [38].

There is a tendency to multicoloration, not just the shades of tan but variegated black, brown, red, blue, and white (Fig. 3.1a, c, d). Melanoma in situ is usually a macule with an irregular border and variable size, including diameters <5 mm (Fig. 3.1b). Compared with the unaided eye, dermoscopy reveals several additional structural features, which are typical of melanoma, including blue-white weil, irregular pigmentation and irregular dots/globules at the periphery (Fig. 3.1e). Melanoma may arise de novo or in association with a preexisting nevus. Areas of color change within a nevus, especially dark areas that extend beyond the border of the remainder

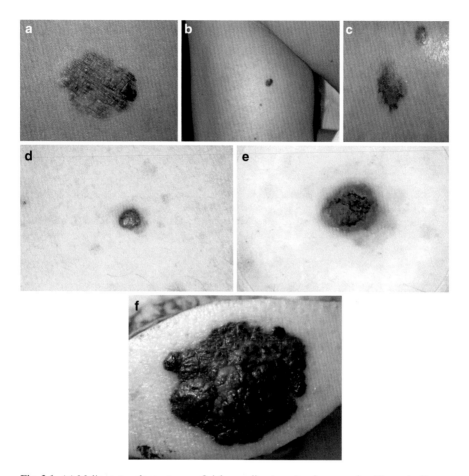

Fig. 3.1 (**a**) Malignant melanoma, superficial spreading type, trunk, measuring 15 mm in diameter, illustrating border asymmetry and color variation. (**b**) A small approximately 5 mm in diameter melanoma in situ, leg, illustrating subtle asymmetry and scalloped border. (**c**) A large melanoma, superficial spreading type of the arm exhibiting the ABCDs and plaque-like elevation centrally. (**d**) Melanoma – superficial spreading type. A slowly growing papule with eccentric hyperpigmentation, leg, illustrating color variation and asymmetry. (**e**) Melanoma – superficial spreading type. On dermoscopic examination there is *blue-whitish* veil in *center* and *black* globules with intermingled *whitish lines* (reticular depigmentation) at periphery. (Original magnification ×10). (**f**) Melanoma – superficial spreading type. This large 2.8 cm plaque with nodule formation on the trunk exhibits the ABCDs, although more advanced. It is associated with a poor prognosis

of the lesion, are suspicious for melanoma arising in a nevus. As a vertical growth phase develops, a papule or nodule usually appears [39].

Melanoma lacking clinically evident pigment is termed "amelanotic." The lesion is pink, erythematous, or flesh colored and commonly mimics basal cell carcinoma (Fig. 3.2). The clinical diagnosis is challenging because it may mimic benign or malignant melanocytic and non-melanocytic neoplasms and inflammatory skin diseases [40].

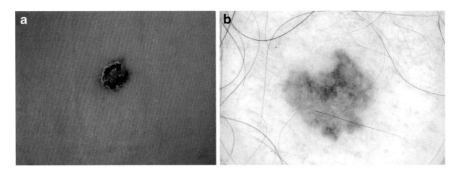

Fig. 3.2 (a) Amelanotic melanoma. An isolated 6 mm *bright pink* scaly nodule on the left upper arm. (b) This *light-colored* lesion illustrates the positive dermoscopic features of amelanotic melanoma: having predominant central vessels, more than 1 shade of *pink, dotted* and linear irregular vessels, and irregularly shaped depigmentation

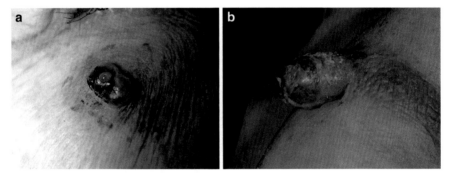

Fig. 3.3 (a) Pedunculated amelanotic 26-mm diameter nodular melanoma lesion with 6.5-mm Breslow thickness on face. (b) Melanoma – nodular type. A tricolored nodule surrounded by erythema and induration on the arm

3.2.2   Nodular Melanoma

Nodular melanoma (NM) is the second most common type of cutaneous melanoma in the fair-skinned population, which tends to occur in slightly older patients than SSM (median age: 7th decade). It occurs twice as often in men as in women. It accounts for approximately 15–30 % of all melanomas and occurs at any location as a rapidly expanding nodule that may show ulceration and hemorrhage [41]. The lesions arise without a clinically apparent radial growth phase. The tumors may be smooth and dome-shaped, fungating, friable, or ulcerated. Bleeding is usually a late sign (Fig. 3.3a, b).

Clinically, they may be confused with basal cell carcinomas, particularly if they are amelanotic, and with nodules occurring in SSM [42].

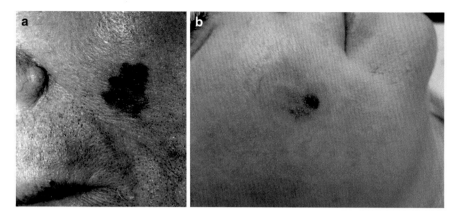

Fig. 3.4 (a) Melanoma – lentigo maligna type. This 2.3 cm irregularly shaped, asymmetric *brown* plaque had its beginning with the uniformly pigmented lesion at the *right lower* portion of this clinical photograph. (b) Melanoma – lentigo maligna type. The neoplasm is broad, poorly circumscribed and shows eccentric hyperpigmentation inferiorly

3.2.3 Lentigo Maligna (Lentiginous Melanoma on Sun-Damaged Skin)

Lentigo maligna melanoma (LMM) represents a minority of cutaneous melanoma (up to 15 %) diagnosed in elderly patients (median age 8th decade). It involves chronically sun-damaged skin, most commonly on the face, with a preference for the nose and cheek (Fig. 3.4a, b).

LM begins as a tan macule that extends peripherally, with gradual uneven darkening over the course of years. The spread and darkening are usually so slow that the patient pays little attention to this insidious lesion. After a radial growth period of 5–20 years, a vertical growth phase of invasive melanoma can develop. The term lentigo maligna is used to mean melanoma in situ of sun-exposed skin (radial growth only), and LMM is used for those with dermal invasion (vertical growth). A palpable nodule within the original macular lesion is the best evidence that this has occurred, though there may be darkening or bleeding as well [43]. Lentiginous types of melanoma also give rise to desmoplastic melanoma, which may appear as a papule, firm plaque, or inconspicuous area of induration.

3.2.4 Acral Lentiginous Melanoma

Acral lentiginous melanoma is the most common type of melanoma in dark-skinned and Asian population [44]. This is because the frequency of the other types is low in these patients, not because the incidence of ALM is any higher than in white persons.

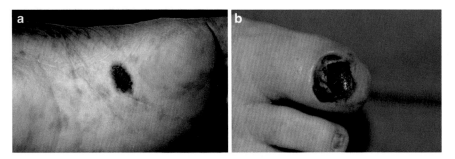

Fig. 3.5 (a) Acral lentiginous melanoma illustrating asymmetry, centrifugal spread and color variation. (b) *Left* hallux of patient with subungual melanoma. Nail plate is eroded and replaced by hemorrhagic crust. Proximal and lateral nail folds are swollen and erythematous

The medial age of patients is 50 years, with equal sex distribution. The most common site of melanoma in black persons is the foot, with 60 % of patients having subungual or plantar lesions. All lentiginous melanomas demonstrate a junctional growth pattern and tend to have indistinct margins. Over time, a vertical growth phase develops. Periungual hyperpigmentation, a distinct black discoloration of the proximal nail fold at the end of a pigmented streak (Hutchinson's sign), is an ominous sign suggesting melanoma in the matrix of the nail (Fig. 3.5a, b).

The early changes of ALM may be light brown and uniformly pigmented. The thumb and hallux are more frequently involved than other digits. In time, the lesion becomes darker and nodular and may ulcerate. Metastases to the epitrochlear and axillary nodes are common, because there is often a delay in diagnosis. Subungual melanoma accounts for 1–3 % of all melanomas and is typically classified as a variant of ALM. Persistent pigmentation of the nail apparatus should raise concern for melanoma as it may be misdiagnosed as onychomycosis, verruca vulgaris, chronic paronychia, subungual hyperkeratosis, pyogenic granuloma, glomus tumor, Kaposi sarcoma, or subungual hematoma.

3.3 Other Melanoma Variants

3.3.1 Desmoplastic Melanoma

Desmoplastic melanoma (DM) is an uncommon variant of spindle cell melanoma histologically defined as *pure* (pDM) and *mixed* (mDM) based on the degree of desmoplasia (growth of dense connective tissue or stroma) present in the tumor; pDMs have more and mDMs less than 90 % desmoplasia. The distinction appears to have clinical, prognostic, and therapeutic importance; pDM is associated with better overall survival and less frequent metastasis to regional lymph nodes than mDM. In contrast, mDM appear to display similar biologic behavior to non-desmoplastic melanoma subtypes, including SSM [45].

It most often occurs on the head or neck of older men, many times within a subtle lentigo maligna. The typical clinical lesion consists of a skin-colored, red, brown, or pink nodule or papule, mostly on sun-exposed skin. It is not uncommon for patients to present with a history of a nonspecific or scar-like lesion that developed without any antecedent trauma. The lesions may also occur on the digits in association with a subtle acral lentiginous melanoma. One-third of the cases presents only a palpable dermal irregularity and is amelanotic. The lesions are commonly neurotropic and demonstrate extensive growth along the perineurium beyond the bulk of the tumor.

The molecular profile of DM consists of a decrease in the expression of genes involved in melanin synthesis and increased expression of the glycoprotein, clusterin, which is involved in cell adhesion, tissue, and fibrous remodeling.

Deep tissue biopsies are necessary to establish the diagnosis as superficial portions of the tumor show subtle or non-diagnostic findings which may be mistaken for scars or spindle cell neoplasms.

3.3.2   Ocular Melanoma

Ocular melanoma is the second most common type of melanoma after cutaneous and the most common primary intraocular malignant tumor in adults. It can arise within the eye, in the uveal tissue, or in the conjunctiva, orbit, or eyelid. A large majority of ocular melanomas originate from the uvea (iris, choroidal, and ciliary body melanomas), while conjunctival melanomas are far less frequent. Incidence of uveal melanoma has remained stable over the last three decades. Worldwide, it has been estimated that there are 7095 cases of uveal melanoma annually with 4747 in Caucasians, 738 in Hispanics, 1286 in Asians, and 316 in African patients [46].

Light eye color, fair skin color, and inability to tan are well-known risk factors for development of uveal melanoma. Patients with melanosis oculi (nevus of Ota), preexisting choroidal nevus, and type I neurofibromatosis may also be at higher risk for uveal melanoma.

Iris melanoma, ciliary body melanoma, and choroidal melanoma are usually asymptomatic until they reach a large size, at which time it causes pain, floaters, secondary glaucoma, and peripheral or central vision obstruction leading to a visual field defects. Diagnosis is in most cases established by clinical examination with great accuracy.

Melanoma of the uvea appears clinically as a dome-shaped mass, pigmented in most cases (55 %). Nonpigmented (15 %) and mixed pigmented/nonpigmented (30 %) of uveal melanomas have been described. Iris melanoma occurs primarily in the inferior quadrant of the eye and it shows pigment in 82 % of the cases. Ciliary body melanoma tends to be diagnosed as a large mass because it hides behind the iris until symptoms of retinal detachment or lens displacement are noted.

Choroidal melanoma appears as a deep mass to the retina, often producing retinal detachment. Local treatment of uveal melanoma has improved, with increased use of conservative methods and preservation of the eye, but survival rates have remained unchanged. Prognosis of patients with metastasis remains poor, and metastatic disease remains the leading cause of death among patients with uveal melanoma. Current standard treatment for conjunctival melanoma is wide local excision with adjuvant therapy, including brachytherapy, cryotherapy, and topical application of chemotherapeutic agent.

3.3.3   Mucosal Melanoma

Melanomas may occur in the mouth, larynx, nasopharynx, vagina, and anus. These tumors are rare (1 % of all melanoma cases) but tend to be advanced, likely because early detection is difficult. Mucosal melanomas most commonly contain mutations in the CKIT gene [47].

Primary melanoma of the mucous membranes is rare but typically demonstrates a lentiginous (junctional) growth pattern. In the mouth, especially the palate, the lesion is usually pigmented and may be ulcerated. It may occur in the nasal mucosa as a polypoid tumor. On the lip can present as an indolent ulcer. Melanoma of the vulva is manifested by a tumor, often ulcerated, with bleeding and pruritus. It is most often detected after metastasis to the groin has occurred.

3.3.4   Clear-Cell Sarcoma (Melanoma of the Soft Parts)

Primary soft tissue melanomas (clear-cell sarcoma, melanoma of the soft parts) occur most frequently on the lower extremities of young people. The average age onset is 27. The history is of an enlarging often painful mass on an extremity, with the foot and ankle involved 43 % of the time. The lesion appears to arise from neural crest cells. Frequently translocations of chromosomes 12 and 22 are present [48].

The tumors arise in and are bound to tendons or fascia and only uncommonly invade the overlying skin. Metastases are often present at first diagnosis, and the prognosis is poor. Local recurrence or distant metastases after the initial excision are frequent and result in death in more than 50 % of reported cases. Treatment is with wide excision and lymph node dissection. Radiotherapy and chemotherapy are used as an adjunct in some cases.

3.3.5   Animal-type Melanoma/Pigmented Epithelioid Melanocytoma

Animal-type melanoma/pigmented epithelioid melanocytoma (PEM) is a rare distinct melanoma subtype, characterized by proliferation of heavily pigmented epithelioid and spindled melanocytes with pleomorphic nuclei, dendritic cells, numerous melanophages and sometimes an inflammatory infiltrate of lymphocytes. Clinically, it presents as blue to jet black plaques or nodules usually located on the lower legs. It has a propensity for regional lymphatic metastasis and is rarely capable of disseminated metastatic disease and death. Younger patients have a more indolent disease [49].

References

1. Altekruse S, Kosary C, Krapcho M et al (2010) SEER cancer statistics review, 1975–2007. National Cancer Institute, Bethesda, MD
2. American Cancer Society (2015) cancer.org
3. Weinstock MA (2001) Epidemiology, etiology, and control of melanoma. Med Health R I 84(7):234–236
4. Geller AC, Clapp RW, Sober AJ et al (2013) Melanoma epidemic: an analysis of six decades of data from the Connecticut Tumor Registry. J Clin Oncol 31:4172–4178
5. Siegel R, Naishadham D, Jemal A (2013) Cancer statistics, 2013. CA Cancer J Clin 63:11–30
6. Katalinic A, Waldman A, Weinstock MA et al (2012) Does the skin cancer screening save lives?: an observational study comparing trends in melanoma mortality in regions with and without screening. Cancer 118:5395–5402
7. Caini S, Gandini S, Sera F, Raimondi S, Fargnoli MS, Boniol M, Armstrong BK (2009) Meta-analysis of risk factors for cutaneous melanoma according to anatomical site and clinico-pathological variant. Eur J Cancer 45(17):3054–3063
8. Clark LN, Shin DB, Troxel AB, Khan S, Sober AJ, Ming ME (2007) Association between the anatomic distribution of melanoma and sex. J Am Acad Dermatol 56:768–773
9. Butler ST, Fosko SW (2010) Increased prevalence of left-sided skin cancers. J Am Acad Dermatol 63:1006–1010
10. Cockburn MG, Zadnick J, Deapen D (2006) Developing epidemic of melanoma in Hispanic population in California. Cancer 106:1162–1168
11. Pollitt RA, Clarke CA, Swetter SM, Peng DH, Zadnick J, Cockburn M (2011) The expanding melanoma burden in California hispanics: importance of socioeconomic distribution, histologic subtype, and anatomic location. Cancer 117:152–161
12. Clairwood M, Ricketts J, Grant-Kels J, Gonsalves L (2014) Melanoma in skin of color in Connecticut: an analysis of melanoma incidence and stage at diagnosis in non-Hispanic blacks, non-Hispanic whites, and Hispanics. Int J Dermatol 53(4):425–433
13. Myles ZM, Buchanan N, King JB et al (2012) Anatomic distribution of malignant melanoma on the non-Hispanic black patient, 1998–2007. Arch Dermatol 148:797–801
14. Shaikh WR, Xiong M, Weinstock MA (2012) The contribution of nodular subtype to melanoma mortality in the United States, 1978 to 2007. Arch Dermatol 148:30–36
15. Berwick M, Armstrong BK, Ben-Porat L et al (2005) Sun exposure and mortality from melanoma. J Natl Cancer Inst 97(3):195–199
16. Rigel DS (2008) Cutaneous ultraviolet exposure and its relationship to the development of skin cancer. J Am Acad Dermatol 58(5 Suppl 2):S129–S132
17. Swerdlow AJ, English J, MacKie RM (1986) Benign melanocyte nevi as a risk factor for malignant melanoma. BMJ 292:1555–1559
18. Bataille V, Bishop JA, Sasieni P et al (1996) Risks of cutaneous melanoma in relation to the numbers, types, and sites of naevi: a case-control study. Br J Cancer 73:1605–1611
19. Udayakumar D, Mahato B, Gabree M, Tsao H (2010) Genetic determinants of cutaneous melanoma predisposition. Semin Cutan Med Surg 29(3):190–195
20. Vourc'h-Jourdain M, Martin L, Barbarot S et al (2013) Large congenital melanocytic nevi: therapeutic management and melanoma risk: a systematic review. J Am Acad Dermatol 68(3):493–498.e1–14

21. Tucker MA (2009) Melanoma epidemiology. Hematol Oncol Clin North Am 23(3):383–395
22. Garbe C, Leiter U (2009) Melanoma epidemiology and trends. Clin Dermatol 27(1):3–9
23. Boniol M, Autier P, Boyle P et al (2012) Cutaneous melanoma attributable to sunbed use: systematic review and meta-analysis. BMJ 345:e4757
24. Austin MT, Xing Y, Hayes-Jordan AA, Lally KP, Cormier JN (2013) Melanoma incidence rises for children and adolescents: an epidemiologic review of pediatric melanoma in the United States. J Pediatr Surg 48(11):2207–2213
25. Oeffinger KC, Mertens AC, Sklar CA et al (2006) Chronic health conditions in adult survivors of childhood cancer. N Engl J Med 355(15):1572–1582
26. Mayer JE et al (2014) Screening, early detection, education, and trends for melanoma: current status (2007–2013) and future directions: Part I. Epidemiology, high-risk groups, clinical strategies, and diagnostic technology. J Am Acad Dermatol 71(4):599.e1–599.e12, quiz 610, 599.e12
27. Mayer JE, Swetter SM, Fu T, Geller AC (2014) Screening, early detection, education, and trends for melanoma: current status (2007–2013) and future directions: Part II. Screening, education, and future directions. J Am Acad Dermatol 71(4):611.e1–611.e10, quiz 621–2
28. Demenais F et al (2010) Melanoma genetics consortium. Association of MC1R variants and host phenotypes with melanoma risk in CDKN2A mutation carriers: a GenoMEL study. J Natl Cancer Inst 102(20):1568–1583
29. Cust AE et al (2012) MC1R genotypes and risk of melanoma before age 40 years: a population-based case-control-family study. Int J Cancer 131(3):E269–E281
30. Kubica AW, Brewer JD (2012) Melanoma in immunosuppressed patients. Mayo Clin Proc 87(10):991–1003
31. Brewer JD et al (2011) Malignant melanoma in solid transplant recipients: collection of database cases and comparison with surveillance, epidemiology, and end results data for outcome analysis. Arch Dermatol 147(7):790–796
32. Hollenbeak CS, Todd MM, Billingsley EM, Harper G, Dyer AM, Lengerich EJ (2005) Increased incidence of melanoma in renal transplantation recipients. Cancer 104(9): 1962–1967
33. Silverberg MJ, Chao C, Leyden WA et al (2011) HIV infection, immunodeficiency, viral replication, and the risk of cancer. Cancer Epidemiol Biomarkers Prev 20(12):2551–2559
34. Nikolaou V, Stratigos AJ (2014) Emerging trends in the epidemiology of melanoma. Br J Dermatol 170(1):11–19
35. Terushkin V, Halpern AC (2009) Melanoma early detection. Hematol Oncol Clin North Am 23:481–500
36. Geller AC, Swetter SM, Brooks K, Demierre MF, Yaroch AL (2007) Screening, early detection, and trends for melanoma: current status (2000–2006) and future directions. J Am Acad Dermatol 57:555–572
37. Marzuka-Alcalá A, Gabree MJ, Tsao H (2014) Melanoma susceptibility genes and risk assessment. Methods Mol Biol 1102:381–393
38. Scolyer RA, Long GV, Thompson JF (2011) Evolving concepts in melanoma classification and their relevance to multidisciplinary melanoma patient care. Mol Oncol 5(2):124–136
39. Forman SB, Ferringer TC, Peckham SJ, Dalton SR, Sasaki GT, Libow LF, Elston DM (2008) Is superficial spreading melanoma still the most common form of malignant melanoma? J Am Acad Dermatol 58(6):1013–1020
40. Napolitano M, Didona B, Passarelli F, Annessi G, Bono R (2014) Amelanotic melanoma mimicking cutaneous epitheliomas. J Am Acad Dermatol 70(4):e75–e76
41. Mar V, Roberts H, Wolfe R, English DR, Kelly JW (2013) Nodular melanoma: a distinct clinical entity and the largest contributor to melanoma deaths in Victoria. Aust J Am Acad Dermatol 68(4):568–575
42. Moreau JF, Weinstock MA, Geller AC, Winger DG, Ferris LK (2014) Individual and ecological factors associated with early detection of nodular melanoma in the United States. Melanoma Res 24(2):165–171
43. Tiodorovic-Zivkovic D et al (2015) Age, gender, and topography influence the clinical and dermoscopic appearance of lentigo maligna. J Am Acad Dermatol 72:801–808

44. Marchetti MA, Chung E, Halpern AC (2015) Screening for acral lentiginous melanoma in dark-skinned individuals. JAMA Dermatol 151:1055–1056
45. Chen LL, Jaimes N, Barker CA, Busam KJ, Marghoob AA (2013) Desmoplastic melanoma: a review. J Am Acad Dermatol 68(5):825–833
46. Shields JA, Shields CL (2008) Intraocular tumors. In: Shields JA, Shields CL (eds) An Atlas and textbook, 2nd edn. Lippincott Williams and Wilkins, Philadelphia
47. Patrick RJ, Fenske NA, Messina JL (2007) Primary mucosal melanoma. J Am Acad Dermatol 56(5):828–834
48. Bianchi G et al (2014) Clear cell sarcoma of soft tissue: a retrospective review and analysis of 31 cases treated at Istituto Ortopedico Rizzoli. Eur J Surg Oncol 40(5):505–510
49. Ludgate MW, Fullen DR, Lee J, Rees R, Sabel MS, Wong SL, Johnson TM (2010) Animal-type melanoma: a clinical and histopathological study of 22 cases from a single institution. Br J Dermatol 162(1):129–136

Chapter 4
Pathology of Melanoma

Victor G. Prieto and Christopher R. Shea

Abstract Melanoma results in a significant social impact due to its relatively high mortality and young age of affected patients. During the last decade there have been several crucial advances providing insight to the molecular alterations responsible for melanoma development. Thus, as an example, we now know that most melanomas carry a mutation of the *BRAF* gene that can be targeted by several therapeutic agents. However, in 2016, the most important evaluation tool to predict prognosis and guide patient management continues to be histologic examination. Thus, this chapter describes the most important histologic factors that allow to render a diagnosis of melanoma and related lesions, with special emphasis to the AJCC/CAP classification of melanoma.

Keywords Histologic evaluation • Melanoma subtypes • Differential diagnosis CAP • AJCC

4.1 Introduction

Although far from being the most common cancer in humans, it is clear that cutaneous melanoma is becoming more and more of a health problem. The incidence of melanoma cases has risen strikingly over the past several decades. Although part of this increment may be due to increased awareness or changes in diagnostic criteria, there appears to be a real increase in incidence [1]. Melanoma has a relatively high mortality and affects patients at a younger age than most other skin cancers, thus resulting in a very high social impact. Among the list of risk factors associated with melanoma, of great significance is a history of exposure to ultraviolet radiation (UVR), particularly in childhood and in bursts associated with severe sunburns [2].

V.G. Prieto, MD, PhD (✉)
Department of Pathology and Department of Dermatology, The University of Texas,
MD Anderson Cancer Center, Houston, TX, USA
e-mail: vprieto@mdanderson.org

C.R. Shea, MD
Department of Medicine, University of Chicago Medicine, Chicago, IL, USA

© Springer Science+Business Media New York 2016
C.A. Torres-Cabala, J.L. Curry (eds.), *Genetics of Melanoma*, Cancer Genetics,
DOI 10.1007/978-1-4939-3554-3_4

Related to sensitivity to sun exposure are fair skin, red hair, and blue or green eyes. Also associated with development of cutaneous melanoma are the number of nevi (typical acquired, congenital, or dysplastic) and of ephelides and lentigines. Some rare syndromes associated with decreased capacity for DNA repair (e.g., xeroderma pigmentosum) lead to increased rates of melanoma [3, 4]. Immunosuppression and personal or family history of melanoma are also associated with increased risk of melanoma.

In this chapter we will review some of the most important histopathologic features of melanoma and associated lesions.

Melanomas Arising in Nevi The number of nevi that a person has is an independent risk factor for melanoma [5]. However, because nevi are so prevalent while melanomas are much less common, only very rarely will a nevus develop into a melanoma [6]. Up to 10–35 % of melanoma cases show nevi in the immediately adjacent skin, including some sort of melanocytic "dysplasia" in up to about 40 % [7–9]. It is conceivable that in some additional cases a precursor nevus may have been completely overrun by the subsequent melanoma.

Particular types of nevus are especially likely to give rise to melanoma. The atypical/dysplastic/Clark nevus is discussed below. Large (>20 cm) congenital nevi have a 10 % or more lifetime risk of developing melanoma [10]. Notably, melanoma may arise from the intradermal component of congenital nevi [11, 12], whereas de novo melanoma usually originates from the epidermis and only later invades the dermis. Unlike large congenital lesions, small- and medium-sized congenital nevi only rarely develop melanoma [13].

Histopathologically, congenital lesions show melanocytes arranged as nests or single cells deep in the dermis, especially around skin adnexa and vessels. Involvement of the arrector pili muscle by nevus cells is very common. Some congenital nevi, particularly in areas exposed to trauma, may have single-cell growth and focal cytologic atypia in the superficial portion, thus resembling melanoma [14].

Some congenital nevi have focally nodular appearance, sometimes called proliferative nodules. These nodules generally occur in the first year of life within large congenital nevi; on the other hand, this diagnosis should be made only with great caution in older patients since it may reflect the development of a melanoma arising in that nevus. Histopathologically, they contain a discrete nodule with expansile architecture, mitotic figures, and some cytologic atypia. Distinction from melanoma arising in congenital nevus rests on a gradual transition to the typical nevus areas at the periphery and lack of extensive necrosis, atypical mitotic figures, or associated inflammatory infiltrate. All proliferative nodules require close clinical follow-up, because of the possibility of childhood melanoma, a rare but important tumor [15–17], usually arising from a congenital nevus. Metastases may rarely occur even from relatively thin primary childhood melanomas [15].

4.2   Nevi Simulating Melanoma

Atypical/Dysplastic/Clark Nevus These terms are synonymous; the NIH Consensus Conference in 1992 recommended dropping the term "dysplastic nevus" due to the controversy surrounding the term "dysplasia" and proposed instead "nevus with architectural disorder and cytologic atypia" [18]. The concept is simple: it is a nevus that resembles melanoma, clinically and histopathologically. Points of clinical similarity between dysplastic nevus and melanoma include large size (generally >5 mm), poor circumscription, border irregularity, color variegation, and asymmetry. Newer techniques, such as dermoscopy (magnifying lens directly applied to the skin surface) [19], telespectrophotometry (analysis of color variation) [20], ultrasonic imaging [21], macroscopic spectral imaging [22], Melafind®, confocal laser microscopy, etc., may help clinicians distinguish dysplastic nevi from melanoma and thus avoid unnecessary biopsies. Atypical nevi occur at a prevalence of 2–9 % in unselected white populations in most series. One outlying study reported that 53 % of white adults had such lesions, probably because the inclusion criteria for diagnosis were broad, including even small lesions lacking cytologic atypia [23]. Nevi with clinical and histopathologic atypia, as traditionally defined, represent a strong, independent risk factor for development of melanoma [24] whether they occur sporadically or in the context of a melanoma-prone familial predisposition (dysplastic nevus syndrome) [25]. Moreover, this melanoma risk rises proportionately with number of atypical nevi present and the degree of atypia as diagnosed histopathologically. The higher the degree (mild, moderate, and severe), the more likely that the patient has had or will develop melanoma [26]. Another report [27] studied couples in which one of the two individuals had had a recent diagnosis of melanoma; then, both were examined clinically, and the most clinically atypical lesion was biopsied in either individual. When compared, the degree of dysplasia seen was higher in the patient with recent diagnosis of melanoma, compared with the spouse's biopsy. Apart from this role as a risk factor, atypical nevi may act as a precursor lesion to melanoma in some cases; molecular studies have demonstrated similar genetic changes in both atypical nevi and melanoma, as discussed below.

The histopathologic features of atypical nevi comprise abnormalities in architecture, host response, and cytology. There exists a broad consensus on architectural criteria [28], which include bridging of rete ridges, lateral extension of the junctional component ("shoulder"), and location of nests along sides of rete ridges. Regarding cytologic features, some authors insist that cytologic atypia is an absolute requirement [29], while others disagree [30]. In our view, both the degree of cytologic atypia and the extent of architectural disorder vary widely and tend to be highly correlated. Thus the architecture-versus-cytology controversy may reflect a false dichotomy. In a series of 166 consecutive atypical nevi, we found that about

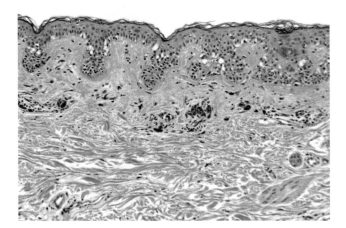

Fig. 4.1 Dysplastic (Clark) nevus: Notice the fusion of the epidermal rete ridges ("bridging"), dermal fibrosis, dermal vessels, and lymphocytic infiltrate (hematoxylin and eosin, x200)

85 % of lesions fell into the mild-moderate categories with regard to both cytologic atypia and architectural disorder; the remainder had a higher degree of atypical features suggesting (but falling short of full diagnostic criteria for) melanoma [31] (Fig. 4.1).

Atypical nevi may occur due to abnormalities in DNA repair in response to UVR, as shown in vitro [32]. Patients with dysplastic nevus syndrome have chromosomal instability, documented in normal skin, atypical nevi, and blood lymphocytes. Atypical nevi contain increased amounts of pheomelanin compared with common nevi, and this might increase their susceptibility to UVR damage [33]. Shifts among these melanin types may reflect changes in pigment regulatory genes such as that for the melanocortin-1 receptor [34].

Recurrent nevi regrow following partial surgical removal [35] due to recolonization of the epidermis by melanocytes from follicles, eccrine ducts, adjacent epidermis, or dermis [36]. Histopathologically, they may simulate melanoma, showing strikingly confluent growth of junctional melanocytes, focal suprabasal (pagetoid) spread of melanocytes, and dermal fibrosis reminiscent of regression (Fig. 4.2) [35]. In such cases it is important to detect the possible presence of remnants of nests of benign melanocytes immediately beneath the scar and confinement of the disorderly architecture to the area directly overlying the scar. In problematic cases, immunohistochemistry can be helpful [37] (analysis of maturation with HMB-45 and anti-Ki67, see below).

Suprabasal (pagetoid) melanocytosis simulating melanoma has also been described in nevi following UVR exposure [38]. The presence of suprabasal dyskeratinocytes

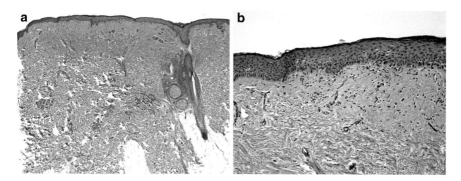

Fig. 4.2 Recurrent nevus: (**a**) Beneath an area of flat epidermis, there is fibrotic dermis (hematoxylin and eosin, x40). (**b**) The epidermis contains large, single-celled melanocytes, circumscribed to the area of fibrosis (hematoxylin and eosin, x100)

(sunburn cells) and the lack of high-grade atypia are helpful clues. Nevi of *acral skin* (e.g., palms, soles) [39–41] and genital (*vulvar*) nevi may contain confluent, basal, single melanocytes and focal suprabasal (pagetoid) melanocytosis, an architectural pattern that simulates melanoma. Diagnosis of acral/mucosal melanoma requires significant cytologic atypia, asymmetry, inflammatory infiltrates, and dermal mitotic figures. Clinical-pathologic correlation is also important; a high index of suspicion for melanoma is appropriate for acral lesions of recent onset in older patients, or those over 1 cm in diameter. Conservative, complete excision should be considered for atypical acral, pigmented lesions.

Desmoplastic nevus may mimic dermatofibroma, because of the prominent fibrosis of the stroma, and also resembles desmoplastic melanoma, both having dermal atypical cells. However, desmoplastic nevi are infrequently located on the head or neck (a common site for desmoplastic melanoma), lack mitotic figures, have significantly fewer Ki-67-reactive cells, and exhibit a gradient in HMB-45 expression, diminishing toward the deep area of the lesions (see below, immunohistochemistry) [42].

Spitz (spindled and epithelioid cell) nevus (Fig. 4.3). Spitz first introduced this lesion under the name "melanoma of childhood," and one of her initial cases actually was a malignant melanoma that metastasized fatally [43]. However, Spitz nevi can usually be distinguished from melanoma by their relative symmetry, sharp circumscription, scant pagetoid spread, Kamino bodies [44], cohesiveness of nests with peripheral clefts, minimal melanin pigment, vertical orientation of junctional nests ("raining down" or "bunches of bananas"), cytologic maturation, "breaking up" of nests to disperse as single cells among deeper collagen bundles, and edema and telangiectasia of the dermis. Lesions lacking the above features, or exhibiting necrosis, biphasic pattern (nevus), or deep mitotic figures, raise the possibility of spitzoid melanoma [45, 46], a very difficult diagnostic area in which consensus is often elusive [47]. Complete excision of all atypical spitzoid lesions seems prudent. Moreover, we recommend conservative but complete primary excision of even

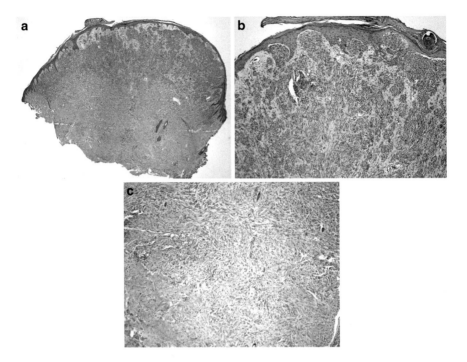

Fig. 4.3 Spitz nevus: (**a**) Large, symmetrical proliferation of melanocytes, arranged mostly in nests in the superficial dermis, with diminution in size with depth (maturation) (hematoxylin and eosin, x20). (**b**) Large nests close to the epidermis (hematoxylin and eosin, x100). (**c**) In the deep dermis, cells disperse as single cells among collagen fibers (hematoxylin and eosin, x100)

routine-appearing Spitz nevi if clinically feasible, because key features including circumscription and symmetry cannot be reliably evaluated in lesions extending to the margins and because in the event of recurrence it may be truly impossible to distinguish them from melanoma.

The term *ancient nevus* has been proposed for unusual, biphasic, intradermal pigmented lesions exhibiting asymmetry at scanning magnification [48], due to the presence of a biphenotypic melanocytic proliferation of both common nevus cells and of cells with large, pleomorphic nuclei, scattered deep mitotic figures, and "degenerative" sclerosis and hemorrhage. The main histopathologic differential diagnosis is with melanoma arising in an intradermal nevus. Since at least one of the original cases reportedly developed metastasis (communication at the Annual Meeting of the American Society of Dermatopathology), it follows that distinction between ancient nevus and melanoma is not straightforward.

Pigmented epithelioid melanocytomas have been described as a proliferation of heavily pigmented epithelioid or spindled melanocytes. These lesions share many features with cellular blue nevi and deep penetrating nevi. They are more common on the extremities. They may be ulcerated and present central necrosis. Since lymph node metastasis may occur in up to 50 % of the cases and there are rare cases with liver metastases [49], these lesions should be considered to have at least low-grade malignant potential.

4.3 Melanoma

4.3.1 Melanomas Simulating Nevi

The term *nevoid melanoma* has been used for melanomas deceptively composed of relatively small tumor cells, at first glance seeming to be nevus cells, but exhibiting nuclear atypia and deep mitotic figures. Lesions exhibiting strong HMB-45 labeling in the deep dermal component, especially when combined with evidence of cell proliferation (e.g., Ki-67 or PCNA expression; see below), may be nevoid melanomas rather than nevi [50]. Some melanomas exhibit a *maturation* pattern mimicking benign nevi. When compared with conventional melanoma and common compound nevi, this group of melanomas with maturation has intermediate features [51]. That is, with increasing depth, paradoxically maturing melanomas have smaller nuclear and cellular areas and decreased expression of Ki-67, gp100 (with HMB-45), and tyrosinase. In addition, in contrast with compound nevi, mitotic figures and melanin pigment can be detected in the deep portions of this type of melanoma.

Certain metastatic melanomas closely resemble nevi. This is particularly true of *epidermotropic metastases* [52, 53], including epidermotropic metastatic melanoma also with *paradoxical maturation* [51], and *dermal metastases simulating blue nevi* [54].

Early melanoma has been arbitrarily defined as those lesions with Breslow thickness ≤1 mm. Some such lesions also are in so-called radial growth phase (RGP), considered to have little if any potential for metastasis, with overall survival exceeding 90 % at 5 years after complete excision. By definition, all MIS (Clark level I) and some superficially invasive (most Clark level II lesions) are in RGP. After this point, some authors consider that melanoma enters a tumorigenic phase [vertical growth phase (VGP)] with significant capability for metastasis [55].

Melanoma in situ (MIS) is defined as melanoma confined to the epidermis and adnexal epithelium. It has an excellent prognosis, since it can almost always be cured by simple excision. Since MIS has a very low rate of metastasis, and to reduce the psychological charge that a diagnosis of melanoma conveys to the patient, some authors have proposed the use of other terms, such as *atypical melanocytic proliferation*. An expert panel from the UK examined interobserver agreement in the diagnosis of 95 melanocytic neoplasms, including many "borderline" lesions [56], and attempted to develop common definitions. There was a good overall agreement regarding benignity versus malignancy, but subclassifications as to degree of atypia or depth of invasion were more problematical. Specifically, the distinction between severe junctional atypia and MIS could not be made reliably. The authors therefore recommended combining these two diagnoses into one category of melanocytic intraepidermal neoplasia, in analogy to the practice used for severe cervical dysplasia/carcinoma in situ. However, not all authors agree with this terminology [57]. In our practice we routinely use the term MIS when appropriate, as it seems to convey an appropriate sense of therapeutic urgency to most clinicians, without necessarily implying a dismal outcome for the patient.

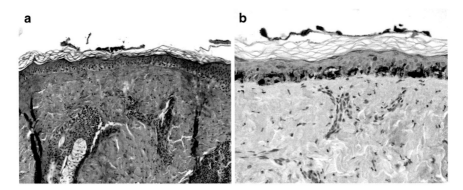

Fig. 4.4 Lentigo maligna melanoma: (**a**) Notice the large melanocytes scattered along the dermal-epidermal junction. The flat contour of the epidermis is usually associated with chronic actinic (solar) damage (hematoxylin and eosin, x200). (**b**) A pan-melanocytic cocktail highlights the presence of large melanocytes along the dermal-epidermal junction (HMB-45, anti-MART-1 [A 103], and anti-tyrosinase with diaminobenzidine [DAB] and hematoxylin, x400)

MIS may exhibit the histopathologic patterns of lentigo maligna, superficial spreading, and acral lentiginous (see below). Lentigo maligna-type MIS occurs in sun-exposed areas, mostly in elderly individuals. It is characterized by dendritic, large or small, round melanocytes with hyperchromatic nuclei, either as single cells or in nests, involving predominantly the basal layer of the epidermis and adnexa (Fig. 4.4). A useful clue to the diagnosis is that the epidermis itself is usually atrophic (flat) and there is actinic elastosis in the dermis.

It is important to examine the dermis beneath lesions of MIS to determine the possible presence of regression (defined as fibrosis, a lymphocytic infiltrate, and melanophages). Such lesions may correspond to previously invasive melanomas in which the dermal component regressed to a point where no melanoma cells are identified in the dermis. Such regressive changes can impart a risk of metastasis to even thin melanomas [58].

Since most MIS of the lentigo maligna type occur in sun-exposed skin, it sometimes becomes difficult to distinguish between a background phenomenon of actinic damage with atypical melanocytes and frank MIS. In specimens with solar elastosis (morphologic indication of actinic damage), the presence of a confluent growth of melanocytes (either with large nuclei and prominent nucleoli or with small, hyperchromatic nuclei) along the dermal-epidermal junction also involving the skin adnexa is indicative of MIS [59]. Also, since many specimens from elderly individuals are taken from the face (e.g., to rule out basal cell carcinoma, actinic keratosis, etc.), one should keep in mind that the specimen may also contain MIS, lentigo maligna type. Therefore, in such situations, it is essential to examine the epidermis adjacent to the main lesion for the presence of concurrent MIS.

Invasive melanomas are usually classified into more major histopathologic groups: nodular, lentigo maligna type, superficial spreading type, and acral lentiginous. Although this subclassification does not provide independent prognostic information, we still recommend including it in pathology reports. Furthermore,

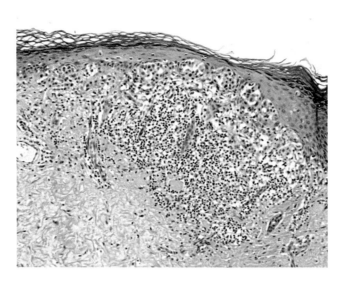

Fig. 4.5 Superficial spreading melanoma: Large melanocytes involve all layers of the epidermis, both as nests and as single cells (pagetoid upward migration) (hematoxylin and eosin, x200)

recent studies indicate that there are different oncogenic pathways for these subtypes (see molecular pathogenesis). Apart from providing epidemiological information (e.g., lentigo maligna usually occurs in sun-damaged skin), it may be helpful at the time of evaluation of re-excision specimens (e.g., lentigo maligna usually is associated with a peripheral proliferation of melanoma cells arranged as single cells that may be difficult to distinguish in routine hematoxylin and eosin slides). Superficial spreading melanoma is by far the most common type (75 %) and shows a predominantly nested growth pattern, usually with prominent pagetoid upward migration (Fig. 4.5). Nodular melanoma lacks an RGP; conceptually, this most likely reflects the rapid enlargement of the dermal tumor, overrunning an in situ component that previously existed. Lentigo maligna melanoma is associated with flat, atrophic (sun-damaged) epidermis and solar elastosis. Acral-lentiginous melanoma occurs in the acral regions (feet and hands, with a predilection for subungual and periungual regions) and is characterized by dendritic cells with extensive pagetoid upward migration (Fig. 4.6); similar features may also be seen in melanomas arising on mucosal sites such as vulva.

4.3.2 Histopathologic Evaluation of Melanoma: Prognostic Factors

Histopathologic examination of melanocytic lesions provides the best assessment for prognosis and also impacts subsequent management and treatment. The American Joint Committee on Cancer (AJCC) has published a list of histopathologic features that reportedly have an impact on prognosis [60], being the main three ones Breslow thickness, ulceration, and dermal mitotic figures.

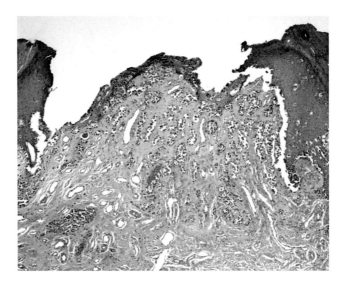

Fig. 4.6 Acral-lentiginous melanoma: Markedly pigmented melanoma cells involve the epidermis. As a feature characteristic of acral location, notice the thick stratum corneum overlying the epidermis (*top*) (hematoxylin and eosin, x40)

In addition, at our institutions we provide the list of multiple prognostic factors as requested/suggested by the collage of american pathologists (CAP) [61].

Breslow thickness is measured from the top of the granular layer to the deepest melanoma cell (Fig. 4.7), using a calibrated ocular micrometer; Breslow thickness is usually reported in millimeters and tenths of millimeters (some authors recommend to provide it as hundredths of millimeters; we follow this method for those lesions thinner than 2 mm).

Ulceration is defined as full-thickness loss of epidermis overlying the melanoma; traumatic mechanisms such as a previous biopsy should be excluded.

Mitotic figures are quantified as a number of mitotic figures identified in dermal melanocytes, as mitotic figures per square mm, and not as an average, but rather by the counting in the "hot spot" (see below). Due to their importance for patient management, these three (Breslow thickness, ulceration, and number of dermal mitotic figures) are the features that are considered mandatory in the pathology report. Thus, the AJCC classification includes:

- pT1a (invasive melanoma, ≤ 1.00 mm, without ulceration or mitotic figures)
- pT1b (invasive melanoma, ≤ 1.00 mm, with ulceration *or* mitotic figures; see also below Clark level)
- pT2a (invasive melanoma, ≥1.01 mm and <2.00 mm, without ulceration)
- pT2b (invasive melanoma, ≥1.01 mm and <2.00 mm, with ulceration)
- pT3a (invasive melanoma, ≥2.01 mm and <4.00 mm, without ulceration)
- pT3b (invasive melanoma, ≥2.01 mm and <4.00 mm, with ulceration)

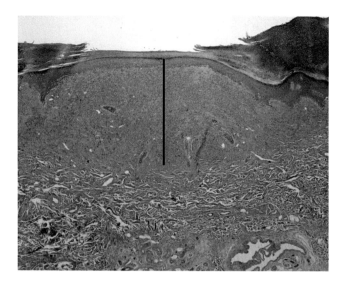

Fig. 4.7 The measurement of the Breslow thickness is usually performed with an ocular having a built-in ruler or reticule (ocular micrometer). Skin sections should be cut perpendicularly to the epidermal surface to avoid skewed measurements. Breslow thickness is defined as the distance between the top of the granular layer (the layer immediately beneath the stratum corneum of the epidermis) and the deepest-located melanocyte. In case of ulceration, the measurement is performed from the base of the ulcer. Nests of tumor cells within vessels (vascular invasion), immediately adjacent to skin adnexa, or satellite lesions are not included in the measurement (hematoxylin and eosin, x20)

- pT4a (invasive melanoma, >4.00 mm, without ulceration)
- pT4b (invasive melanoma, >4.00 mm, with ulceration)

- *Clark levels* are defined as: I, melanoma limited to the epidermis (melanoma in situ); II, focally involving the papillary dermis; III, filling and expanding the papillary dermis; IV, involving the reticular dermis; and V, involving the subcutaneous tissue (Fig. 4.8). The Clark level is highly correlated with the Breslow thickness, is a relatively subjective and poorly reproducible measure, and has only minor independent prognostic import except in the case of level IV or V invasion in melanomas less than 1 mm thick. For these reasons, in the current AJCC classification, Clark level is no longer used for staging, except in such thin melanomas. Vascular invasion has been reported to have an adverse effect, on relapse rate and mortality [62]; immunohistochemistry, e.g., with detection of D2-40, may help detecting the vascular invasion [63].

  Mainly for research purposes, we recommend the pathology report should also contain other histopathologic features that may or may not have prognostic significance: RGP, VGP, regression, perineural invasion, degree of lymphocytic infiltrate, satellitosis, the presence of associated melanocytic nevus, type of cytology, and adequacy of margins.

- *Radial growth phase* (RGP) is defined as the presence of melanoma cells in the epidermis at least three rete ridges (vertical extensions of the epidermis into the

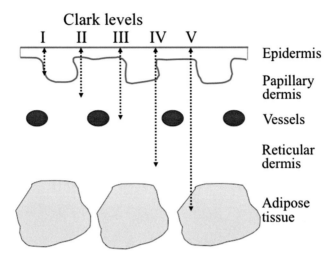

Fig. 4.8 Clark levels: (I) melanoma in situ, (II) focally involving the papillary dermis, (III) filling and expanding the papillary dermis, (IV) involving the reticular dermis, and (V) involving the subcutaneous tissue

dermis) beyond the most lateral dermal component. In some studies, melanomas in pure RGP (without associated VGP) have a much better prognosis (very low metastatic rate).

- *Vertical growth phase* (VGP) can be most simply defined by the presence of dermal nest(s) of melanoma larger than any nest in the epidermis or dermal-epidermal junction, by the presence of any mitotic figures in the dermal component, or by both criteria.
- *Regression* is defined as the presence of dense fibrosis, and a lymphocytic infiltrate with fibrosis and melanophages, often with increased vascularity. This combination of features likely represents an area of melanoma in which melanoma cells have been destroyed by an inflammatory infiltrate. Paradoxically, in most studies regression is a negative prognostic factor, probably because it permits "undercounting" of the true (previous) Breslow thickness (Fig. 4.9). It has been suggested that measurement of the thickness of the area of regression may be a surrogate to determine the extent of the original level of invasion.
- *Vascular invasion* is defined as detection of melanoma cells within vascular spaces, regardless if they are lymphatic or blood vessels and, as noted above, it may become part of the staging scheme from the AJCC in the next classification (Fig. 4.10).
- *Perineural invasion* is the presence of melanoma cells within or around dermal nerves.
- The *degree of lymphatic infiltrate* is classified as minimal (only scattered lymphocytes), non-brisk (focal lymphocytic infiltrate), and brisk (dense, band-like lymphocytic infiltrate throughout the base of the entire dermal component; tumor-infiltrating lymphocytes, TILs); according to some studies, a brisk response is associated with better prognosis.

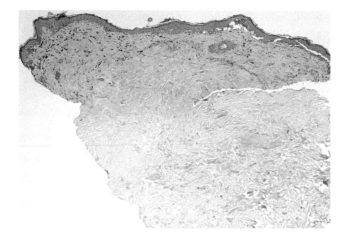

Fig. 4.9 Melanoma with regression. Notice that the dermis immediately beneath the epidermis has a pink color (fibrosis) with dilated vessels and focal melanin pigment, consistent with dermal regression (hematoxylin and eosin, x20)

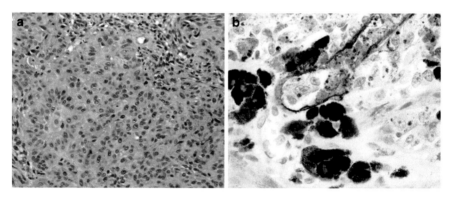

Fig. 4.10 Vascular invasion: (**a**) There is cluster of melanoma cells within a vessel (the space is lined by flat, endothelial cells) (hematoxylin and eosin, x100). (**b**) Anti-D2–40 highlights the endothelial cells lining the vessel (Anti-D2–40 with diaminobenzidine (DAB) and hematoxylin, x400)

– *Microscopic satellites* are nests of melanoma cells located away from the main lesion. There is no clear-cut definition of microsatellites; some authors define them as located more than three collagen bundles from the main lesion or else, clearly separated from the main lesion. In our practice we diagnose microsatellites as tumor nests surrounded by normal dermis rather than surgical scar from the previous specimen or fibrotic changes characteristic of melanoma stroma. These clusters of tumor cells probably represent in-transit metastasis, accounting for the negative impact on survival.

– *Cytology:* Most melanomas have *epithelioid* (round) or *spindle cells* (elongated or fusiform); other less common types are rhabdoid (large, round, with eccentric nuclei) and nevoid (small cells resembling nevus cells). Cytomorphology is not an independent risk factor in most studies, but should be reported as an aid to the pathologist who may be confronted with a re-excision, recurrence, or metastasis; in particular, spindle-cell desmoplastic variants of melanoma may simulate scar tissue, eluding detection in re-excision specimens.

– *Margins*, both peripheral and deep, should be reported as either free or involved by melanoma. It is currently the standard of clinical care to perform a wide re-excision of all invasive melanomas primarily removed with narrow (<1 cm) margins. Since the gold standard is the clinical determination of the distance of the tumor to the margin, there is no agreement in reporting the distance of the tumor to the margin as performed on the histopathologic slides. In general, most clinicians determine the clinical margin necessary for the re-excision based upon the Breslow thickness: MIS, 0.5 cm margin; less than 1 mm, 1 cm margin; more than 1 mm, 2 cm margin (recommendation of the NIH Consensus Conference, Washington, D.C., 1992 [18]). Although there is no apparent difference in survival, a 1-cm re-excision in thick melanomas (greater than 2 mm Breslow thickness) results in higher rate of local recurrences than when larger margins are sought [64].

4.4 Examination of Lymph Nodes

The concept of sentinel lymph node (SLN) has profoundly changed the management of many solid tumors, including melanoma (see elsewhere in this book). Regarding histopathologic evaluation of SLN, since this is the lymph node or nodes most likely to contain melanoma cells, every effort should be made to maximize the sensitivity and specificity of histopathologic techniques.

There are two main ways of processing SLNs. One method bisects the lymph node along the long axis, cutting through the lymph node hilum [65]. In contrast, in our institutions, we routinely breadloaf SLNs (sectioning of the node perpendicular to the long axis, similar to a loaf of bread) because it allows examination of a large surface of the lymph node in the initial sections (Fig. 4.11) and avoids the problem of trying to find the hilum in small lymph nodes [66].

If the first routine hematoxylin and eosin section is negative for melanoma, we cut a section deeper in the paraffin block (~200 μm) and then examine another routine section along with two immunohistochemical slides labeled with a cocktail containing anti-MART-1, anti-tyrosinase, and HMB-45 (Fig. 4.12). Regarding lymphatic metastasis, when examining lymph nodes, the report should contain the number of positive lymph nodes and total number of lymph nodes examined. In our experience, factors correlating with survival include the size of the largest tumor deposit, the location (subcapsular better than intraparenchymal), and the presence or absence of extracapsular extension. Thus, these three parameters should probably be included in the pathology report.

Regarding examination of completion lymphadenectomy specimens, due to the complexity of the method employed for the examination of SLNs, non-SLNs are to

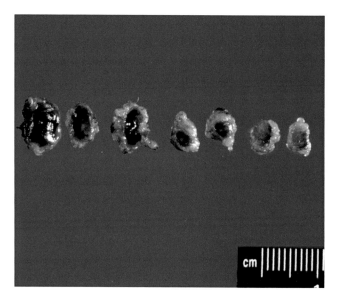

Fig. 4.11 Breadloafing of a lymph node with pigment tattoo

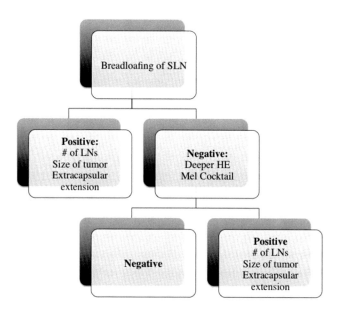

Fig. 4.12 Algorithm for diagnosis of sentinel lymph nodes. If the initial hematoxylin and eosin section is negative, we cut three additional sections deeper in the block (approximately 200 μm in the block). The first one is stained with hematoxylin and eosin, and the second is labeled with a pan-melanocytic cocktail (HMB-45, anti-tyrosinase, and anti-MART-1). The third slide is left in reserve in case examination of additional markers is needed (e.g., HMB-45 alone, S100 protein, SOX10)

be examined histopathologically in a simpler manner, identical to that used for other lymph nodes in the body. Briefly, the entire lymph node is processed and examined in hematoxylin and eosin sections. Occasionally, if there are any cells suspicious to be metastatic melanoma, immunohistochemical studies may be used, but this is not performed in every single case.

4.5 Immunohistochemistry

Immunohistochemistry is based on the use of antigens directed against appropriate protein targets (antibodies). This method allows the determination of the phenotype (antigen expression) of the selected cells. The use of antibodies against antigens usually expressed in melanocytes, such as S100 protein, gp100 (detected with HMB-45), MART-1 (melanoma antigen recognized by T cells), or tyrosinase, permits confirmation that a given neoplasm exhibits melanocytic differentiation. S100 protein is a nuclear and cytoplasmic calcium-binding protein, which is expressed by most melanocytes. However, other cells (e.g., Langerhans cells, dendritic cells in dermis and lymph nodes, neural cells) also express it. Therefore, although very sensitive, this marker is relatively nonspecific. In our hands, the most important use of anti-S100 protein is the detection of melanocytic differentiation in desmoplastic and spindle cell melanomas. MART-1 is an antigen expressed by most melanocytes and both benign (nevus cells) and melanoma cells. It is very specific, since only steroid-producing tumors (such as adrenal and some ovarian neoplasms) and, rarely, macrophages will also express it [67]. Since it is more sensitive than HMB-45, we routinely use anti-MART-1 to support a diagnosis of melanocytic differentiation in non-desmoplastic melanomas. Another application is to help in the distinction between desmoplastic melanoma and spindle cell nevus; the former is usually negative or only focally positive, while the latter is strongly and diffusely positive [68]. gp100 (HMB-45 antigen) is a glycoprotein associated with immature melanosomes; in the lymph nodes, only melanoma cells express this antigen. We routinely use this marker to help in the differential diagnosis between nevus and melanoma (see below). Tyrosinase, an enzyme associated with melanin synthesis, has a pattern of expression similar to that of gp100. Expression of microphthalmia transcription factor (MiTF) or SOX10 can aid in the diagnosis of desmoplastic melanoma when other specific melanoma markers are negative.

There are several applications for immunohistochemistry in the examination of pigmented lesions. These "lineage-specific" uses of immunohistochemistry are widely accepted as diagnostic adjunct. For example, in small biopsies, immunohistochemistry may be helpful in distinguishing pigmented basal cell carcinoma from small cell melanoma [69]. Also, when examining sentinel node specimens, immunohistochemistry may help detect small clusters of or even single melanoma cells within the lymph node [70, 71] (Fig. 4.13). Detection of such small deposits of melanoma cells is important since the AJCC classification considers cases with any melanoma cell in the lymph node (whether detected by hematoxylin and eosin or by

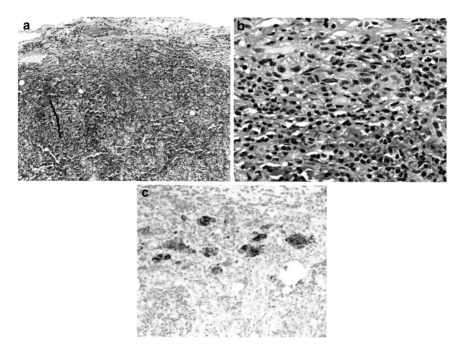

Fig. 4.13 Sentinel lymph node with micrometastatic melanoma. (**a**) Routine hematoxylin and eosin stain appears negative at this low power (hematoxylin and eosin, x100). (**b**) High power shows only a few suspicious mononuclear cells in the subcapsular area, which may correspond to melanoma or lymphoid cells (hematoxylin and eosin, x400). (**c**) These cells are labeled with a pan-melanocytic cocktail, therefore supporting the diagnosis of metastatic melanoma (HMB-45, anti-MART-1 [A 103], and anti-tyrosinase with diaminobenzidine (DAB) and hematoxylin, x400)

immunohistochemistry) as stage 3a lesions (metastatic melanoma to a regional lymph node).

An exciting but more controversial field is the use of immunohistochemistry for the differential diagnosis of melanoma and nevus [72, 73]. Although some pathologists would disagree, we strongly feel that, in *selected* cases and when considered in the *context of clinical and histopathologic data*, immunohistochemical findings can be of considerable utility in the diagnosis of melanocytic lesions. An example is the assessment of maturation in the dermal component of melanocytic lesions. In benign lesions, superficial, round, type A nevus cells immunohistochemically resemble neurons, whereas the deep, spindle, type C nevus cells more closely resemble Schwann cells [74, 75]. This morphology is reflected in the decreased ("maturational") expression of gp100 by those melanocytes at the base of the nevus, as opposed to the persistent expression observed in most melanomas [42, 76]. Furthermore, the almost universal lack of mitotic figures in the deep regions of nevi correlates with the very sparse expression of proliferation markers (such as Ki-67 or Ki-S5) by the deeper neoplastic cells in nevi. In a study of 384 melanocytic lesions [77], the common, dysplastic, and Spitz nevi exhibited reactivity in <6 % of cells, which tended to be located at the dermal-epidermal junction or superficial dermis. In contrast, melanomas exhibited a mean proliferative fraction of 16.4 %, especially in the deeper aspect. Based on Ki-S5 (Ki-67) expression, Rudolf et al. reclassified 112 problematic pigmented lesions and went on to demonstrate systemic progression in 70.7 % of the cases reclassified as melanoma but in no cases reclassified as nevi. This highly significant result indicates the potential clinical utility of immunohistochemical methods as one aspect of diagnosis of difficult melanocytic lesions.

The group of melanocytic lesions with marked fibrous stroma includes desmoplastic nevus and desmoplastic melanoma. As mentioned above, melanomas, including those with desmoplastic stroma, show increased cellular proliferation as measured with anti-Ki-67 [42]. Also useful is the common loss of expression of many melanocytic markers (gp100, MART-1) in desmoplastic melanoma but not in desmoplastic nevus. Thus, a melanocytic lesion lacking MART-1 expression but preserving S100 and SOX10 would likely be malignant. The only exception to this rule is the sometimes reduced expression of MART-1 in some neurotized nevi [78].

4.6 Concept of Melanoma Progression

As in other fields of oncology, in melanoma there is presumed to be a progression of molecular and cellular events that accompany the cellular transformation from benignity to malignancy. A similar process has been well documented in squamous lesions of the genitalia (progression of epithelial dysplasia, through carcinoma in situ, to invasive carcinoma) and in the large intestine (adenomatous polyp, adenocarcinoma "in situ," and invasive adenocarcinoma) [79], and it is likely to be a general model of oncogenesis. Although some authors steadfastly refuse this concept as applied to melanoma [9], it seems likely to us that there exists a spectrum of lesions between obviously benign nevi and frank melanoma. However, just by looking at the large numbers of benign nevi and the relatively much lower number of melanomas, it is obvious that a majority of nevi never transform into melanoma. Melanocytes in the epidermis proliferate, forming benign nevic lesions (either common or atypical). A small number of those may transform into MIS, proliferate, and ultimately invade the dermis. There they may undergo a further qualitative change from tumorigenic to non-tumorigenic growth and ultimately attain competency for metastasis. When the melanoma cells form nests in the dermis that are larger than any given intraepidermal nest or when any mitotic figures are detected in the dermis, those thin melanomas are classified as being in VGP. Although this is a somewhat arbitrary distinction, it is true that most of the early melanomas that subsequently develop metastasis fulfill the criteria for VGP.

The risk of progression of any nevus to invasive melanoma is extremely low. Even clinically atypical nevi are generally stable, as assessed by serial photography; on the other hand, a persistent change in a pigmented lesion's size, shape, or color is a high-risk marker for melanoma. The major exception is the expected life-cycle pattern of common nevi, believed to undergo a change from junctional to compound to intradermal location, as discussed above. To further complicate this topic, at least 50 % of melanomas may appear de novo and not within a preexisting nevus, and a number of melanomas appear within the *dermis* of congenital nevi.

Despite the existence of a spectrum of melanocytic atypia, ranging from banal nevi to outright melanoma, the experienced pathologist should be able to render a confident diagnosis of nevus versus melanoma in the great majority of cases encountered in routine practice. This opinion is not deterred by the results of a study [80] in which eight experts reviewed 37 cases of melanoma or of nevus sharing features with melanoma and were asked to classify them as malignant, indeterminate, or benign. The expert panel achieved only moderate concordance, with complete agreement obtained in only 30 % of cases. In part, the discordance may have reflected the selection of particularly problematic cases at the high end of the spectrum. Moreover, semantic differences among participants about whether dysplastic/ atypical lesions should be considered benign, indeterminate, or malignant may have exaggerated the reported disagreements.

4.6.1 Molecular Pathogenesis of Melanocytic Dysplasia and Melanoma

Several genetic changes are associated with the proposed melanoma progression [81–87]. Anomalies in chromosome 1 (1p36) occur in some patients with the dysplastic nevus syndrome/familial melanoma [88]. Such families also exhibit abnormalities in at least a second gene, on chromosome 9, that encodes an inhibitor of a kinase involved in the cell cycle, named p16^{INK4a} [89] or cyclin-dependent kinase inhibitor-2 (CDKN2A). Loss of p16 expression correlates with melanoma progression [90]. Loss of heterozygosity for p16 occurs early in the proposed progression sequence, having been reported also in atypical nevi; this finding supports a common pathogenesis of atypical nevi with melanoma. In families carrying mutations in the gene for p16, the presence of clinically atypical nevi was correlated with an earlier onset of melanoma [91]. Molecular studies confirm that the different histopathologic subtypes of melanoma are related to different pathogenic pathways [92]. The addition of activating mutations in N-ras to melanoma cells already containing mutations in p16 may induce the VGP phenotype [93]. Such N-ras mutations are common in melanomas from chronically sun-exposed skin but rare in mucosal melanomas [94]. c-Kit mutations are more common in acral and mucosal melanomas. GNAQ and GNA11 are more commonly mutated in heavily pigmented melanomas ("blue nevus-like") and uveal melanomas.

Several genes are mutated relatively consistently in thick melanomas, correlating with a decreased survival. These include c-myc (nuclear protein required for transition from G_1 to S phase), p53 (gatekeeper protein preventing cell proliferation after DNA damage), bcl-2 (anti-apoptotic factor), transforming growth factor-β (TGF-β, protein involved in angiogenesis and wound healing), CD40 (receptor inducing escape from apoptosis), MDA-7 (a melanoma-differentiation antigen), and the cyclin-dependent kinase inhibitors p27 and p21 (KIP1 and Waf-1/SDI-1, respectively) [95–97]. Enzymes that degrade collagen may facilitate permeation of the dermis and access to blood vessels. Among those, collagenases 1 and 3 are expressed in invasive and metastatic but not in in situ melanomas [98]. Similarly, some integrins (molecules involved in cell-to-cell recognition), such as the beta 3 subunit of the vitronectin receptor, are first detected in VGP melanomas [99], as is interleukin-8 (IL-8) [100]. Since tumors must recruit new vessels in order to grow, there must be secretion of angiogenic factors at some point. Some studies have shown increased vascularity in VGP versus RGP melanomas [101]. Two candidate proteins for this angiogenesis are vascular endothelial growth factor [102, 103] and basic fibroblastic growth factor (b-FGF), which have mitogenic effects on endothelial cells. By immunohistochemistry and in situ hybridization, b-FGF is expressed in invasive but not in situ melanomas [104]. Related to angiogenesis, there is a relationship between numbers of mast cells (which contain high quantities of angiogenic factors) and invasiveness in melanomas [104]. An exciting new field is the detection of markers that may serve as therapeutic targets. Some melanomas express c-kit and other tyrosine kinases (PDGF alpha and beta receptors, abl, abl-related gene protein), which are known targets for Gleevec® [105] and other anti-tyrosine kinases. Also melanomas express akt [106], a target of several small synthetic molecules that may prove useful for treatment of patients with melanoma.

Generally, only small quantities of tissue are available for analysis in common nevi, atypical nevi, and early melanoma. Therefore, most genetic changes have been described in either deeply invasive primary lesions or metastatic lesions or in cell lines. Breakthrough techniques such as laser microdissection now allow removal and analysis of minute quantities of tissue [107], potentially allowing molecular analysis of the earliest stages of incipient melanoma. After the particular tissue regions, cells, or even subcellular structures of interest are separated by a laser-based method, appropriate techniques such as comparative genomic hybridization (CGH) can be applied to analyze different molecular changes. This approach has been used to detect mutations in the *BRAF* gene [108] or chromosomal differences between RGP and VGP melanoma. These studies have demonstrated losses of chromosomes 9 and 10 early in melanoma progression and gains of chromosome 7 later in melanoma progression [109, 110].

There are several techniques that have been applied to the analysis of melanoma lesions. CGH has enabled comparison between the DNA derived from the melanoma and labeled with a fluorochrome and a reference DNA labeled with a different fluorochrome (Fig. 4.14a). Chromosomal gains or losses are detected as predominance of one or another fluorochrome [110, 111]. Those studies identified that primary melanomas were typified by multiple gains and losses in discrete regions of the genome (Fig. 4.14b). Whereas greater than 95 % of melanomas demonstrated some degree of chromosomal copy number aberration, only a rare subset of melanocytic nevi (Spitz nevi) demonstrated isolated gain of short arm of chromosome 11. CGH also demonstrated differences among melanomas of varying histopathologic subtypes, related to their anatomic location and the degree of antecedent UVR exposure [112].

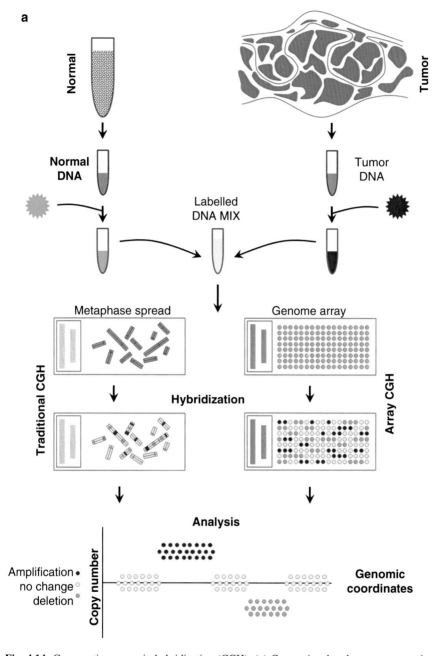

Fig. 4.14 Comparative genomic hybridization (CGH). (**a**) Conventional and array comparative genomic hybridization. Genomic DNA is extracted from tumor and normal tissues. It is then labeled with *green* and *red* fluorochromes. The DNA samples are denatured and then hybridized to normal metaphase chromosomes or to a microarray platform of cloned genomic DNA. The ratios of fluorescence intensities of the *red* and *green* signals are proportional to the ratios of copy numbers of the loci in the chromosomes or arrays. (**b**) CGH analysis. The fluorescent signals are translated into diagrams showing the entire karyotype and location of gains (indicated as *green lines* and areas next to chromosomes) and losses (*red lines* and areas) of chromosomal copy numbers. This example shows, among others, gain in 6p and losses in 6q, found in melanoma (adapted from Bauer J, Bastian B. Dermatol Therapy 2006 (19) 40–6; courtesy of Dr. Priyadharsini Nagarajan)

b

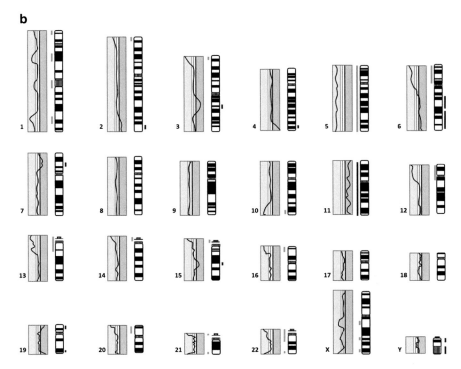

Fig. 4.14 (continued)

Although these data suggest the possible diagnostic utility of CGH when distinguishing melanoma from nevus, it requires a relatively large amount of pure tumor cells (without stroma, vessels, or inflammatory cells), and the abnormality must be present in a sufficient number of tumor cells to be detectable in the analysis.

Fluorescence in situ hybridization (FISH) utilizes fluorescently labeled probes corresponding to discrete areas in chromosomes with alterations known to be present in melanoma. By counting the number of fluorescent signals per nucleus, aberrations are described as a percentage of tumor nuclei carrying greater or fewer than two signals. Since FISH uses formalin-fixed, paraffin-embedded sections, it thus offers the ability to evaluate which cells display the changes. In that way it is possible to determine that if only an area of the lesion has abnormalities, it may correspond to a melanoma arising in association with a nevus.

The original FISH studies included four probes: RREB1 (6p25), CEN6 (centromere 6), MYB (6q23), and CCND1 (11q13). Since all cells should contain two signals of the centromere 6 probe, its counts were used to determine the ratio of gains or losses. The new generation test includes probes for RREB1, CCND1, p16 (9p21), MYC (8q24), and CEN9 (centromere 9) (Fig. 4.15a). Depending on the laboratory, there are different algorithms for the best percentage cutoffs to distinguish melanoma from nevus [113–116]. A possible pitfall is interpretation of a positive FISH

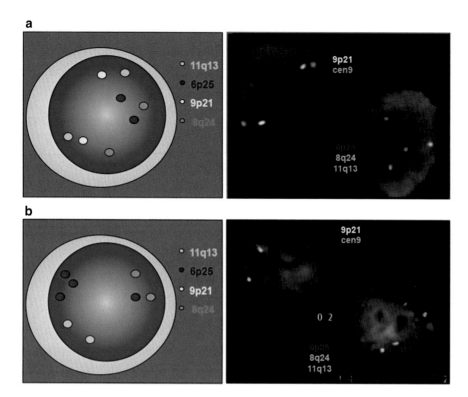

Fig. 4.15 FISH in melanoma. (**a**) Normal cell displaying two signals per tested probe. This result is interpreted as negative and is not supportive of melanoma. (**b**) Lack of the two gold signals (9p21) is interpreted as homozygous deletion of 9p21 (p16), a finding associated with melanoma, specifically spitzoid type. Notice the two signals corresponding to centromere 9, confirming the biallelic loss. Along with the right histopathological and immunohistochemical findings, this result supports the diagnosis of melanoma (Courtesy of Dr. Michael Tetzlaff)

in polyploidy (typically tetraploid) spitzoid lesions since such spitzoid lesions behave in a benign fashion [117].

Overall, it has been reported that FISH has a sensitivity of ~80 % and specificity of >90 % when distinguishing melanoma from nevus. However, when the FISH assay is applied to ambiguous lesions, i.e., lesions in which the dermatopathologist is not able to render a definite diagnosis of melanoma or nevus [118], a number of FISH-positive lesions did not develop recurrence or metastasis, a finding that can be interpreted that those lesions were melanomas cured by excision or that had not developed metastasis yet. Furthermore other studies with positive FISH results lacked confirmation of the findings when examined by array CGH [116, 119]. It seems that the combination of expert dermatopathology diagnosis and FISH generates the optimum results [120].

There have been recent FISH studies indicating that spitzoid lesions with homozygous deletion of 9p21 behave in a malignant fashion (i.e., as spitzoid melanomas) [121] (Fig. 4.15b) and that amelanotic melanomas with amplification of *c-myc* (8q24) present an aggressive clinical course [122].

In summary we, as others, consider that FISH results should only be considered in the context of an expert histopathologic examination and that, by itself, positive FISH does not equal a diagnosis of melanoma and that a negative FISH does not equal a diagnosis of nevus. Further studies are necessary to determine if detection of homozygous deletion of 9p21 or amplification of 8q24 is sufficient, on themselves, to establish a diagnosis of melanoma.

Matrix-assisted laser desorption ionization (MALDI) imaging mass spectrometry has recently been applied to try to detect protein differences between Spitz nevi and spitzoid melanomas [123]. This study has shown promising results since it was able to show significant differences between Spitz nevus and spitzoid melanoma, just by analyzing the peptide contents of the tumor and comparing it with the normal control of the same patient. Interestingly, the discriminating model included five peptides, among them actin and vimentin. Furthermore, the same study indicated that analyzing the peptide contents of the peritumoral stroma also allowed distinguishing between benign and malignant spitzoid lesions. Further studies are needed to determine the practical application of this technique to the diagnosis of melanocytic lesions.

References

1. Dennis LK (1999) Analysis of the melanoma epidemic, both apparent and real – Data from the 1973 through 1994 surveillance, epidemiology, and end results program registry. Arch Dermatol 135(3):275–280
2. de Gruijl FR (1999) Skin cancer and solar UV radiation. Eur J Cancer 35(14):2003–2009
3. Stern JB, Peck GL, Haupt HM, Hollingsworth HC, Beckerman T (1993) Malignant melanoma in xeroderma pigmentosum: search for a precursor lesion. J Am Acad Dermatol 28(4):591–594
4. Prieto VG, Kanik A, Salob S, McNutt NS (1994) Primary cutaneous myxoid melanoma: immunohistologic clues to a difficult diagnosis. J Am Acad Dermatol 30(2 Pt 2):335–339
5. Holly EA, Kelly JW, Shpall SN, Chiu SH (1987) Number of melanocytic nevi as a major risk factor for malignant melanoma. J Am Acad Dermatol 17(3):459–468
6. Rhodes AR, Harrist TJ, Day CL, Mihm MC Jr, Fitzpatrick TB, Sober AJ (1983) Dysplastic melanocytic nevi in histologic association with 234 primary cutaneous melanomas. J Am Acad Dermatol 9(4):563–574
7. Maize JC, Ackerman AB (1987) Malignant melanoma. In: Maize JC, Ackerman AB (eds) Pigmented lesions of the skin. Clinicopathologic correlations. Lea & Febiger, Philadelphia, p 165
8. Elder DE, Clark WH Jr, Elenitsas R, Guerry D, Halpern AC (1993) The early and intermediate precursor lesions of tumor progression in the melanocytic system: common acquired nevi and atypical (dysplastic) nevi. Semin Diagn Pathol 10:18–35
9. Ackerman AB, Cerroni L, Kerl H. Melanoma in association with a nevus. In: Pitfalls in histopathologic diagnosis of malignant melanoma. Philadelphia: Lea & Febiger; 1994, p. 142–143.
10. DeDavid M, Orlow SJ, Provost N et al (1997) A study of large congenital melanocytic nevi and associated malignant melanomas: review of cases in the New York University Registry and the world literature. J Am Acad Dermatol 36:409–416
11. Rhodes AR, Wood WC, Sober AJ, Mihm MC Jr (1981) Nonepidermal origin of malignant melanoma associated with a giant congenital nevocellular nevus. Plast Reconstr Surg 67(6):782–790

12. Tajima Y, Nakahima T, Sugano I, Nagao K, Kondo Y (1994) Malignant melanoma within an intradermal nevus. Am J Dermatopathol 16:301–306
13. Sahin S, Levin L, Kopf AW et al (1998) Risk of melanoma in medium-sized congenital melanocytic nevi: a follow-up study. J Am Acad Dermatol 39(3):428–433
14. Hurwitz RM, Buckel LJ (1997) Superficial congenital compound melanocytic nevus. Another pitfall in the diagnosis of malignant melanoma. Dermatol Surg 23(10):897–900
15. Scalzo DA, Hida CA, Toth G, Sober AJ, Mihm MC Jr (1997) Childhood melanoma: a clinicopathological study of 22 cases. Melanoma Res 7(1):63–68
16. Ruiz-Maldonado R, Orozco-Covarrubias M (1997) Malignant melanoma in children. A review. Arch Dermatol 133(3):363–371
17. Ceballos PI, Ruiz-Maldonado R, Mihm MCJ (1995) Melanoma in children. N Engl J Med 332:656–662
18. Health NIO (1992) NIH consensus conference. Diagnosis and treatment of early melanoma. JAMA 268:1314–1319
19. Andreassi L, Perotti R, Rubegni P et al (1999) Digital dermoscopy analysis for the differentiation of atypical nevi and early melanoma – a new quantitative semiology. Arch Dermatol 135(12):1459–1465
20. Bono A, Tomatis S, Bartoli C et al (1999) The ABCD system of melanoma detection: a spectrophotometric analysis of the asymmetry, border, color, and dimension. Cancer 85(1):72–77
21. Solivetti FM, Thorel MF, Di Luca SA, Bucher S, Donati P, Panichelli V (1998) Role of high-definition and high frequency ultrasonography in determining tumor thickness in cutaneous malignant melanoma. Radiol Med 96(6):558–561
22. Yang P, Farkas DL, Kirkwood JM, Abernethy JL, Edington HD, Becker D (1999) Macroscopic spectral imaging and gene expression analysis of the early stages of melanoma. Mol Med 5(12):785–794
23. Piepkorn M, Meyer LJ, Goldgar D et al (1989) The dysplastic melanocytic nevus: a prevalent lesion that correlates poorly with clinical phenotype. J Am Acad Dermatol 20(3):407–415
24. Tucker MA, Halpern A, Holly EA et al (1997) Clinically recognized dysplastic nevi. A central risk factor for cutaneous melanoma. JAMA 277:1439–1444
25. Clark WHJ, Reimer RR, Greene M, Ainsworth AM, Mastrangelo MJ (1978) Origin of familial melanomas from heritable melanocytic lesions. 'The B-K mole syndrome'. Arch Dermatol 114(5):732–738
26. Arumi-Uria M, McNutt NS, Finnerty B (2003) Grading of atypia in nevi: correlation with melanoma risk. Mod Pathol 16(8):764–771
27. Shors A, Kim S, White E et al (2006) Naevi with moderate to severe histological dysplasia: a risk factor for melanoma. Br J Dermatol 155:988–993
28. Hastrup N, Clemmensen OJ, Spaun E, Søndergaard K (1994) Dysplastic naevus; histological criteria and their inter-observer reproducibility. Histopathology 24:503–509
29. Barnhill RL, Roush GC, Duray PH (1990) Correlation of histologic architectural and cytoplasmic features with nuclear atypia in atypical (dysplastic) nevomelanocytic nevi. Hum Pathol 21(1):51–58
30. Rivers JK, Cockerell CJ, McBride A (1990) Quantification of histologic features of dysplastic nevi. Am J Dermatopathol 12:42–50
31. Shea CR, Vollmer RT, Prieto VG (1999) Correlating architectural disorder and cytologic atypia in Clark (dysplastic) melanocytic nevi. Hum Pathol 30(5):500–505
32. Moriwaki SI, Tarone RE, Tucker MA, Goldstein AM, Kraemer KH (1997) Hypermutability of UV-treated plasmids in dysplastic nevus/familial melanoma cell lines. Cancer Res 57(20):4637–4641
33. Salopek TG, Yamada K, Ito S, Jimbow K (1991) Dysplastic melanocytic nevi contain high levels of pheomelanin: quantitative comparison of pheomelanin/eumelanin levels between normal skin, common nevi, and dysplastic nevi. Pigment Cell Res 4(4):172–179
34. Suzuki I, Im S, Tada A et al (1999) Participation of the melanocortin-1 receptor in the UV control of pigmentation. J Invest Dermatol 4(1):29–34

35. Kornberg R, Ackerman AB (1975) Pseudomelanoma: recurrent melanocytic nevus following partial surgical removal. Arch Dermatol 111(12):1588–1590
36. Park HK, Leonard DD, Arrington JH 3rd, Lund HZ (1987) Recurrent melanocytic nevi: clinical and histologic review of 175 cases. J Am Acad Dermatol 17(2 Pt 1):285–292
37. Hoang MP, Prieto VG, Burchette JL, Shea CR (2001) Recurrent melanocytic nevus: a histologic and immunohistochemical evaluation. J Cutan Pathol 28(8):400–406
38. Tronnier M, Smolle J, Wolff HH (1995) Ultraviolet irradiation induces acute changes in melanocytic nevi. J Invest Dermatol 104:475–478
39. Fallowfield ME, Collina G, Cook MG (1994) Melanocytic lesions of the palm and sole. Histopathology 24(5):463–467
40. Clemente C, Zurrida S, Bartoli C, Bono A, Collini P, Rilke F (1995) Acral-lentiginous naevus of plantar skin. Histopathology 27:549–555
41. Boyd AS, Rapini RP (1994) Acral melanocytic neoplasms: a histologic analysis of 158 lesions. J Am Acad Dermatol 31(5):740–745
42. Harris GR, Shea CR, Horenstein MG, Reed JA, Burchette JL Jr, Prieto VG (1999) Desmoplastic (sclerotic) nevus: an underrecognized entity that resembles dermatofibroma and desmoplastic melanoma. Am J Surg Pathol 23(7):786–794
43. Spitz S (1948) Melanomas of childhood. Am J Pathol 24:591–609
44. Kamino H, Flotte TJ, Misheloff E, Greco MA, Ackerman AB (1979) Eosinophilic globules in Spitz's nevi. New findings and a diagnostic sign. Am J Dermatopathol 1:319–324
45. Handfield-Jones SE, Smith NP (1996) Malignant melanoma in childhood. Br J Dermatol 134:607–616
46. Walsh N, Crotty K, Palmer A, McCarthy S (1998) Spitz nevus versus spitzoid malignant melanoma: an evaluation of the current distinguishing histopathologic criteria. Hum Pathol 29(10):1105–1112
47. Barnhill RL, Argenyi ZB, From L et al (1999) Atypical Spitz nevi/tumors: lack of consensus for diagnosis, discrimination from melanoma, and prediction of outcome. Hum Pathol 30(5):513–520
48. Kerl H, Soyer HP, Cerroni L, Wolf IH, Ackerman AB (1998) Ancient melanocytic nevus. Semin Diagn Pathol 15(3):210–215
49. Zembowicz A, Carney JA, Mihm MC (2004) Pigmented epithelioid melanocytoma: a low-grade melanocytic tumor with metastatic potential indistinguishable from animal-type melanoma and epithelioid blue nevus. Am J Surg Pathol 28(1):31–40
50. McNutt NS, Urmacher C, Hakimian J, Hoss DM, Lugo J (1995) Nevoid malignant melanoma: morphologic patterns and immunohistochemical reactivity. J Cutan Pathol 22:502–517
51. Ruhoy SM, Prieto VG, Eliason SL, Grichnik JM, Burchette JL, Shea CR (2000) Malignant melanoma with paradoxical maturation. Am J Surg Pathol 24(12):1600–1614
52. Heenan PJ, Clay CD (1991) Epidermotropic metastatic melanoma simulating multiple primary melanomas. Am J Dermatopathol 13:396–402
53. Abernethy JL, Soyer HP, Kerl H, Jorizzo JL, White WL (1994) Epidermotropic metastatic malignant melanoma simulating melanoma in situ. A report of 10 examples from two patients. Am J Surg Pathol 18(11):1140–1149
54. Busam KJ (1999) Metastatic melanoma to the skin simulating blue nevus. Am J Surg Pathol 23:276–282
55. Elder DE, Guerry D, Epstein MN et al (1984) Invasive malignant melanomas lacking competence for metastasis. Am J Dermatopathol 6(Suppl):55–61
56. Cook MG, Clarke TJ, Humphreys S et al (1996) The evaluation of diagnostic and prognostic criteria and the terminology of thin cutaneous malignant melanoma by the CRC Melanoma Pathology Panel. Histopathology 28(6):497–512
57. Ackerman AB (1998) Melanoma in situ. Hum Pathol 29(11):1328–1329
58. Guitart J, Lowe L, Piepkorn M et al (2003) Metastasizing thin melanoma or multiple primary melanomas? Arch Dermatol 139(3):388–389

59. Ackerman AB (1985) Malignant melanoma in situ: the flat, curable stage of malignant melanoma. Pathology 17(2):298–300
60. Balch CM, Gershenwald JE, Soong SJ, Thompson JF (2011) Update on the melanoma staging system: the importance of sentinel node staging and primary tumor mitotic rate. J Surg Oncol 104(4):379–385
61. Balch CM, Gershenwald JE, Soong SJ et al (2009) Final version of 2009 AJCC melanoma staging and classification. J Clin Oncol 27(36):6199–6206
62. Barnhill RL, Fine JA, Roush GC, Berwick M (1996) Predicting five-year outcome for patients with cutaneous melanoma in a population-based study. Cancer 78(3):427–432
63. Petersson F, Diwan AH, Ivan D et al (2009) Immunohistochemical detection of lymphovascular invasion with D2-40 in melanoma correlates with sentinel lymph node status, metastasis and survival. J Cutan Pathol 36:1157–1163
64. Thomas JM, Newton-Bishop J, A'Hern R et al (2004) Excision margins in high-risk malignant melanoma. N Engl J Med 350(8):757–766
65. Morton DL, Wen DR, Wong JH et al (1992) Technical details of intraoperative lymphatic mapping for early stage melanoma. Arch Surg 127(4):392–399
66. Prieto VG, Clark SH (2002) Processing of sentinel lymph nodes for detection of metastatic melanoma. Ann Diagn Pathol 6(4):257–264
67. Trejo O, Reed JA, Prieto VG (2002) Atypical cells in human cutaneous re-excision scars for melanoma express p75NGFR, C56/N-CAM and GAP-43: evidence of early Schwann cell differentiation. J Cutan Pathol 29(7):397–406
68. Kucher C, Zhang PJ, Pasha T et al (2004) Expression of Melan-A and Ki-67 in desmoplastic melanoma and desmoplastic nevi. Am J Dermatopathol 26(6):452–457
69. Prieto VG, Lugo J, McNutt NS (1996) Intermediate- and low-molecular-weight keratin detection with the monoclonal antibody MNF116. An immunohistochemical study on 232 paraffin-embedded cutaneous lesions. J Cutan Pathol 23(3):234–241
70. White WL, Loggie BW (1999) Sentinel lymphadenectomy in the management of primary cutaneous malignant melanoma. Dermatol Clin 17:645–655
71. Prieto V (2001) Processing of sentinel lymph nodes (SLN) for detection of metastatic melanoma: proposal for an alternative method to serial sectioning. Lab Invest 81(1):66A
72. Prieto VG, Shea CR (2011) Immunohistochemistry of melanocytic proliferations. Arch Pathol Lab Med 135(7):853–859
73. Prieto VG, Shea CR (2008) Use of immunohistochemistry in melanocytic lesions. J Cutan Pathol 35(Suppl 2):1–10
74. Prieto VG, McNutt NS, Lugo J, Reed JA (1997) The intermediate filament peripherin is expressed in cutaneous melanocytic lesions. J Cutan Pathol 24(3):145–150
75. Reed JA, Finnerty B, Albino AP (1999) Divergent cellular differentiation pathways during the invasive stage of cutaneous malignant melanoma progression. Am J Pathol 155(2):549–555
76. Bacchi CE, Bonetti F, Pea M, Martignoni G, Gown AM (1996) HMB-45: a review. Appl Immunohistochem 4:73–85
77. Rudolph P, Schubert C, Schubert B, Parwaresch R (1997) Proliferation marker Ki-S5 as a diagnostic tool in melanocytic lesions. J Am Acad Dermatol 37(2 Pt 1):169–178
78. Henderson SA, Kapil J, Prieto VG (2014) Immunohistochemical expression of neurotized nevi. J Cutan Pathol 41(2):215
79. Fearon ER, Vogelstein B (1990) A genetic model for colorectal tumorigenesis. Cell 61:750–767
80. Farmer ER, Gonin R, Hanna MP (1996) Discordance in the histopathologic diagnosis of melanoma and melanocytic nevi between expert pathologists. Hum Pathol 27(6):528–531
81. Balaban G, Herlyn M, Guerry D et al (1984) Cytogenetics of human malignant melanoma and premalignant lesions. Cancer Genet Cytogenet 11(4):429–439
82. D'Alessandro I, Zitzelsberger H, Hutzler P et al (1997) Numerical aberrations of chromosome 7 detected in 15 microns paraffin-embedded tissue sections of primary cutaneous melanomas by fluorescence in situ hybridization and confocal laser scanning microscopy. J Cutan Pathol 24(2):70–75

83. Isshiki K, Elder DE, Guerry D, Linnenbach AJ (1993) Chromosome 10 allelic loss in malignant melanoma. Genes Chromosomes Cancer 8(3):178–184
84. Isshiki K, Seng BA, Elder DE, Guerry D, Linnenbach AJ (1994) Chromosome 9 deletion in sporadic and familial melanomas in vivo. Oncogene 9(6):1649–1653
85. Millikin D, Meese E, Vogelstein B, Witkowski C, Trent J (1991) Loss of heterozygosity for loci on the long arm of chromosome 6 in human malignant melanoma. Cancer Res 51(20):5449–5453
86. Thompson FH, Emerson J, Olson S et al (1995) Cytogenetics of 158 patients with regional or disseminated melanoma. Subset analysis of near-diploid and simple karyotypes. Cancer Genet Cytogenet 83(2):93–104
87. Wolfe KQ, Southern SA, Herrington CS (1997) Interphase cytogenetic demonstration of chromosome 9 loss in thick melanomas. J Cutan Pathol 24(7):398–402
88. Goldstein AM, Goldin LR, Dracopoli NC, Clark WH Jr, Tucker MA (1996) Two-locus linkage analysis of cutaneous malignant melanoma/dysplastic nevi. Am J Hum Genet 58(5):1050–1056
89. Liggett WHJ, Sidransky D (1998) Role of the p16 tumor suppressor gene in cancer. J Clin Oncol 16:1197–1206
90. Reed JA, Loganzo F Jr, Shea CR et al (1995) Loss of expression of the p16/cyclin-dependent kinase inhibitor 2 tumor suppressor gene in melanocytic lesions correlates with invasive stage of tumor progression. Cancer Res 55(13):2713–2718
91. Hashemi J, Linder S, Platz A, Hansson J (1999) Melanoma development in relation to nonfunctional p16/INK4A protein and dysplastic naevus syndrome in Swedish melanoma kindreds. Melanoma Res 9(1):21–30
92. Bastian BC (2004) Molecular genetics of melanocytic neoplasia: practical applications for diagnosis. Pathology 36(5):458–461
93. Fujita M, Norris DA, Yagi H et al (1999) Overexpression of mutant ras in human melanoma increases invasiveness, proliferation and anchorage-independent growth in vitro and induces tumour formation and cachexia in vivo. Melanoma Res 9(3):279–291
94. Jiveskog S, Ragnarsson-Olding B, Platz A, Ringborg U (1998) N-ras mutations are common in melanomas from sun-exposed skin of humans but rare in mucosal membranes or unexposed skin. J Invest Dermatol 111(5):757–761
95. Bales ES, Dietrich C, Bandyopadhyay D et al (1999) High levels of expression of p27(KIP1) and cyclin E in invasive primary malignant melanomas. J Invest Dermatol 113(6):1039–1046
96. Ekmekcioglu S, Ellerhorst J, Mhashilkar AM et al (2001) Down-regulated melanoma differentiation associated gene (mda-7) expression in human melanomas. Int J Cancer 94(1):54–59
97. Kraehn GM, Utikal J, Udart M et al (2001) Extra c-myc oncogene copies in high risk cutaneous malignant melanoma and melanoma metastases. Br J Cancer 84(1):72–79
98. Airola K, Karonen T, Vaalamo M et al (1999) Expression of collagenases-1 and -3 and their inhibitors TIMP-1 and -3 correlates with the level of invasion in malignant melanomas. Br J Cancer 80(5–6):733–743
99. Hsu MY, Shih DT, Meier FE et al (1998) Adenoviral gene transfer of beta3 integrin subunit induces conversion from radial to vertical growth phase in primary human melanoma. Am J Pathol 153(5):1435–1442
100. Singh RK, Varney ML, Bucana CD, Johansson SL (1999) Expression of interleukin-8 in primary and metastatic malignant melanoma of the skin. Melanoma Res 9(4):383–387
101. Erhard H, Rietveld FJ, van Altena MC, Brocker EB, Ruiter DJ, de Waal RM (1997) Transition of horizontal to vertical growth phase melanoma is accompanied by induction of vascular endothelial growth factor expression and angiogenesis. Melanoma Res 7(Suppl 2):S19–S26
102. Achen MG, Williams RA, Minekus MP et al (2001) Localization of vascular endothelial growth factor-D in malignant melanoma suggests a role in tumour angiogenesis. J Pathol 193(2):147–154
103. Straume O, Akslen LA (2001) Expression of vascular endothelial growth factor, its receptors (FLT-1, KDR) and TSP-1 related to microvessel density and patient outcome in vertical growth phase melanomas. Am J Pathol 159(1):223–235

104. Reed JA, McNutt NS, Albino AP (1994) Differential expression of basic fibroblast growth factor (bFGF) in melanocytic lesions demonstrated by in situ hybridization: implications for tumor progression. Am J Pathol 144(2):329–336

105. Shen SS, Zhang PS, Eton O, Prieto VG (2003) Analysis of protein tyrosine kinase expression in melanocytic lesions by tissue array. J Cutan Pathol 30(9):539–547

106. Dai DL, Martinka M, Li G (2005) Prognostic significance of activated Akt expression in melanoma: a clinicopathologic study of 292 cases. J Clin Oncol 23(7):1473–1482

107. Gupta SK, Douglas-Jones AG, Morgan JM (1997) Microdissection of stained archival tissue. J Clin Pathol 50:218–220

108. Uribe P, Wistuba II, Gonzalez S (2003) BRAF mutation: a frequent event in benign, atypical, and malignant melanocytic lesions of the skin. Am J Dermatopathol 25(5):365–370

109. Wiltshire RN, Duray P, Bittner ML et al (1995) Direct visualization of the clonal progression of primary cutaneous melanoma: application of tissue microdissection and comparative genomic hybridization. Cancer Res 55(18):3954–3957

110. Bastian BC, LeBoit PE, Hamm H, Brocker EB, Pinkel D (1998) Chromosomal gains and losses in primary cutaneous melanomas detected by comparative genomic hybridization. Cancer Res 58(10):2170–2175

111. Bastian BC, Olshen AB, LeBoit PE, Pinkel D (2003) Classifying melanocytic tumors based on DNA copy number changes. Am J Pathol 163(5):1765–1770

112. Curtin JA, Fridlyand J, Kageshita T et al (2005) Distinct sets of genetic alterations in melanoma. N Engl J Med 353(20):2135–2147

113. Gerami P, Mafee M, Lurtsbarapa T, Guitart J, Haghighat Z, Newman M (2010) Sensitivity of fluorescence in situ hybridization for melanoma diagnosis using RREB1, MYB, Cep6, and 11q13 probes in melanoma subtypes. Arch Dermatol 146(3):273–278

114. Morey AL, Murali R, McCarthy SW, Mann GJ, Scolyer RA (2009) Diagnosis of cutaneous melanocytic tumours by four-colour fluorescence in situ hybridisation. Pathology 41(4):383–387

115. Newman MD, Mirzabeigi M, Gerami P (2009) Chromosomal copy number changes supporting the classification of lentiginous junctional melanoma of the elderly as a subtype of melanoma. Mod Pathol 22(9):1258–1262

116. Vergier B, Prochazkova-Carlotti M, de la Fouchardiere A et al (2011) Fluorescence in situ hybridization, a diagnostic aid in ambiguous melanocytic tumors: European study of 113 cases. Mod Pathol 24(5):613–623

117. Isaac AK, Lertsburapa T, Pathria Mundi J, Martini M, Guitart J, Gerami P (2010) Polyploidy in spitz nevi: a not uncommon karyotypic abnormality identifiable by fluorescence in situ hybridization. Am J Dermatopathol 32(2):144–148

118. Gerami P, Jewell SS, Morrison LE et al (2009) Fluorescence in situ hybridization (FISH) as an ancillary diagnostic tool in the diagnosis of melanoma. Am J Surg Pathol 33(8):1146–1156

119. Gaiser T, Kutzner H, Palmedo G et al (2010) Classifying ambiguous melanocytic lesions with FISH and correlation with clinical long-term follow up. Mod Pathol 23(3):413–419

120. Tetzlaff MT, Wang WL, Milless TL et al (2013) Ambiguous melanocytic tumors in a tertiary referral center: the contribution of fluorescence in situ hybridization (FISH) to conventional histopathologic and immunophenotypic analyses. Am J Surg Pathol 37(12):1783–1796

121. Gerami P, Cooper C, Bajaj S et al (2013) Outcomes of atypical spitz tumors with chromosomal copy number aberrations and conventional melanomas in children. Am J Surg Pathol 37(9):1387–1394

122. Pouryazdanparast P, Brenner A, Haghighat Z, Guitart J, Rademaker A, Gerami P (2012) The role of 8q24 copy number gains and c-MYC expression in amelanotic cutaneous melanoma. Mod Pathol 25(9):1221–1226

123. Lazova R, Seeley EH, Keenan M, Gueorguieva R, Caprioli RM (2012) Imaging mass spectrometry—a new and promising method to differentiate Spitz nevi from Spitzoid malignant melanomas. Am J Dermatopathol 34(1):82–90

Part III
Genetics of Melanoma

Chapter 5
Inherited Gene Mutations in Melanoma

Lana N. Pho, Marjan Champine, Sancy A. Leachman, and Wendy Kohlmann

Abstract The future of melanoma prevention and early diagnosis lies in personalized medicine. Patient-tailored management should target processes of initiation, uncontrolled proliferation, and invasion of melanocytes to abort progressive and incurable disease. Our growing knowledge of the somatic mutations in melanogenesis and the hereditary melanoma susceptibility genes is enabling clinicians to manipulate the neoplastic genotypes and develop effective treatments and raise the potential for a cure. Genomic analyses using high-throughput sequencing and comparative genomic hybridization have been instrumental in identifying these key molecules in melanomagenic pathways.

We subcategorize various aspects of the genetics of melanoma into the following updated review: inherited syndromes predisposing to melanoma risk, molecular mechanisms in melanogenesis and metastasis, new tumor-targeted drug therapies, and clinical prevention/management guidelines for high-risk patients. Genetic counseling is an integral service owing to the surmounting evidence for the hereditary nature and genetic pathogenesis of melanoma. Genetic consulting addresses and provides patient education on genetic principles, genetic testing availability, and interpretation of melanoma susceptibility testing. In concert, geneticists, oncologists, and clinicians offer personalized prevention, early detection, and treatment algorithms based on the patient's genetic and environmental influences and to select antitumor therapies aimed at neoplastic genotypic traits with sustainable treatment success.

Keywords Melanoma • *CDKN2A* • *CDK4* • *MC1R* • High risk • Genetics • Genetic counseling • Genetic testing • Somatic mutation • Germline mutation • Inherited syndromes • Cancer prevention • Mitogen-activated protein kinase • Phosphoinositide 3-kinase • Medical management • Risk stratification • *BRAF*

L.N. Pho (✉) • M. Champine • W. Kohlmann
University of Utah Health Sciences, Salt Lake City, UT, USA
e-mail: Lana.Pho@hsc.utah.edu; Wendy.Kohlmann@hci.utah.edu

S.A. Leachman (✉)
Oregon Health and Science University, Portland, OR, USA
e-mail: leachmas@ohsu.edu

© Springer Science+Business Media New York 2016   117
C.A. Torres-Cabala, J.L. Curry (eds.), *Genetics of Melanoma*, Cancer Genetics,
DOI 10.1007/978-1-4939-3554-3_5

5.1 Introduction

Melanoma is an aggressive type of skin cancer, especially when diagnosed in advanced or metastatic stages. Based on US Surveillance, Epidemiology, and End Results (SEER) rates from 2007 to 2009, the lifetime risk of developing melanoma is 1 in 50 in the United States. In the United States, the incidence rate of melanoma in men is 27.2 per 100,000 compared to 16.7 per 100,000 in women. According to recent SEER data, the 5-year relative survival rate significantly drops when melanoma is diagnosed beyond a localized stage (62.4 % for regional stage and 15.1 % for metastatic disease). Compounding the mortality statistics, SEER data reported that the overall incidence of melanoma increased by 2.6 % per year between 1985 and 2009. Deliberate sun-seeking behaviors and ultraviolet (UV) radiation exposure from increasing use of indoor tanning facilities account in part for the observed upward trend [1–3]. Promotion of sun protective behaviors and education on timely screening with full-body dermatologic examinations are essential to the melanoma prevention campaign and early detection for curative treatment. In addition, optimal practice would synthesize the findings on physical exam (i.e., an individual's phenotypic traits—skin pigmentation, hair color, eye color, and nevi count) with an individual's personal and family histories (including previous nonmelanoma and melanoma skin cancers as well as genetic syndromes associated with melanoma predisposition) in order to provide a personalized risk assessment. When patients present with a melanoma diagnosis, the clinical focus is also on the tumor genotype for selection of a medical treatment that targets the tumor's biological activity.

The basis of melanoma development stems from germline and somatic genetic profiles of both the affected individual and his/her melanoma tumor. Melanoma predisposition genes that increase one's susceptibility and the accumulation of several somatic mutational events in the cell cycle of melanocytes underlie tumorigenesis. Extensive studies of somatic genetic aberrations revealed that the critical steps in melanomagenesis are disruptions in extracellular tyrosine kinase receptor function and dysregulation in intracellular signaling mechanisms in cell-cycle control. Melanoma is a disease with genetic heterogeneity and involves several notable intracellular signaling pathways including the mitogen-activated protein kinase (MAPK) pathway, the phosphoinositide 3-kinase (PI3K) signaling pathway, the retinoblastoma (Rb) pathway, and the p53 pathway. Numerous studies to date demonstrate melanoma tumor formation involving these individual or collective pathways that normally regulate cell growth and timely apoptosis [4–6].

Twin studies estimate that 30–55 % of melanoma risk variability lies within hereditary genetic defects, and strong melanoma-prone kindreds represent about 10 % of melanoma cases. These genetic syndromes associated with melanoma predisposition involve highly penetrant germline mutant genes, while lesser penetrant genes encode for pigmentary or phenotypic melanoma traits (e.g., skin pigmentation, hair color, eye color, and nevus count). In other words, multiple genetic factors may interact in determining an individual's risk for melanoma. Similar to the somatic genetic mutations involved in melanogenesis, the high-risk germline mutations are involved in regulating cell-cycle survival and apoptosis [7–12].

Investigation into other genomic pathways in sporadic and inherited melanoma will define other putative genetic molecular signatures ripe for engineering future-targeted therapy. Formerly, clinicopathologic characteristics of melanoma were used when evaluating patients for clinical trials with traditional chemotherapies and immunotherapies. Today, tumor genotyping capitalizes on known molecular pathways implicated in melanoma progression to aid in the development of better targeted therapies for patients with melanoma.

5.2 Somatic Genetic Alterations and Signaling Pathways in Melanoma

Metastatic melanomas are notoriously difficult to treat in advanced stages. Recent progress in the identification of several melanoma oncogenes and tumor suppressor genes has led to development of targeted molecular treatments for metastatic melanoma. Cellular signaling mechanisms are key regulators in the transformation of benign melanocytes to uncontrolled malignant proliferation, carcinogenesis, and invasion. These aberrations occur at the extracellular induction of the tyrosine kinase receptor or in the intracellular network of signaling cascades that promote cancerous growth and anomalous apoptosis. Table 5.1 lists the current promising drugs and their intended targeted pathways in melanogenesis. These pathways may individually or collectively participate in altered cellular growth and survival in melanoma.

BRAF is the activated mammalian homologue of the rapidly accelerated fibrosarcoma (*RAF*) serine–threonine protein kinase family. Other RAF isoforms are *ARAF* and *CRAF*, but currently they are not associated with known mutations in melanoma tumorigenesis. *BRAF* oncogenic mutations are observed in about 50–70 % of melanoma cell lines and human cutaneous melanomas [14, 38–42]. This makes *BRAF* the most commonly defined somatic mutation in melanogenesis. *BRAF*-V600E substitution accounts for 90 % of all *BRAF* mutations [43, 44]. Additionally, somatic *BRAF* mutations occur with high frequency, 82 %, in benign and atypical melanocytic nevi [14, 41, 45, 46]. It is postulated that melanocytic nevi with a *BRAF* mutation evolve into carcinoma when a second mutation occurs in an oncogene or tumor suppressor gene. Thus, *BRAF* mutations play a critical role in tumorigenesis and possibly the progression from benign nevi to melanoma [47].

In the RAS–RAF–MEK–MAPK (also known as the MAPK or mitogen-activated protein kinase) pathway, activating mutant *BRAF* directs downstream mitogen-activated extracellular signal-regulated kinase (MEK) signaling to promote cell growth and survival [15]. The RAF protein normally downregulates cyclin D, which halts cell-cycle progression. Mutations within *RAF* will constitutively upregulate cyclin D and therefore promote oncogenesis.

The RAF inhibitors, vemurafenib, dabrafenib, and trametinib exert antitumor effects on mutant BRAF (*BRAF*-V600E) human melanoma tumors by inhibiting the MAPK pathway and its associated signaling cascade involved in abnormal cellular

Table 5.1 Somatic mutations in melanogenesis and targeted treatment

Gene	Clinical associations	Mutation	Mutation frequency	Pathway	Targeted therapeutic drug(s)	Possible indication
BRAF	Non-chronic sun-damaged skin [13]	Val600Glu *BRAF* mutant (account for 90 % of all BRAF-mutated melanoma tumors) [13–16]	~50–75 % [17, 18]	Activates mitogen-activated protein kinase (MAPK) pathway	Vemurafenib, dabrafenib, and trametinib [19, 20]	Metastatic melanoma
NRAS	Non-chronic sun-damaged skin [13]	Codon 61 (exon 2) or codons 12 or 13 (exon 1) [21, 22]	15–30 % [13, 23–25]	Activates RAF kinase and PI3K (phosphoinositide 3 kinase) pathway	Tipifarnib, phase II trial completed [26]	Metastatic melanoma
PTEN	Late-stage melanoma?	Various genetic alterations on chromosome 10q	<5–20 % [27–30]	AKT inhibitor in PI3K pathway	Perifosine, phase II trial completed [31]	Metastatic or recurrent melanoma
c-KIT	Chronic sun-damaged skin and mucosal and acral melanomas [5]	Exon 11, Leu576Pro (most common) but also exons 9, 11, 13, 17, 18 in *c-KIT* [32, 33] or amplification of *c-Kit* gene [32]	<1 % [34]	Activates KIT transmembrane receptor tyrosine kinase	Imatinib, nilotinib, and dasatinib [35–37]	Metastatic melanoma

division and propagation. Vemurafenib is FDA approved for patients with unresectable or metastatic melanoma and who have a proven *BRAF*-V600E mutation. In a multicenter phase II trial involving 132 patients, vemurafenib was associated with a response rate (as scored by the standardized response evaluation criteria in solid tumors or RECIST) of 53 % (44–62 %, 95 % confidence interval, CI). Eight patients (6 %) experienced complete remission (defined as disappearance of tumor for at least 1 month) and 47 % showed a partial response (defined as demonstrating ≥30 % of tumor regression). The response was observed early (at first radiologic assessment at 6 weeks) [48]. Similarly, in a multicenter phase III trial that enrolled a total of 250 eligible patients, 47 % of patients on dabrafenib showed a partial response and 3 % demonstrated complete remission. Recently, dabrafenib in combination with trametinib appears to be more effective than monotherapy and display similar side effect profiles. All of these patients had melanoma tumors expressing *BRAF*-V600E mutations and had advanced disease despite prior treatment with traditional IL-2 immunotherapy [19].

NRAS is the human oncogene of the RAS (rat sarcoma) family and activates the MAPK signaling pathway. *RAS* directly stimulates intracellular *RAF* kinases. RAS is a family of GTP-binding proteins with several isoforms (HRAS, KRAS, and NRAS) and is found on the inner surface of the cell membrane. Thus, *RAS* serves as the intermediary in the transduction of intracellular signaling triggered from extracellular growth factors. *NRAS* mutations are not as frequent as *BRAF* mutations (present in 15–25 % of human cutaneous melanomas and cell lines) [44, 49, 50]. On the other hand, *NRAS* mutations are present in 30 % of amelanotic nodular melanomas, which is similar to the frequency of *BRAF* mutations [51]. Unlike the high frequency of *BRAF* mutations seen in atypical nevi as noted above, *NRAS* mutations are observed in 56 % of congenital nevi compared to dysplastic nevi, suggesting that *NRAS* may be a genetic risk factor for malignant melanoma formation in this type of nevi [23, 52, 53].

To date, *NRAS* and *BRAF* mutations are mutually exclusive and are rarely seen concomitantly in sporadic primary melanoma tumors [13, 21, 22, 49, 54]. The finding that both affect the MAPK pathway suggests that mutations in either *NRAS* or *BRAF* may obliterate cell survival or represent an evolutionary functional redundancy.

CDKN2A protein participates in the pathway, *p53*, involved in cell-cycle control. In 25 affected members from six unrelated Swedish kindreds with established *CDKN2A* germline mutations, 95 % of primary melanomas and metastatic melanomas demonstrated somatic *NRAS* mutations compared to 10 % of sporadic melanomas [55]. The specific activating mutation in codon 61 of *NRAS* exhibited UV-inducible mutations and was also detected in melanoma in situ and dysplastic nevi from these affected individuals with *CDKN2A* germline mutations. This study reveals the complex interaction of germline hereditary *CDKN2A* mutation and somatic activating *RAS* mutation influenced by environmental UV radiation and proposes a mechanism for both hereditary and somatic genetic mutations as causative in melanogenesis.

An NRAS antitumor drug known as R115777, or tipifarnib, may have potential in aborting the signal transduction in melanoma tumors. In RAS-based signaling, farnesylation is crucial in the posttranslational modification of *RAS* for localization to membrane compartments to activate cellular transcription. Tipifarnib was used in a phase II clinical trial as an inhibitor of farnesylation and demonstrated no clinical improvement in a cohort of melanoma patients. However, tipifarnib inhibited 85–95 % farnesyltransferase activity in tumor tissue [26]. The lack of a significant clinical tumor response suggests that a more complete blockage of other signaling pathways is required or an alternative, salvage mechanism exists. Other pitfalls include dose-limiting toxicities and thus, potential subtherapeutic dosage. Nevertheless, there may still be a role for tipifarnib in the melanoma treatment algorithm as an adjuvant agent, since selective inhibition of farnesyltransferase activity can potentially target *RAS* mutant activating specific melanoma tumor genotype.

NRAS activates another distinct mechanism in melanogenesis in addition to the MAPK pathway. The RAS family members can activate the lipid kinase phosphatidylinositol 3′-kinsase (PI3K) pathway. Upon mutant activation, PI3K phosphorylates and signals downstream serine–threonine kinase (AKT) molecule function, which is involved in proliferation, survival, invasion, and angiogenesis [56, 57]. A specific isoform distinctive in melanoma, *AKT3*, demonstrated overexpression in 63 sporadic human melanomas and resulted in loss of AKT3-dependent cellular apoptosis [57]. *AKT* is oncogenic in that elevated protein levels of AKT3 correlated adversely with patient survival and was detected in >60 % of melanomas from patients with advanced disease [56, 57].

Unlike *RAS* and *RAF* mutations, *AKT* somatic mutations are rare and seen in only 3 % of cutaneous melanomas [34, 58, 59]. However, somatic mutations in the *PTEN* tumor suppressor gene have been demonstrated in melanoma tumors. *PTEN* encodes for a lipid and protein phosphatase and negatively regulates growth factors that can activate *AKT3*. Mutations in the *PTEN* gene lead to aberrant AKT3 oncogenic stimulation by uninhibited growth factors and drive carcinogenesis. *PTEN* mutations are reported in <5–20 % of primary and metastatic melanomas [27–30] and in 30–60 % of melanoma cell lines [27–29, 60]. No cases of mutations were observed in 28 melanoma samples from affected patients belonging to melanoma-prone families (i.e., multiple cases of melanoma) [28]. The low *PTEN* mutation frequency observed in uncultured melanomas compared to the high frequency of *RAS*- and *RAF*-activating mutations suggests that *PTEN* mutation may be rare and/or a late event in melanogenesis [27, 61]. *PTEN* somatic mutations have been observed in concert with *BRAF*-activating mutations (in the MAPK pathway), but not *NRAS*, consistent with redundant abrogation of the PI3K pathway [6, 28, 62]. A phase II study of perifosine, an alkylphosphocholine analogue, in 18 patients with melanoma found that the agent was associated with stable disease in 21 % of patients but progression of disease in 61 % [31]. Current utility of *PTEN*-activating mutation inhibitors remains uncertain in the armamentarium of targeted therapy for melanoma.

The extracellular signaling protein proposed as a potential therapeutic target in melanoma is the *c-Kit* receptor tyrosine kinase membrane receptor (also known as *KIT*). Extracellular KIT ligand induction of c-KIT receptor protein leads to a signaling cascade within both the MAPK and PI3K pathways. In patients with melanoma tumors harboring an activating mutation or amplification of *c-KIT* gene, KIT inhibition drugs such as imatinib mesylate (a tyrosine kinase inhibitor), nilotinib, and dasatinib have shown significant clinical response in early clinical trials [35–37]. The loss of KIT protein expression is observed in the sequential progression from benign melanocyte to metastatic melanoma. Mutated *c-KIT* is reported in 39 % of mucosal melanomas, 36 % of acral melanomas, and 28 % of chronically sun-damaged skin but has not been demonstrated in melanomas arising from anatomic sites without sun damage [5]. For comparison, *BRAF* mutations at these same anatomic sites were less frequent and reported in 3 % of mucosal melanomas, 21 % of acral melanomas, and 6 % of chronically sun-damaged skin. On the other hand, *BRAF* mutations were seen in 56 % of non-chronically damaged skin. This suggests that patients with *c-KIT* mutations or melanoma tumor with these clinical characteristics (i.e., mucosal, acral, and/or sun-damaged body surfaces) may be more responsive to targeted therapy using imatinib. In a phase II clinical trial, one patient with metastatic acral melanoma on imatinib mesylate achieved near complete response sustained beyond 1 year [63]. Other similar cases have been reported in the literature [64, 65]. In a larger phase II clinical trial, patients with metastatic melanoma and either a *c-KIT* mutation or amplification were treated with imatinib mesylate. Of the 43 patients enrolled in the clinical trial, 41.9 % demonstrated tumor regression. Twenty-three percent (10.2–36.4 %, 95 % CI) showed partial response and 30.2 % (16–44.4 %, 95 % CI) showed stable disease [35]. Other similar studies support melanoma harboring *c-KIT* mutations are sensitive to KIT inhibitors [66, 67].

5.3   Germline Mutations in Melanoma Predisposition Genes

While the majority, or 90 %, of melanomas develop sporadically during one's lifetime, 10 % are due to an inherited genetic proclivity [68, 69]. Any familial clustering of melanoma is a strong predictor of personal melanoma risk. In a meta-analysis, an individual's risk is increased 2.24-fold based on having one first-degree relative affected with melanoma [70, 71]. This increased risk likely comes from shared genetic variants that encode for fair skin, blond or red hair, and blue eyes which will be discussed in the next section [71–73]. These pigmentary traits are considered less penetrant, and the relative risk is elevated up to fivefold compared to those with darker skin types and hair color. Rare families with multiple cases of melanoma may have mutations in high-penetrance susceptibility genes. Individuals who inherit mutations in one of two known high-penetrance melanoma predisposition genes (*CDKN2A* and *CDK4*) have a 30- to 70-fold lifetime risk of developing melanoma or 50–80 % risk of developing melanoma by age 80 years old [74–76].

The chances of harboring a germline mutation in *CDKN2A* increases from 1 % in sporadic melanomas to 30–40 % when more than three cases of melanoma is identified in a melanoma-prone kindred [77].

The highly penetrant genes are cyclin-dependent kinase 4 (*CDK4*) located on human chromosome 12q14 and cyclin-dependent kinase inhibitor 2A (*CDKN2A*) located on human chromosome 9p21 [78–80]. Kamb and colleagues as well as Nobori and colleagues found homozygous *CDKN2A* deletions in 60–75 % of somatic primary melanoma tumors [80, 81]. The disease-related *CDKN2A* germline mutations were soon after identified in families whose affected members showed linkage to 9p21 [80–83]. These studies collectively support *CDKN2A* genetic alterations and can participate in both germline and somatic melanoma carcinogenesis.

CDKN2A encodes for two tumor suppressor proteins, p16 (also known as INK4A or p16[INK4A]) and ARF (also known as p14[ARF] or p14). The protein product p16 is transcribed from exons 1α, 2α, and 3α. ARF protein product is transcribed from the alternate reading frame of exons 1β, 2β, and 3β in *CDKN2A*. Mutations affecting either the p16 or ARF or both proteins have been associated with melanoma susceptibility. Mutations in *CDKN2A* account for approximately 20–40 % of families with a hereditary pattern of melanoma. Germline mutations in exon 1β, which only affect the ARF protein, account for only 1–2 % of high-risk families [84–87]. See Table 5.2, which summarizes the hereditary melanoma syndromes.

CDKN2A is a critical regulatory gene in the cell cycle involving the retinoblastoma (Rb) pathway. Normally, p16 activates a tumor suppressor gene, retinoblastoma (*Rb*), by direct protein binding and negative regulation of Cdk4/6 [11, 81, 104]. This halts cell-cycle progression from G_1 to S phase and arrests cellular proliferation. If there are deletions, mutations, or silencing of *CDKN2A*, there is upregulation of Cdk4, which has been observed in both sporadic and familial melanomas, and reentry into the cell cycle [81, 105, 106].

The alternative reading frame encoding ARF protein product controls another pathway, p53, in the cell cycle. The p53 protein is a transcription factor that targets downstream functional genes involved in accelerated DNA repair, inhibition of cell-cycle progression, and cellular apoptosis. In the skin, UV radiation is the most damaging external cellular stressor that activates *p53*. ARF protein product inhibits MDM2 (a ubiquitin–protein ligase) and prevents p53 proteasomal degradation. Genetic aberrations in *ARF* release inhibition on MDM2, thereby allowing MDM2 to tightly bind to *p53*. MDM2 targets *p53* for ubiquitin-mediated proteasomal degradation and, therefore, blocks *p53* transcriptional activity. When exposed to UV, vulnerable melanocytes with *ARF* mutations undergo unrepaired DNA propagation, escape from apoptosis, and cellular survival which lead to carcinogenesis [8, 9, 12]. *ARF* germline mutations are rare in melanoma-prone kindreds, and similarly somatic homozygous or heterozygous *p53* gene mutations are rare in human melanoma (<1–25 %) [4, 107–113]. However, in patients with xeroderma pigmentosa, type C (XPC), who have defective DNA repair, the frequency of somatic *p53* mutations in melanoma tumors is as high as 60 % [114]. The majority of melanomas were of the subtype lentigo maligna melanoma (LMM) and clinically similar to LMM located on chronic sun-exposed body surface areas observed in the elderly population. This suggests that a common pathway of melanogenesis may exist for LMM development in individuals with XPC and the general population that develop LMM on sun-exposed anatomical sites [114].

CDK4 encodes for a kinase also involved in the Rb pathway. As explained above, *p16* normally targets Cdk4 kinase in order to activate tumor suppression. The inability of Cdk4 kinase to bind to *p16* due to mutations in *CDK4* leads to oncogenic stimulation and cell-cycle progression [7, 115–117]. Only 1–2 % of high-risk melanoma families carry *CDK4* deleterious mutations [7, 88, 116–119].

Table 5.2 Genodermatoses associated with melanoma susceptibility and cancer surveillance

Name	OMIM	Mode of inheritance	Gene	Gene function	Lifetime melanoma risk	Surveillance
Familial atypical multiple mole melanoma syndrome (FAMMM)	155601	Autosomal dominant	CDKN2A [78]	Cyclin-dependent kinase inhibitor of CDK4 protein	60–90 % [76, 88, 89]	Full-body skin exam every 6–12 months starting at age 10. Baseline whole-body photography every 6–12 months beginning at age 10. Monthly self-skin exams beginning in childhood. Photoprotection with sunblock, protective clothing, and limit UV exposure [74, 90–92]
Melanoma-prone familial syndromes	600160	Autosomal dominant	p16INK4A (INK4A on CDKN2A locus)	Cyclin-dependent kinase inhibitor of CDK4 protein	50–80 % (which varies by geography) [75, 88]	Full-body skin exam every 6–12 months starting at age 10. Baseline whole-body photography every 6–12 months beginning at age 10. Monthly self-skin exams beginning in childhood. Photoprotection with sunblock, protective clothing, and limit UV exposure [74, 90–92]
	600160	Autosomal dominant	p14ARF (ARF on CDKN2A locus)	Protein stabilizer of p53	50–80 % [75, 88]	Full-body skin exam every 6–12 months starting at age 10. Baseline whole-body photography every 6–12 months beginning at age 10. Monthly self-skin exams beginning in childhood. Photoprotection with sunblock, protective clothing, and limit UV exposure [74, 90–92]
	123829	Autosomal dominant	CDK4	Protein kinase target of p16	50–80 % [75, 88]	Full-body skin exam every 6–12 months starting at age 10. Baseline whole-body photography every 6–12 months beginning at age 10. Monthly self-skin exams beginning in childhood. Photoprotection with sunblock, protective clothing, and limit UV exposure [74, 90–92]

(continued)

Table 5.2 (continued)

Name	OMIM	Mode of inheritance	Gene	Gene function	Lifetime melanoma risk	Surveillance
	608035	Autosomal dominant	1p22 locus [93]	Unknown, possible tumor suppressor [94]	Undefined	Not yet defined
	155600	Autosomal dominant	1p36	Unknown, possible tumor suppressor [95, 96]	Undefined	Not yet defined
	613099	Autosomal dominant	16q24.3	Unknown [97]	Undefined	Not yet defined
Melanoma-pancreatic cancer syndrome	606719	Autosomal dominant	CDKN2A [88]	Cyclin-dependent kinase inhibitor of CDK4 protein	60–90 % [76, 88, 89]	Full-body skin exam every 6–12 months starting at age 10. Baseline whole-body photography every 6–12 months beginning at age 10. Monthly self-skin exams beginning in childhood. Photoprotection with sunblock, protective clothing, and limit UV exposure [74, 90–92]
Melanoma-astrocytoma syndrome	155755	Autosomal dominant	CDKN2A gene [86]	Cyclin-dependent kinase inhibitor of CDK4 protein	Undefined	Full-body skin exam every 6–12 months. Monthly self-skin exams. Photoprotection with sunblock, protective clothing, and limit UV exposure. MRI advised if neurologic symptoms present [74]
Uveal melanoma syndrome	603089	Autosomal dominant	BAP1 gene [98, 99]	Ubiquitin carboxy-terminal hydrolase	Undefined	Full-body skin exam every 6–12 months. Monthly self-skin exams. Photoprotection with sunblock, protective clothing, and limit UV exposure. Baseline and periodic ophthalmologic exam [74]

Xeroderma pigmentosa	278700 (XP-A), 133510 (XP-B), 278720 (XP-C), 278730 (XP-D), 278740 (XP-E), 29882 (XP-F), 278780 (XP-G), 278750 (XP-V)	Autosomal recessive	XPA, XPB, XPC, XPD, DDB2, ERCC4, RAD2, POLH	DNA repair	2000-fold	Full-body skin exam every 3–12 months. Monthly self-skin exams. Absolute photoprotection with sunblock, protective clothing, and avoid UV exposure. Avoid tobacco use. Periodic ophthalmologic exam, neurologic exam, and audiograms [74]
Oculocutaneous albinism type 2	203200	Autosomal recessive	OCA2	Tyrosinase transport	Odds ratio 1.31	Full-body skin exam every 6–12 months. Monthly self-skin exams. Absolute photoprotection with sunblock, protective clothing, and avoid UV exposure Annual ophthalmologic exam [74]
Hereditary retinoblastoma	180200	Autosomal dominant	RB1	Functions in proliferation, DNA replication, DNA repair, cell-cycle checkpoint control	Up to 80-fold [100–102]	Full-body skin exam every 6–12 months. Monthly self-skin exams. Absolute photoprotection with sunblock, protective clothing, and avoid UV exposure Every 1–2 months ophthalmologic exam for first year of life, followed by every 2–3 months for next year, then every 3 months until 3 years of age, and every 4–6 months until 6 years [74, 103]

5.4 Clinical Features of Melanoma-Associated Genodermatoses

The most well-characterized melanoma predisposition genes are *CDKN2A* (OMIM#600160) and *CDK4* (OMIM#123829) as previously described, but other discovered genetic loci lend support to the genetic heterogeneity of melanoma susceptibility. Cutaneous malignant melanoma with features of multiple dysplastic nevi has been called hereditary dysplastic nevus syndrome or familial multiple mole and melanoma syndrome (FAMMM, OMIM#155600) [120, 121]. The first family described showed an autosomal dominant inheritance of 10–100 dysplastic nevi (size ranging from 5 to 15 mm) and early-onset melanoma occurrences [121, 122]. About 25–40 % (60–75 % do not have a known *CDKN2A* mutation) of families harbor a *CDKN2A* mutation with a gene penetrance as high as 60–90 % [76, 88]. Affected individuals develop melanoma ranging from 20 to 45 years old and sometimes can develop multiple primary melanomas [88, 120]. Multiple dysplastic nevi develop by late childhood or at onset of puberty [123, 124]. While some *CDKN2A* mutation carrying families exhibit sufficient clinically atypical or dysplastic nevi to meet the clinical diagnostic criteria of FAMMM, it is likely that nevus development is regulated by separate loci as several studies have found that nevus phenotype is an unreliable predictor of carrying a *CDKN2A* mutation [68, 125, 126]. Linkage studies have demonstrated potential nevi predisposition loci on 1p36 (OMIM#155600), locus 1p22 (OMIM#608035), and locus 16q24.3 (OMIM#613099).

Lynch et al. described eight families with *CDKN2A* mutations who had melanoma and pancreatic cancers but also with the atypical multiple mole phenotype (≥50 dysplastic nevi). Families with the melanoma-pancreatic cancer syndrome (also known as familial atypical multiple mole melanoma-*pancreatic* carcinoma syndrome, or FAMMM-P, OMIM#606719) are characterized by familial clustering of melanoma and pancreatic cancers. Approximately 25 % of families with *CDNK2A* mutations include a relative with pancreatic cancer, and mutations in the gene have been associated with a 13- to 22-fold, or 17 % lifetime, pancreas cancer risk [127, 128]. Studies have found that the presence of pancreatic cancer in families with multiple cases of melanoma significantly increases the likelihood of the cancer risk in the family being attributed to a *CDKN2A* mutation [88, 127, 129]. However, outside of populations which carry the *p16-Leiden* founder mutation, most studies have found that familial pancreatic cancer in the absence of melanoma to rarely be associated with *CDKN2A* mutations [128, 130, 131]. Schutte et al. showed somatic inactivation of the Rb/p16 tumor suppressor pathway in nearly 100 % of sporadic pancreatic carcinomas which suggests that *CDKN2A* gene appears to be a mutual regulator in carcinogenesis of pancreatic cancer and malignant melanoma [10]. As in sporadic pancreatic cancer, cigarette smoking is an important risk modifier [132]. Cigarette smoking is associated with earlier onset of pancreatic cancer by 10 years in pancreatic-prone families [133]. Pancreatic cancer screening is not included in the recommendations for any of the conditions associated with CDKN2A mutation carriers [134]. At this time the optimal patient approach of pancreatic cancer screening remains uncertain. But some studies have proposed endoscopic ultrasound, high-resolution pancreatic protocol CT, endoscopic retrograde cholangiopancreatography, or MRI to assess for pancreatic mass starting at age 50 or 10 years younger than the earliest family member with pancreatic cancer (with no clinically reliable sensitive test available) [134–137].

The melanoma-astrocytoma syndrome (OMIM#155755) is characterized by two highly increased cancer risks. Studies to date have described rare families with melanoma and the more common nervous system malignancy, astrocytoma, as well as other nervous system tumors including medulloblastoma, glioblastoma multiforme, ependymoma, glioma, meningioma, and acoustic neurilemmoma [86, 138]. The original kindreds described by Kaufman et al. and Bahuau et al. showed linkage to 9p21.3 and affected members demonstrated deletions within 9p locus [139–141]. Randerson-Moor et al. described a large family with a germline deletion of exon 1β specific to $p14^{ARF}$ gene [86]. Tachibana et al. identified a heterozygous germline deletion in $p16$ gene [142]. Therefore, some families exhibiting a clustering of melanoma and nervous system tumors have been attributed to *CDKN2A* mutations, but large studies of *CDKN2A* mutation carrier have not demonstrated a significantly increased risk for brain tumor in mutation carriers [88].

Uveal melanoma syndrome (OMIM#155720) is an autosomal dominantly inherited condition that predisposes to ocular melanoma [98, 143]. Recently, a truncating genetic defect in *BAP1* segregated a three-generational kindred of family members affected with uveal melanoma, cutaneous melanoma, and numerous atypical nevi [144, 145]. Possible genetic heterogeneity exists for this syndrome as three unrelated large Danish families with cutaneous melanoma and uveal melanoma phenotypes demonstrated linkage to 9p21 but no identifiable candidate gene [146]. Harbour et al. showed that somatic *BAP1* mutations were present in about 50 % of uveal melanoma tumors and >84 % in metastatic uveal disease [144]. The function of *BPA1* is not well defined but thought to be a tumor suppressor in the cell cycle [147]. Current studies identify *BPA1* as a functional ubiquitin carboxy-terminal hydrolase important in regulating proliferation [147, 148].

Xeroderma pigmentosa (XP) (OMIM#278700, 610651, 278720, 278730, 278740, 278760, 278780, 278750) is a rare heritable disorder characterized by photosensitivity and increased risk of early-onset melanoma and nonmelanoma skin cancers. XP is inherited in an autosomal recessive manner and is genetically and clinically heterogenous. There are several complementation groups of XP (XP-A, XP-B, XP-C, XP-D, XP-E, XP-F, XP-G, and XP-V) which involve several genes and the most common subtype is XP-A [149]. Fibroblasts from an affected individual can be cultured to identify the specific subtype and defective DNA repair gene. Individuals with XP have a genetic defect that prevents a cell's ability to repair UV-induced DNA photoproducts. Thus, about 60 % of XP report a history of severe blistering sunburn from minimal UV exposure. Other clinical phenotypes include high density of freckles and poikilodermatous changes (hypopigmentation, hyperpigmentation, lentigines, skin atrophy, telangiectasias, and freckles) on a sun-exposed skin. Melanoma risk in these affected individuals are 1000- to 2000-fold increased compared to the general population risk and have a younger median age of onset at 22 years old [150]. Ocular melanoma has also been reported in these affected individuals [151, 152].

The oculocutaneous albinism type 2 gene (OCA2, also known as the *P* gene) (OMIM#203200) functions in transporting copper-containing enzyme, tyrosinase, into melanosomes for melanin production. *OCA2* is reportedly responsible for 50 % of pigmentation in the eyes in the general population [97, 153, 154]. Hereditary OCA2 is an autosomal recessive disorder whereby mutations in *OCA2* results in failure to synthesize melanin which leads to light skin color, yellow hair, and blue-gray irides and an increased risk for UV-induced melanoma [155–157]. The odds ratio of developing melanoma is reported to be 1.31 in these individuals [158].

Hereditary retinoblastoma (OMIM#180200) is an autosomal dominant syndrome characterized by a predominately 90 % risk for unilateral or bilateral retinoblastoma which occurs within the first 3 years of age. However, these individuals, by virtue of an inactivated copy of the *Rb* gene, also have an increased risk for melanoma and other malignancies. Since the *Rb* pathway is one of the known mechanisms of dysregulation in the melanocytic cell cycle as previously discussed, it is not surprising that studies have reported an increase risk of melanoma as high as 80-fold compared to the general population risk [100–102]. In one study, melanoma demonstrated a high standardized mortality ratio of 23.29 (2.82–84.11, 95 % CI) when compared to survivors with sporadic retinoblastoma [102]. Other lifetime risks of cancer among the survivors include lung cancer, bladder cancer, and sarcomas. Most of the excessive cancer risks can be prevented by limiting exposures to UV light, radiotherapy, tobacco use, and other known environmental carcinogens.

5.5   Germline Polymorphisms in Pigmentary Genes

We have discussed several germline genes whose deleterious mutations confer significant lifetime melanoma risk ranging from 50–80 % in melanoma-prone kindreds worldwide. A recent study reported that 30–50 % of melanoma risk variations observed among known hereditary melanoma kindreds are due to shared genetic polymorphisms in low- to moderate-risk genes encoding for hair, eye, and skin color [159]. A population-based study of Australian twins estimates that 55 % of melanoma risk lies within genetic influences rather than shared environmental traits [160]. This large twin study showed a higher concordance compared to nonidentical twins for melanoma with an overall 9.8 likely chance of having melanoma compared to 1.8 times by chance alone. While the high-penetrance genes are essential in controlling cell growth, programming apoptosis, and regulating signaling pathways in the cell cycle, the low- to moderate-penetrance genes encode for mechanisms responsible for pigmentary and nevi phenotypes associated with melanoma susceptibility. Alleles associated with a melanoma phenotype increase melanoma risk on their own, and they also have an additive affected with high-risk genes and increase penetrance when co-inherited. These moderate- to low-penetrance genes exert small disease effect; however, they comprise the larger proportion of melanoma-predisposing genes in the population and, thus, are as important in melanoma risk assessment. In fact, investigation into an individual's pigmentary phenotype has provided research insight into other genetic mechanisms that transforms individual melanocytes into malignant tumor. Discovery of these moderate-to low-penetrance genes have been accomplished by using genome-wide association studies (GWAS). GWAS entails a systematic search of genetic loci throughout the human genome to find associations with cutaneous melanoma. These candidate genes are subjected to case–control datasets to analyze for statistical significance between the susceptibility locus and melanoma risk.

The most commonly known moderate-risk penetrance gene is the melanocortin-1 receptor (*MC1R*), and variants in this gene confer a 1.1- to 3.7-fold risk for melanoma [161, 162]. The *MC1R* gene is a 7-transmembrane G-protein-coupled receptor expressed on the surface of melanocytes that is inducible by α-melanocyte-stimulating hormone (α-MSH) [163, 164]. The final effect switches from red/yellow (pheomelanins) to brown/black (eumelanins) photoprotective melanin production. Various polymorphic mutations within the *MC1R* gene lead to receptor dysfunction and result in reduced eumelanin and increased pheomelanin content. The corresponding phenotypes include red hair and fair skin phenotypes that are vulnerable to UV-induced oxidative stress and a relative risk of developing cutaneous melanoma with reported 2.99–8.10 for red hair color, 1.47 for blue eye color, 2.06 for fair skin, 2.09 for skin type I, and 2.10 for freckles [71, 165–168]. Common *MC1R* homozygous or heterozygous alleles are Arg160Trp, His260Pro, Asp294His, Asp84Glu, Arg142His, and Arg151Cys which predispose to red hair, fair skin, and ultraviolet light sensitivity along with melanoma development. Homozygous or heterozygous variants such as Val60Leu, Val92Met, Ile155Thr, and Arg163Gln are associated with melanoma development but not necessarily the *MC1R* phenotype [165, 169]. The gene penetrance of the *CDKN2A* mutations increased from 50 to 84 % when the mutation was co-inherited with a *MC1R* variant [161].

Microphthalmia-associated transcription factor (*MITF*) is a moderate-penetrance melanoma susceptibility gene. *MITF* is a transcription factor regulating cell-cycle control and melanocyte differentiation. MITF is downstream of the MAPK pathway. Upon UV-induced DNA damage, melanocyte-stimulating hormone (*MSH*) derived from the precursor proopiomelancortin gene (*POMC*) binds to receptor on melanocytes. Subsequent induction and expression of intracellular *MITF* result in transport to nucleus and transcription of upregulatory genes controlling for melanocyte differentiation, melanosome formation, melanin production, and melanocyte survival. Germline mutations theoretically could inactivate *MITF*, could decrease in melanin production, and could dysregulate cell-cycle control leading to melanogenesis. Yokoyama et al. identified a Glu318Lys variant in *MITF* in a family with multiple cases of melanoma. The variant was found to track with three out of seven cases of melanoma in the family. Analysis of this variant in large case–control cohorts from the United Kingdom and Australia found an odds ratio of 2.09 (95 % CI, 1.14–3.94). Like Yokoyama et al., Ghiorzo et al. also showed that carriers of *MITF* Glu318Lys variant had a 6.40-fold increase in developing multiple primary melanomas. The odds ratio of developing melanoma in *MITF* Glu318Lys germline mutation carriers was up to threefold in sporadic and familial cases. The odds ratios for developing melanoma carriers with a strong family history (first- and second-degree relatives) of pancreatic cancer or renal cancer were 31- and 58-fold, respectively [129, 170]. These studies support *MITF* as a moderate-penetrance melanoma susceptibility gene that can also predispose to other malignancies.

MITF regulates the solute carrier family 45 member 2 gene (*SLC45A2*) [171]. SLC45A2 (also known as *MATP* gene) is mapped to 5p13.2 and is a sodium–hydrogen transporter protein that mediates melanin synthesis. Germline mutations in *SLC45A2* have been linked to oculocutaneous albinism, type 4, while germline polymorphisms are associated with skin and hair pigmentation. In several studies, the *SLC45A2* variants, particularly Phe374Leu and Glu272Lys, have been demonstrated to be protective for melanoma (odds ratio ranging from 0.35 to 0.75, 95 % CI, 0.24–0.95) [156, 157, 159, 171–173]. These studies also demonstrate that *SLC45A2* are significantly associated with olive and dark skin pigmentation, black to blond hair, and ability to tan.

GWAS-based approach also found an association with agouti signaling protein (*ASIP*) mutation carriage and risk of melanoma [157, 174–176]. *ASIP* gene is an antagonist of *MC1R* and, thus, participates in the melanocortin pathway for pigmentary-related melanoma risk. Overexpression of the ASIP protein product leads to yellow pheomelanin production. The allelic polymorphisms in *ASIP* locus region result in red hair phenotype and facial freckling [175].

Missense variants in both the tyrosinase gene (*TYR*) and tyrosinase-related protein 1 (*TYRP1*) encoding for melanosomal enzymes have been associated with increase melanoma risk [157, 175, 177]. *TYRP1* normally functions in the eumelanin pathway, but rare mutations are responsible for oculocutaneous albinism, type 3. Heterozygous compound mutant alleles in *TYR* result in ocular albinism (also known as oculocutaneous albinism, type 2). The increased risk for melanoma from each of these moderate to low-penetrance genes are highlighted in Table 5.3.

5.6   Family and Personal History Risks

Inheriting genetic polymorphisms in low- to moderate-penetrance genes confer a modest risk of developing melanoma compared to the high-penetrance genes, *CDKN2A* and *CDK4*, as discussed above. A thorough physical exam and ascertainment of family pedigree of malignancies can guide the probability of finding a mutation in one of these known genes. However, in some families, there are yet unknown hereditary risks. For these families, the risk is significant based on the number of family members affected and personal history of cutaneous malignancy. Based on a large meta-analysis study, an individual's relative risk is increased at 1.74 if one belongs to a family history with either a first- or second-degree relative affected with melanoma [71].

A recent prospective cohort study reported that a personal history of nonmelanoma skin cancers increases one's own risk of melanoma and observed a relative

Table 5.3 Moderate- and low-penetrance germline mutations affecting phenotype and melanoma risk

Gene	Locus	Penetrance	Function	Phenotype	Melanoma risk (RR = relative risk and OR = odds ratio)
MC1R	16q24.3	Moderate	Melanin production	Red hair and poor UVR-induced tanning response	RR: 2.2–3.9 [71–73, 159]
OCA2	15q13.1	Moderate	Regulatory	Determinant of blue eye color	OR: 1.31 [159]
MITF	3p14-p13	Moderate	Melanin production and cell-cycle control	Increased nevi count and non-blue eye color	OR: 2.95–30 [129, 170, 178]
ASIP	20q11.22	Low	Pheomelanin production	Red hair, high density of freckling, and sun sensitivity	RR: 1.09–1.72 [157, 174, 175, 179]
TYR	11q14.3	Low	Melanogenic enzyme	Ocular albinsim	RR: 1.13–1.21 [159, 179]
TYRP1 (also known as OCA3)	9p23	Low	Melanogenic enzyme that stabilizes TYR	Red hair and blue eye color	RR: 0.77–1.15 [157, 175, 179]
SLC45A2 (also known as OCA4)	5p13.3-13.2	Low	Hydrogen–sodium exchanger	Blond hair, blue eyes, and high density of freckling, and sun sensitivity	RR: 0.35–0.75 [157, 159]
Nevi count (≥101–120)	–	Low	–	Multiple dysplastic nevi	RR: 6.89 [72]
Dysplastic nevi	–	Low	–	Dysplastic nevi (≥5 mm, irregular or poorly defined borders, variable shades of brown, sometimes with reddish or pink hue)	RR: 6.36 [72]

risk of 1.99 in men and 2.58 in women [180]. Other previous studies have similarly reported that a personal history of nonmelanoma skin cancers, also including precancerous actinic keratosis, carries a relative risk of 2.8–17 [71, 181–184]. A personal history of melanoma alone elevates one's 5-year risk of developing a second primary melanoma to 11.4 %, and this risk is further increased to 30.9 % in individuals with a third primary melanoma [185]. A personal phenotypic trait of multiple nevi count not associated with a known genetic syndrome is strongly associated with a relative risk of 1.18–1.32 and a higher relative risk of 6.89 if nevi count ≥101 [72, 186].

Several studies ascertained that 17–25 % of melanoma arise from atypical or dysplastic nevi [187–191]. The relative risk is 3.63 (2.85–4.62, 95 % CI) [192]. Melanoma risk also rose with increasing number of dysplastic nevi but a more profound melanoma risk may be associated with a personal nevi count greater than 50 [189, 192].

Other personal history risk factors include large (>20 cm) congenital melanocytic nevi with a reported melanoma incidence estimated at 2.3 per 1000 patient-years and Parkinson disease diagnosis associated with a melanoma relative risk of 1.95 (1.44–2.59, 95 % CI) [193, 194].

5.7 The Role of Genetic Testing in Melanoma Risk Assessment

To complete an optimal cancer risk assessment, the individual's personal and familial cancer histories should always be carefully documented, confirmed whenever possible, and reviewed as this information may be useful in determining the appropriateness of genetic testing. Currently, genetic testing is clinically available for the highly penetrant genes CDKN2A and CDK4, mutations in either of which confers a molecular diagnosis of hereditary melanoma. However, owing to the rarity of mutations in CDK4, most research on genetic testing has focused on CDKN2A [195]. Therefore, we will focus on genetic testing of the CDKN2A gene in this chapter.

The information gathered from genetic testing of CDKN2A may help delineate an individual's level of risk for melanoma and/or pancreatic cancer and may also be useful in providing appropriate management recommendations for his/her relatives. Criteria have been suggested for when to appropriately offer genetic testing for hereditary melanoma. The probability of detecting a genetic mutation is lower in high melanoma-incidence areas and greater in low melanoma-incidence areas. In regions with a high melanoma incidence (>10/100,000), three incidences of melanoma and/or pancreatic cancer on the same side of the family warrant a sufficient probability of harboring a mutation; therefore, testing should be considered. However, in areas in which melanoma is less common, two incidences of melanoma or melanoma and pancreatic cancer on the same side of the family are sufficient for consideration of testing [195]. Clinicians must note that these are general guidelines that should not supersede clinical judgment. Many regions will have both high- and low-risk populations and ultimately the decision to offer genetic testing should rely on the individual's personal and family history rather than solely on where they reside.

When first evaluating a family for hereditary melanoma, genetic testing should ideally begin in a family member who has a personal history of either melanoma or pancreatic cancer. This increases the likelihood of detecting a mutation if one is present in the family [196]. The results from genetic testing should be interpreted within the context of the individual's personal and family history. There are three possible results from genetic testing [196]:

1. *A positive genetic test result may be obtained.* This indicates that a mutation in the *CDKN2A* gene has been identified, conferring an increased lifetime risk for melanoma of 60–90 % and an approximately 17 % lifetime risk of developing pancreatic cancer [75, 76, 88, 89, 197]. Owing to these increased risks, more careful screening and photoprotection measures are recommended, as listed in Table 5.2. Furthermore, due to the autosomal dominant pattern of inheritance, an individual who carries a deleterious mutation in *CDKN2A* has a 50 % chance of passing this mutation down to each of his or her offspring. Spontaneous mutations in *CDKN2A* are rare, meaning that most individuals have inherited the mutation from a parent. Therefore, the individual's siblings are considered at 50 % risk of also carrying the familial mutation and testing should be offered to them. Site-specific genetic testing is also indicated for extended family members who may be at risk. Relatives who test positive, but were previously unaware of their increased cancer risks, can begin screening and implementing sun protection practices in order to maximize opportunities for early detection and risk reduction.

2. *A variant of uncertain significance (VUS) is identified.* While the family should still be considered high risk, predictive testing for family members cannot be offered until the significance of the variant is established. Oftentimes genetic testing of the VUS may be available for other family members who are affected with melanoma or pancreatic cancer to help determine if the cancers are tracking with the identified alteration. Until the variant is classified as either deleterious or a polymorphism, individuals with a VUS should be followed based on their personal and family history, alone, and not on the status of this unknown alteration.

3. *No mutation is identified.* This does not mean that an inherited component is not present or that these patients are not at increased risk for developing melanoma. On the contrary, these patients may have the phenotypic variant described earlier, which may still confer a moderately increased melanoma risk. Moreover, studies have suggested that individuals testing negative for a familial mutation may still have up to a 1.7-fold increased risk compared to the general population [198]. Therefore, for these individuals, careful sun protection is recommended and annual dermatological screening should be considered based on their phenotype. Their risk for pancreatic cancer would likely be based on their family history, alone.

It is important to note that mutations in the *CDKN2A* gene account for less than 40 % of familial melanomas [88]. Therefore, the majority of individuals who are the first person in their family to proceed with genetic testing will have a negative test result, meaning that no mutation is identified. This test result does not rule out an increased risk of melanoma in the family and unaffected relatives should still be counseled to adhere to recommendations for increased screening and photoprotection based on their personal and family history.

5.8   Impact of Genetic Testing

Recent studies have emphasized the benefits of *CDKN2A* genetic test reporting on both photoprotective behavioral and psychological outcomes. These studies have looked at *CDKN2A* genetic testing for a known familial mutation, and positive implications have been reported in individuals irrespective of their final genetic test result. The results of a longitudinal study by Aspinwall et al. showed that anxiety and depression were low following *CDKN2A* genetic testing for both carriers and noncarriers. Levels of anxiety decreased during the 2-year follow-up, and depression and melanoma worry also showed decreases in the short term. Worry regarding pancreatic cancer was also low and decreased significantly over time [199]. In an analysis from the same center on the impact of melanoma genetic testing and counseling on photoprotective behaviors, 33 % of study participants, regardless of carrier status, reported incorporating one or more new photoprotective behavior into their lives following results disclosure and post-counseling appointment. Finally, perceived knowledge and health behaviors or plans for increased photoprotection increased, especially among carriers but also in noncarriers as well [200]. In an Australian study, Kasparian and colleagues evaluated the uptake and psychological, behavioral, and cognitive outcomes of genetic testing for individuals with known familial *CDKN2A* mutations. Among the 21 % of participants who underwent genetic testing, carriers reported significantly reduced anxiety scores short term and reduced depression at 12 months [201]. However, there were too few noncarriers in this study to evaluate the impact of genetic testing on their psychological outcomes. While additional research is still needed in this area, these preliminary results indicate that the process of performing genetic testing in the context of pre- and posttest genetic counseling may carry the potential for improved adherence to recommended screening and photoprotective behaviors regardless of the individual's test result without causing significant long- or short-term negative psychological outcomes.

5.9   The Importance of Providing Genetic Counseling

Outside of dermatology, genetic testing and/or referral for genetics evaluation have become much more routine for individuals considered at increased risk for a hereditary cancer syndrome based on their personal and/or family histories. Genetic testing for hereditary melanoma is gradually gaining more acceptance in the clinic as a greater number of studies are published showing the efficacy and positive behavioral implications following the disclosure of genetic test results, as introduced in the previous section. However, the research studies which have demonstrated positive outcomes of genetic testing have all specifically included extensive pre- and posttest counseling and education. Therefore, partnerships between dermatologists and genetics professionals will likely be necessary to realize the same benefits as hereditary melanoma genetic testing continues to move into clinical practices. In the instances in which genetic testing in oncology is recommended by the American Society of Clinical Oncology (ASCO) and the National Comprehensive Cancer

Network (NCCN), these organizations also recommend that it be accompanied by pre- and posttest counseling. This helps to ensure that patients can provide informed consent for genetic testing and that they are well informed and seemingly more prepared to understand the implications of their results and the options available to them and their families [202] (NCCN 2013).

Genetic counselors are becoming increasingly more frequent and relied upon as genetic professionals and as members of many multidisciplinary oncology care teams nationwide [203]. They are specifically trained to provide risk assessment, genetic counseling, and interpretation of genetic test results in the context of the individual's personal and family histories. This helps to ensure that the patient is receiving appropriate recommendations for future follow-up and has support in how to share this important information with at-risk relatives. A typical genetic counseling appointment consists of a review of the individual's personal and family medical and cancer history. The genetic counselor will then use this information to provide the individual with a personalized risk assessment and discuss options for risk reduction and cancer prevention. The acquisition of the family history is not a trivial task. The ability of the genetic counselor to obtain and review medical records for reported medical and family history is a crucial step as this information may be the deciding factor in determining whether or not genetic testing would be informative. Family history is not entirely reliable when obtained solely from an individual's self-report. A study conducted in Queensland, Australia, measured the validity of reported family history and found that up to 40 % of reported histories of melanoma may be inaccurate [204]. Therefore, confirmation of reported cancers by medical records, death certificates, etc., may be critical whenever possible as this may change the management and/or genetic testing recommendations made for an individual and his or her family. With the help of a multidisciplinary team including genetic professionals, accurate information can be readily collected and utilized to provide the patient with superior care.

In addition to reviewing family history, genetic counselors engage in risk management and genetic testing discussions with their patients. However, genetic testing may not always be appropriate for the individual who is initially referred or who is personally seeking information regarding his/her melanoma risk. Regardless of the appropriateness of genetic testing, with a significant family history of melanoma and/or pancreatic cancer, a genetic consultation may still be warranted in helping the patient better grasp his/her level of cancer risk and in learning the screening and photoprotection options available to them. If genetic testing is medically appropriate and will be informative, it will be offered. If elected, informed consent will be obtained. The genetic counselor who orders this test is responsible for its interpretation and disclosure. If this test identifies a VUS, the genetic counselor will institute follow-up discussions with the individual to allow for as much clarification as possible regarding this alteration. The genetic counselor is also typically available to guide the individual in how to inform his or her family about any medically relevant information learned through genetic testing. Therefore, through the process of both pre- and posttest counseling, a genetic counselor in collaboration with the individual's multidisciplinary health-care team can provide a comprehensive and personalized risk assessment and short-term support to patients and their families. This resource can be of great assistance especially when utilized by clinicians functioning in a busy practice.

5.10 Management of Individuals at High Risk for Melanoma

Prevention, routine screening, and early diagnosis are key components in the medical management of individuals at high risk for developing melanoma. In the role of primary prevention, numerous studies have shown that UV light contributes to development of both nonmelanoma and melanoma skin cancers. Even more provoking, other studies show cutaneous malignancies are preventable when UV light exposure is limited [205–208]. With such strong evidence-based medicine, the US Preventive Services Task Force recommends counseling patients on sun protective strategies [209]. Other national organizations including the American Academy of Dermatology, American Cancer Society, and American Academy of Family Physicians have implemented similar positions and recommendations with regard to limiting excessive ultraviolet exposure through sunlight or artificial tanning beds [210–212]. Photoprotection strategies should also include applying sunblock prior and during engagement in outdoor activities and wearing protective, tightly woven clothing and a hat with a wide brim. Other known risk factors should also be emphasized to the patient (e.g., no tobacco use for individuals with *CDKN2A*).

Routine dermatologic screening encompasses both monthly self-skin examinations and regular full-body skin examinations by clinicians trained in providing these exams [213]. A full-body skin would often include examination of the scalp, ocular irides, oral mucosa, genital, and anus. The clinician can show patients how best to perform self-skin examinations during their first visit. Having a partner or family member help with the patient's skin examination at home can also be beneficial and aid in visually challenging body areas (e.g., the back).

Secondary prevention through early diagnosis relies heavily on both patient and clinical provider to establish dermatologic screening schedules tailored from a patient's clinical examination findings (e.g., nevi count, dysplastic nevi, Fitzpatrick skin type), personal history of melanoma and other nonmelanoma skin cancers, and family history. The American Academy of Dermatology recommends routine skin examinations by a dermatologist and monthly self-examinations in individuals classified as high risk as outlined Table 5.2. Those individuals at low to moderate risk can start screening at age 40 years old with annual dermatologic skin examinations [214].

5.11 Future

In the future it is likely that somatic and germline genetic characteristics of melanoma (and of patients who are at risk for melanoma) will become more and more important in the development of individualized and tailored care. Genetic characteristics of tumors will continue to drive targeted and immunologic therapies for the disease, and it is likely that combination therapies, utilizing complete molecular profiling data from a tumor, will guide the selection of agents. It is also likely that molecular profiling of primary tumors will provide an increasingly objective method for diagnosing difficult tumor subtypes as well as providing better prognostic information. Improved prognostication can guide the decisions for additional procedures such as sentinel lymph node biopsy or adjuvant therapy. Comprehensive evaluation of the patient's germline genome, particularly with integration of mRNA and protein expression data, will permit increasingly accurate risk assessment so that personalized prevention programs can be designed. As these large data sets become available, it will also be necessary to analyze the genetic and genomic data quickly and effectively so that clinical decisions can be made in real time for the benefit of the patient. Finally, it should be appreciated that advances in molecular medicine must be accompanied by the development of educational tools and behavioral strategies in order to have impact on patient's lives. Genetic counselors will almost certainly play a central role as a liaison between physicians, scientists, and the patients. The spectrum of possibilities and needs in this rapidly advancing field is extremely broad, and multidisciplinary team approaches will be crucial for ultimate success.

References

1. Robinson JK, Rigel DS, Amonette RA (1997) Trends in sun exposure knowledge, attitudes, and behaviors: 1986 to 1996. J Am Acad Dermatol 37(2 Pt 1):179–186
2. Kwon HT, Mayer JA, Walker KK, Yu H, Lewis EC, Belch GE (2002) Promotion of frequent tanning sessions by indoor tanning facilities: two studies. J Am Acad Dermatol 46(5): 700–705
3. Dellavalle RP, Parker ER, Cersonsky N et al (2003) Youth access laws: in the dark at the tanning parlor? Arch Dermatol 139(4):443–448
4. Albino AP, Vidal MJ, McNutt NS et al (1994) Mutation and expression of the p53 gene in human malignant melanoma. Melanoma Res 4(1):35–45
5. Curtin JA, Busam K, Pinkel D, Bastian BC (2006) Somatic activation of KIT in distinct subtypes of melanoma. J Clin Oncol 24(26):4340–4346
6. Goel VK, Lazar AJ, Warneke CL, Redston MS, Haluska FG (2006) Examination of mutations in BRAF, NRAS, and PTEN in primary cutaneous melanoma. J Invest Dermatol 126(1):154–160
7. Zuo L, Weger J, Yang Q et al (1996) Germline mutations in the p16INK4a binding domain of CDK4 in familial melanoma. Nat Genet 12(1):97–99
8. Kamijo T, Weber JD, Zambetti G, Zindy F, Roussel MF, Sherr CJ (1998) Functional and physical interactions of the ARF tumor suppressor with p53 and Mdm2. Proc Natl Acad Sci USA 95(14):8292–8297
9. Pomerantz J, Schreiber-Agus N, Liegeois NJ et al (1998) The Ink4a tumor suppressor gene product, p19Arf, interacts with MDM2 and neutralizes MDM2's inhibition of p53. Cell 92(6):713–723
10. Schutte M, Hruban RH, Geradts J et al (1997) Abrogation of the Rb/p16 tumor-suppressive pathway in virtually all pancreatic carcinomas. Cancer Res 57(15):3126–3130
11. Serrano M, Hannon GJ, Beach D (1993) A new regulatory motif in cell-cycle control causing specific inhibition of cyclin D/CDK4. Nature 366(6456):704–707
12. Stott FJ, Bates S, James MC et al (1998) The alternative product from the human CDKN2A locus, p14(ARF), participates in a regulatory feedback loop with p53 and MDM2. EMBO J 17(17):5001–5014
13. Curtin JA, Fridlyand J, Kageshita T et al (2005) Distinct sets of genetic alterations in melanoma. N Engl J Med 353(20):2135–2147
14. Pollock PM, Harper UL, Hansen KS et al (2003) High frequency of BRAF mutations in nevi. Nat Genet 33(1):19–20

15. Davies H, Bignell GR, Cox C et al (2002) Mutations of the BRAF gene in human cancer. Nature 417(6892):949–954
16. Amanuel B, Grieu F, Kular J, Millward M, Iacopetta B (2012) Incidence of BRAF p.Val600Glu and p.Val600Lys mutations in a consecutive series of 183 metastatic melanoma patients from a high incidence region. Pathology 44(4):357–359
17. Liu W, Kelly JW, Trivett M et al (2007) Distinct clinical and pathological features are associated with the BRAF(T1799A(V600E)) mutation in primary melanoma. J Invest Dermatol 127(4):900–905
18. Long GV, Menzies AM, Nagrial AM et al (2011) Prognostic and clinicopathologic associations of oncogenic BRAF in metastatic melanoma. J Clin Oncol 29(10):1239–1246
19. Hauschild A, Grob JJ, Demidov LV et al (2012) Dabrafenib in BRAF-mutated metastatic melanoma: a multicentre, open-label, phase 3 randomised controlled trial. Lancet 380(9839): 358–365
20. Flaherty KT, Puzanov I, Kim KB et al (2010) Inhibition of mutated, activated BRAF in metastatic melanoma. N Engl J Med 363(9):809–819
21. Akslen LA, Angelini S, Straume O et al (2005) BRAF and NRAS mutations are frequent in nodular melanoma but are not associated with tumor cell proliferation or patient survival. J Invest Dermatol 125(2):312–317
22. Edlundh-Rose E, Egyhazi S, Omholt K et al (2006) NRAS and BRAF mutations in melanoma tumours in relation to clinical characteristics: a study based on mutation screening by pyrosequencing. Melanoma Res 16(6):471–478
23. Jafari M, Papp T, Kirchner S et al (1995) Analysis of ras mutations in human melanocytic lesions: activation of the ras gene seems to be associated with the nodular type of human malignant melanoma. J Cancer Res Clin Oncol 121(1):23–30
24. van't Veer LJ, Burgering BM, Versteeg R et al (1989) N-ras mutations in human cutaneous melanoma from sun-exposed body sites. Mol Cell Biol 9(7):3114–3116
25. van Elsas A, Zerp SF, van der Flier S et al (1996) Relevance of ultraviolet-induced N-ras oncogene point mutations in development of primary human cutaneous melanoma. Am J Pathol 149(3):883–893
26. Gajewski TF, Salama AK, Niedzwiecki D et al (2012) Phase II study of the farnesyltransferase inhibitor R115777 in advanced melanoma (CALGB 500104). J Transl Med 10:246
27. Pollock PM, Walker GJ, Glendening JM et al (2002) PTEN inactivation is rare in melanoma tumours but occurs frequently in melanoma cell lines. Melanoma Res 12(6):565–575
28. Tsao H, Zhang X, Benoit E, Haluska FG (1998) Identification of PTEN/MMAC1 alterations in uncultured melanomas and melanoma cell lines. Oncogene 16(26):3397–3402
29. Teng DH, Hu R, Lin H et al (1997) MMAC1/PTEN mutations in primary tumor specimens and tumor cell lines. Cancer Res 57(23):5221–5225
30. Celebi JT, Shendrik I, Silvers DN, Peacocke M (2000) Identification of PTEN mutations in metastatic melanoma specimens. J Med Genet 37(9):653–657
31. Ernst DS, Eisenhauer E, Wainman N et al (2005) Phase II study of perifosine in previously untreated patients with metastatic melanoma. Invest New Drugs 23(6):569–575
32. Beadling C, Jacobson-Dunlop E, Hodi FS et al (2008) KIT gene mutations and copy number in melanoma subtypes. Clin Cancer Res 14(21):6821–6828
33. Lin YC, Chang YM, Ho JY et al (2012) C-kit expression of melanocytic neoplasm and association with clinicopathological parameters and anatomic locations in Chinese people. Am J Dermatopathol
34. Curtin JA, Stark MS, Pinkel D, Hayward NK, Bastian BC (2006) PI3-kinase subunits are infrequent somatic targets in melanoma. J Invest Dermatol 126(7):1660–1663
35. Guo J, Si L, Kong Y et al (2011) Phase II, open-label, single-arm trial of imatinib mesylate in patients with metastatic melanoma harboring c-Kit mutation or amplification. J Clin Oncol 29(21):2904–2909
36. Cho JH, Kim KM, Kwon M, Kim JH, Lee J (2012) Nilotinib in patients with metastatic melanoma harboring KIT gene aberration. Invest New Drugs 30(5):2008–2014

37. Kluger HM, Dudek AZ, McCann C et al (2011) A phase 2 trial of dasatinib in advanced melanoma. Cancer 117(10):2202–2208
38. Maldonado JL, Fridlyand J, Patel H et al (2003) Determinants of BRAF mutations in primary melanomas. J Natl Cancer Inst 95(24):1878–1890
39. Uribe P, Wistuba II, Gonzalez S (2003) BRAF mutation: a frequent event in benign, atypical, and malignant melanocytic lesions of the skin. Am J Dermatopathol 25(5):365–370
40. Daniotti M, Oggionni M, Ranzani T et al (2004) BRAF alterations are associated with complex mutational profiles in malignant melanoma. Oncogene 23(35):5968–5977
41. Kumar R, Angelini S, Snellman E, Hemminki K (2004) BRAF mutations are common somatic events in melanocytic nevi. J Invest Dermatol 122(2):342–348
42. Libra M, Malaponte G, Navolanic PM et al (2005) Analysis of BRAF mutation in primary and metastatic melanoma. Cell Cycle 4(10):1382–1384
43. Dong J, Phelps RG, Qiao R et al (2003) BRAF oncogenic mutations correlate with progression rather than initiation of human melanoma. Cancer Res 63(14):3883–3885
44. Takata M, Saida T (2006) Genetic alterations in melanocytic tumors. J Dermatol Sci 43(1):1–10
45. Yazdi AS, Palmedo G, Flaig MJ et al (2003) Mutations of the BRAF gene in benign and malignant melanocytic lesions. J Invest Dermatol 121(5):1160–1162
46. Saldanha G, Purnell D, Fletcher A, Potter L, Gillies A, Pringle JH (2004) High BRAF mutation frequency does not characterize all melanocytic tumor types. Int J Cancer 111(5):705–710
47. Wajapeyee N, Serra RW, Zhu X, Mahalingam M, Green MR (2008) Oncogenic BRAF induces senescence and apoptosis through pathways mediated by the secreted protein IGFBP7. Cell 132(3):363–374
48. Sosman JA, Kim KB, Schuchter L et al (2012) Survival in BRAF V600-mutant advanced melanoma treated with vemurafenib. N Engl J Med 366(8):707–714
49. Jovanovic B, Egyhazi S, Eskandarpour M et al (2010) Coexisting NRAS and BRAF mutations in primary familial melanomas with specific CDKN2A germline alterations. J Invest Dermatol 130(2):618–620
50. Milagre C, Dhomen N, Geyer FC et al (2010) A mouse model of melanoma driven by oncogenic KRAS. Cancer Res 70(13):5549–5557
51. Hocker T, Tsao H (2007) Ultraviolet radiation and melanoma: a systematic review and analysis of reported sequence variants. Hum Mutat 28(6):578–588
52. Papp T, Pemsel H, Zimmermann R, Bastrop R, Weiss DG, Schiffmann D (1999) Mutational analysis of the N-ras, p53, p16INK4a, CDK4, and MC1R genes in human congenital melanocytic naevi. J Med Genet 36(8):610–614
53. Albino AP, Nanus DM, Mentle IR et al (1989) Analysis of ras oncogenes in malignant melanoma and precursor lesions: correlation of point mutations with differentiation phenotype. Oncogene 4(11):1363–1374
54. Long GV, Stroyakovskiy D, Gogas H et al (2015) Dabrafenib and trametinib versus dabrafenib and placebo for Val600 BRAF-mutant melanoma: a multicentre, double-blind, phase 3 randomised controlled trial. Lancet 386(9992):444–451
55. Eskandarpour M, Hashemi J, Kanter L, Ringborg U, Platz A, Hansson J (2003) Frequency of UV-inducible NRAS mutations in melanomas of patients with germline CDKN2A mutations. J Natl Cancer Inst 95(11):790–798
56. Dai DL, Martinka M, Li G (2005) Prognostic significance of activated Akt expression in melanoma: a clinicopathologic study of 292 cases. J Clin Oncol 23(7):1473–1482
57. Stahl JM, Sharma A, Cheung M et al (2004) Deregulated Akt3 activity promotes development of malignant melanoma. Cancer Res 64(19):7002–7010
58. Omholt K, Krockel D, Ringborg U, Hansson J (2006) Mutations of PIK3CA are rare in cutaneous melanoma. Melanoma Res 16(2):197–200
59. Davies MA, Stemke-Hale K, Tellez C et al (2008) A novel AKT3 mutation in melanoma tumours and cell lines. Br J Cancer 99(8):1265–1268

60. Guldberg P, thor Straten P, Birck A, Ahrenkiel V, Kirkin AF, Zeuthen J (1997) Disruption of the MMAC1/PTEN gene by deletion or mutation is a frequent event in malignant melanoma. Cancer Res 57(17):3660–3663

61. Tsao H, Mihm MC Jr, Sheehan C (2003) PTEN expression in normal skin, acquired melanocytic nevi, and cutaneous melanoma. J Am Acad Dermatol 49(5):865–872

62. Tsao H, Goel V, Wu H, Yang G, Haluska FG (2004) Genetic interaction between NRAS and BRAF mutations and PTEN/MMAC1 inactivation in melanoma. J Invest Dermatol 122(2):337–341

63. Kim KB, Eton O, Davis DW et al (2008) Phase II trial of imatinib mesylate in patients with metastatic melanoma. Br J Cancer 99(5):734–740

64. Antonescu CR, Busam KJ, Francone TD et al (2007) L576P KIT mutation in anal melanomas correlates with KIT protein expression and is sensitive to specific kinase inhibition. Int J Cancer 121(2):257–264

65. Satzger I, Kuttler U, Volker B, Schenck F, Kapp A, Gutzmer R (2010) Anal mucosal melanoma with KIT-activating mutation and response to imatinib therapy—case report and review of the literature. Dermatology 220(1):77–81

66. Carvajal RD, Antonescu CR, Wolchok JD et al (2011) KIT as a therapeutic target in metastatic melanoma. JAMA 305(22):2327–2334

67. Hodi FS, Friedlander P, Corless CL et al (2008) Major response to imatinib mesylate in KIT-mutated melanoma. J Clin Oncol 26(12):2046–2051

68. Florell SR, Boucher KM, Garibotti G et al (2005) Population-based analysis of prognostic factors and survival in familial melanoma. J Clin Oncol 23(28):7168–7177

69. Hayward NK (2003) Genetics of melanoma predisposition. Oncogene 22(20):3053–3062

70. Ford D, Bliss JM, Swerdlow AJ et al (1995) Risk of cutaneous melanoma associated with a family history of the disease. The International Melanoma Analysis Group (IMAGE). Int J Cancer 62(4):377–381

71. Gandini S, Sera F, Cattaruzza MS et al (2005) Meta-analysis of risk factors for cutaneous melanoma: III. Family history, actinic damage and phenotypic factors. Eur J Cancer 41(14):2040–2059

72. Gandini S, Sera F, Cattaruzza MS et al (2005) Meta-analysis of risk factors for cutaneous melanoma: I. Common and atypical naevi. Eur J Cancer 41(1):28–44

73. Gandini S, Sera F, Cattaruzza MS et al (2005) Meta-analysis of risk factors for cutaneous melanoma: II Sun exposure. Eur J Cancer 41(1):45–60

74. Kefford RF, Newton Bishop JA, Bergman W, Tucker MA (1999) Counseling and DNA testing for individuals perceived to be genetically predisposed to melanoma: a consensus statement of the Melanoma Genetics Consortium. J Clin Oncol 17(10):3245–3251

75. Bishop DT, Demenais F, Goldstein AM et al (2002) Geographical variation in the penetrance of CDKN2A mutations for melanoma. J Natl Cancer Inst 94(12):894–903

76. Berwick M, Orlow I, Hummer AJ et al (2006) The prevalence of CDKN2A germ-line mutations and relative risk for cutaneous malignant melanoma: an international population-based study. Cancer Epidemiol Biomarkers Prev 15(8):1520–1525

77. de Snoo FA, Hayward NK (2005) Cutaneous melanoma susceptibility and progression genes. Cancer Lett 230(2):153–186

78. Cannon-Albright LA, Goldgar DE, Meyer LJ et al (1992) Assignment of a locus for familial melanoma, MLM, to chromosome 9p13-p22. Science 258(5085):1148–1152

79. Kamb A, Shattuck-Eidens D, Eeles R et al (1994) Analysis of the p16 gene (CDKN2) as a candidate for the chromosome 9p melanoma susceptibility locus. Nat Genet 8(1):23–26

80. Nobori T, Miura K, Wu DJ, Lois A, Takabayashi K, Carson DA (1994) Deletions of the cyclin-dependent kinase-4 inhibitor gene in multiple human cancers. Nature 368(6473): 753–756

81. Kamb A, Gruis NA, Weaver-Feldhaus J et al (1994) A cell cycle regulator potentially involved in genesis of many tumor types. Science 264(5157):436–440

82. Hussussian CJ, Struewing JP, Goldstein AM et al (1994) Germline p16 mutations in familial melanoma. Nat Genet 8(1):15–21

83. Cannon-Albright LA, Goldgar DE, Neuhausen S et al (1994) Localization of the 9p melanoma susceptibility locus (MLM) to a 2-cM region between D9S736 and D9S171. Genomics 23(1):265–268
84. Harland M, Taylor CF, Chambers PA et al (2005) A mutation hotspot at the p14ARF splice site. Oncogene 24(28):4604–4608
85. Hewitt C, Lee Wu C, Evans G et al (2002) Germline mutation of ARF in a melanoma kindred. Hum Mol Genet 11(11):1273–1279
86. Randerson-Moor JA, Harland M, Williams S et al (2001) A germline deletion of p14(ARF) but not CDKN2A in a melanoma-neural system tumour syndrome family. Hum Mol Genet 10(1):55–62
87. Rizos H, Puig S, Badenas C et al (2001) A melanoma-associated germline mutation in exon 1beta inactivates p14ARF. Oncogene 20(39):5543–5547
88. Goldstein AM, Chan M, Harland M et al (2006) High-risk melanoma susceptibility genes and pancreatic cancer, neural system tumors, and uveal melanoma across GenoMEL. Cancer Res 66(20):9818–9828
89. Tucker MA, Fraser MC, Goldstein AM et al (2002) A natural history of melanomas and dysplastic nevi: an atlas of lesions in melanoma-prone families. Cancer 94(12):3192–3209
90. Aspinwall LG, Leaf SL, Dola ER, Kohlmann W, Leachman SA (2008) CDKN2A/p16 genetic test reporting improves early detection intentions and practices in high-risk melanoma families. Cancer Epidemiol Biomarkers Prev 17(6):1510–1519
91. Santillan AA, Cherpelis BS, Glass LF, Sondak VK (2009) Management of familial melanoma and nonmelanoma skin cancer syndromes. Surg Oncol Clin N Am 18(1):73–98, viii
92. Robinson JK, Fisher SG, Turrisi RJ (2002) Predictors of skin self-examination performance. Cancer 95(1):135–146
93. Gillanders E, Juo SH, Holland EA et al (2003) Localization of a novel melanoma susceptibility locus to 1p22. Am J Hum Genet 73(2):301–313
94. Walker GJ, Indsto JO, Sood R et al (2004) Deletion mapping suggests that the 1p22 melanoma susceptibility gene is a tumor suppressor localized to a 9-Mb interval. Genes Chromosomes Cancer 41(1):56–64
95. Hussein MR, Roggero E, Tuthill RJ, Wood GS, Sudilovsky O (2003) Identification of novel deletion Loci at 1p36 and 9p22-21 in melanocytic dysplastic nevi and cutaneous malignant melanomas. Arch Dermatol 139(6):816–817
96. Poetsch M, Dittberner T, Woenckhaus C (2003) Microsatellite analysis at 1p36.3 in malignant melanoma of the skin: fine mapping in search of a possible tumour suppressor gene region. Melanoma Res 13(1):29–33
97. Amos CI, Wang LE, Lee JE et al (2011) Genome-wide association study identifies novel loci predisposing to cutaneous melanoma. Hum Mol Genet 20(24):5012–5023
98. Njauw CN, Kim I, Piris A et al (2012) Germline BAP1 inactivation is preferentially associated with metastatic ocular melanoma and cutaneous-ocular melanoma families. PLoS One 7(4):e35295
99. Wiesner T, Obenauf AC, Murali R et al (2011) Germline mutations in BAP1 predispose to melanocytic tumors. Nat Genet 43(10):1018–1021
100. Draper GJ, Sanders BM, Kingston JE (1986) Second primary neoplasms in patients with retinoblastoma. Br J Cancer 53(5):661–671
101. Sanders BM, Jay M, Draper GJ, Roberts EM (1989) Non-ocular cancer in relatives of retinoblastoma patients. Br J Cancer 60(3):358–365
102. Fletcher O, Easton D, Anderson K, Gilham C, Jay M, Peto J (2004) Lifetime risks of common cancers among retinoblastoma survivors. J Natl Cancer Inst 96(5):357–363
103. Chintagumpala M, Chevez-Barrios P, Paysse EA, Plon SE, Hurwitz R (2007) Retinoblastoma: review of current management. Oncologist 12(10):1237–1246
104. Koh J, Enders GH, Dynlacht BD, Harlow E (1995) Tumour-derived p16 alleles encoding proteins defective in cell-cycle inhibition. Nature 375(6531):506–510

105. Flores JF, Walker GJ, Glendening JM et al (1996) Loss of the p16INK4a and p15INK4b genes, as well as neighboring 9p21 markers, in sporadic melanoma. Cancer Res 56(21):5023–5032

106. Walker GJ, Flores JF, Glendening JM, Lin AH, Markl ID, Fountain JW (1998) Virtually 100% of melanoma cell lines harbor alterations at the DNA level within CDKN2A, CDKN2B, or one of their downstream targets. Genes Chromosomes Cancer 22(2):157–163

107. Barnhill RL, Castresana JS, Rubio MP et al (1994) p53 expression in cutaneous malignant melanoma: an immunohistochemical study of 87 cases of primary, recurrent, and metastatic melanoma. Mod Pathol 7(5):533–535

108. Lubbe J, Reichel M, Burg G, Kleihues P (1994) Absence of p53 gene mutations in cutaneous melanoma. J Invest Dermatol 102(5):819–821

109. Gelsleichter L, Gown AM, Zarbo RJ, Wang E, Coltrera MD (1995) p53 and mdm-2 expression in malignant melanoma: an immunocytochemical study of expression of p53, mdm-2, and markers of cell proliferation in primary versus metastatic tumors. Mod Pathol 8(5): 530–535

110. Poremba C, Yandell DW, Metze D, Kamanabrou D, Bocker W, Dockhorn-Dworniczak B (1995) Immunohistochemical detection of p53 in melanomas with rare p53 gene mutations is associated with mdm-2 overexpression. Oncol Res 7(7–8):331–339

111. Akslen LA, Monstad SE, Larsen B, Straume O, Ogreid D (1998) Frequent mutations of the p53 gene in cutaneous melanoma of the nodular type. Int J Cancer 79(1):91–95

112. Soto JL, Cabrera CM, Serrano S, Lopez-Nevot MA (2005) Mutation analysis of genes that control the G1/S cell cycle in melanoma: TP53, CDKN1A, CDKN2A, and CDKN2B. BMC Cancer 5:36

113. Sparrow LE, Soong R, Dawkins HJ, Iacopetta BJ, Heenan PJ (1995) p53 gene mutation and expression in naevi and melanomas. Melanoma Res 5(2):93–100

114. Spatz A, Giglia-Mari G, Benhamou S, Sarasin A (2001) Association between DNA repair-deficiency and high level of p53 mutations in melanoma of xeroderma pigmentosum. Cancer Res 61(6):2480–2486

115. Wolfel T, Hauer M, Schneider J et al (1995) A p16INK4a-insensitive CDK4 mutant targeted by cytolytic T lymphocytes in a human melanoma. Science 269(5228):1281–1284

116. Soufir N, Avril MF, Chompret A et al (1998) Prevalence of p16 and CDK4 germline mutations in 48 melanoma-prone families in France. The French Familial Melanoma Study Group. Hum Mol Genet 7(2):209–216

117. Molven A, Grimstvedt MB, Steine SJ et al (2005) A large Norwegian family with inherited malignant melanoma, multiple atypical nevi, and CDK4 mutation. Genes Chromosomes Cancer 44(1):10–18

118. Helsing P, Nymoen DA, Ariansen S et al (2008) Population-based prevalence of CDKN2A and CDK4 mutations in patients with multiple primary melanomas. Genes Chromosomes Cancer 47(2):175–184

119. Pjanova D, Molven A, Akslen LA et al (2009) Identification of a CDK4 R24H mutation-positive melanoma family by analysis of early-onset melanoma patients in Latvia. Melanoma Res 19(2):119–122

120. Lynch HT, Brand RE, Hogg D et al (2002) Phenotypic variation in eight extended CDKN2A germline mutation familial atypical multiple mole melanoma-pancreatic carcinoma-prone families: the familial atypical mole melanoma-pancreatic carcinoma syndrome. Cancer 94(1):84–96

121. Lynch HT, Frichot BC 3rd, Lynch JF (1978) Familial atypical multiple mole-melanoma syndrome. J Med Genet 15(5):352–356

122. Clark WH Jr, Reimer RR, Greene M, Ainsworth AM, Mastrangelo MJ (1978) Origin of familial malignant melanomas from heritable melanocytic lesions. 'The B-K mole syndrome'. Arch Dermatol 114(5):732–738

123. Kraemer KH, Greene MH, Tarone R, Elder DE, Clark WH Jr, Guerry D (1983) Dysplastic naevi and cutaneous melanoma risk. Lancet 2(8358):1076–1077

124. Lynch HT, Fusaro RM, Pester J, Lynch JF (1980) Familial atypical multiple mole melanoma (FAMMM) syndrome: genetic heterogeneity and malignant melanoma. Br J Cancer 42(1):58–70
125. Goldstein AM, Struewing JP, Chidambaram A, Fraser MC, Tucker MA (2000) Genotype-phenotype relationships in U.S. melanoma-prone families with CDKN2A and CDK4 mutations. J Natl Cancer Inst 92(12):1006–1010
126. Bergman W, Gruis NA (2007) Phenotypic variation in familial melanoma: consequences for predictive DNA testing. Arch Dermatol 143(4):525–526
127. Maubec E, Chaudru V, Mohamdi H et al (2012) Familial melanoma: clinical factors associated with germline CDKN2A mutations according to the number of patients affected by melanoma in a family. J Am Acad Dermatol 67(6):1257–1264
128. Slater EP, Langer P, Fendrich V et al (2010) Prevalence of BRCA2 and CDKN2a mutations in German familial pancreatic cancer families. Fam Cancer 9(3):335–343
129. Ghiorzo P, Pastorino L, Queirolo P et al (2013) Prevalence of the E318K MITF germline mutation in Italian melanoma patients: associations with histological subtypes and family cancer history. Pigment Cell Melanoma Res 26(2):259–262
130. Ghiorzo P, Fornarini G, Sciallero S et al (2012) CDKN2A is the main susceptibility gene in Italian pancreatic cancer families. J Med Genet 49(3):164–170
131. Bartsch DK, Sina-Frey M, Lang S et al (2002) CDKN2A germline mutations in familial pancreatic cancer. Ann Surg 236(6):730–737
132. Fuchs CS, Colditz GA, Stampfer MJ et al (1996) A prospective study of cigarette smoking and the risk of pancreatic cancer. Arch Intern Med 156(19):2255–2260
133. Rulyak SJ, Lowenfels AB, Maisonneuve P, Brentnall TA (2003) Risk factors for the development of pancreatic cancer in familial pancreatic cancer kindreds. Gastroenterology 124(5):1292–1299
134. Canto MI, Harinck F, Hruban RH et al (2013) International cancer of the pancreas screening (CAPS) consortium summit on the management of patients with increased risk for familial pancreatic cancer. Gut 62(3):339–347
135. Brentnall TA (2005) Management strategies for patients with hereditary pancreatic cancer. Curr Treat Options Oncol 6(5):437–445
136. Parker JF, Florell SR, Alexander A, DiSario JA, Shami PJ, Leachman SA (2003) Pancreatic carcinoma surveillance in patients with familial melanoma. Arch Dermatol 139(8):1019–1025
137. Eckerle MD, Bishop M, Resse E, Sluzevich J (2009) Familial atypical multiple mole melanoma syndrome
138. Azizi E, Friedman J, Pavlotsky F et al (1995) Familial cutaneous malignant melanoma and tumors of the nervous system. A hereditary cancer syndrome. Cancer 76(9):1571–1578
139. Kaufman DK, Kimmel DW, Parisi JE, Michels VV (1993) A familial syndrome with cutaneous malignant melanoma and cerebral astrocytoma. Neurology 43(9):1728–1731
140. Bahuau M, Vidaud D, Jenkins RB et al (1998) Germ-line deletion involving the INK4 locus in familial proneness to melanoma and nervous system tumors. Cancer Res 58(11):2298–2303
141. Bahuau M, Vidaud D, Kujas M et al (1997) Familial aggregation of malignant melanoma/dysplastic naevi and tumours of the nervous system: an original syndrome of tumour proneness. Ann Genet 40(2):78–91
142. Tachibana I, Smith JS, Sato K, Hosek SM, Kimmel DW, Jenkins RB (2000) Investigation of germline PTEN, p53, p16(INK4A)/p14(ARF), and CDK4 alterations in familial glioma. Am J Med Genet 92(2):136–141
143. Abdel-Rahman MH, Pilarski R, Ezzat S, Sexton J, Davidorf FH (2010) Cancer family history characterization in an unselected cohort of 121 patients with uveal melanoma. Fam Cancer 9(3):431–438
144. Harbour JW, Onken MD, Roberson ED et al (2010) Frequent mutation of BAP1 in metastasizing uveal melanomas. Science 330(6009):1410–1413

145. Hoiom V, Edsgard D, Helgadottir H et al (2013) Hereditary uveal melanoma: a report of a germline mutation in BAP1. Genes Chromosomes Cancer 52(4):378–384
146. Jonsson G, Bendahl PO, Sandberg T et al (2005) Mapping of a novel ocular and cutaneous malignant melanoma susceptibility locus to chromosome 9q21.32. J Natl Cancer Inst 97(18):1377–1382
147. Jensen DE, Proctor M, Marquis ST et al (1998) BAP1: a novel ubiquitin hydrolase which binds to the BRCA1 RING finger and enhances BRCA1-mediated cell growth suppression. Oncogene 16(9):1097–1112
148. Ventii KH, Devi NS, Friedrich KL et al (2008) BRCA1-associated protein-1 is a tumor suppressor that requires deubiquitinating activity and nuclear localization. Cancer Res 68(17):6953–6962
149. DiGiovanna JJ, Kraemer KH (2012) Shining a light on xeroderma pigmentosum. J Invest Dermatol 132(3 Pt 2):785–796
150. Kraemer KH, Lee MM, Scotto J (1987) Xeroderma pigmentosum. Cutaneous, ocular, and neurologic abnormalities in 830 published cases. Arch Dermatol 123(2):241–250
151. Ramkumar HL, Brooks BP, Cao X et al (2011) Ophthalmic manifestations and histopathology of xeroderma pigmentosum: two clinicopathological cases and a review of the literature. Surv Ophthalmol 56(4):348–361
152. Dollfus H, Porto F, Caussade P et al (2003) Ocular manifestations in the inherited DNA repair disorders. Surv Ophthalmol 48(1):107–122
153. Donnelly MP, Paschou P, Grigorenko E et al (2012) A global view of the OCA2-HERC2 region and pigmentation. Hum Genet 131(5):683–696
154. Mengel-From J, Wong TH, Morling N, Rees JL, Jackson IJ (2009) Genetic determinants of hair and eye colours in the Scottish and Danish populations. BMC Genet 10:88
155. Jannot AS, Meziani R, Bertrand G et al (2005) Allele variations in the OCA2 gene (pink-eyed-dilution locus) are associated with genetic susceptibility to melanoma. Eur J Hum Genet 13(8):913–920
156. Guedj M, Bourillon A, Combadieres C et al (2008) Variants of the MATP/SLC45A2 gene are protective for melanoma in the French population. Hum Mutat 29(9):1154–1160
157. Nan H, Kraft P, Hunter DJ, Han J (2009) Genetic variants in pigmentation genes, pigmentary phenotypes, and risk of skin cancer in Caucasians. Int J Cancer 125(4):909–917
158. Hawkes JE, Cassidy PB, Manga P et al (2013) Report of a novel OCA2 gene mutation and an investigation of OCA2 variants on melanoma risk in a familial melanoma pedigree. J Dermatol Sci 69(1):30–37
159. Duffy DL, Zhao ZZ, Sturm RA, Hayward NK, Martin NG, Montgomery GW (2010) Multiple pigmentation gene polymorphisms account for a substantial proportion of risk of cutaneous malignant melanoma. J Invest Dermatol 130(2):520–528
160. Shekar SN, Duffy DL, Youl P et al (2009) A population-based study of Australian twins with melanoma suggests a strong genetic contribution to liability. J Invest Dermatol 129(9):2211–2219
161. Box NF, Duffy DL, Chen W et al (2001) MC1R genotype modifies risk of melanoma in families segregating CDKN2A mutations. Am J Hum Genet 69(4):765–773
162. Williams PF, Olsen CM, Hayward NK, Whiteman DC (2011) Melanocortin 1 receptor and risk of cutaneous melanoma: a meta-analysis and estimates of population burden. Int J Cancer 129(7):1730–1740
163. Tsatmali M, Ancans J, Yukitake J, Thody AJ (2000) Skin POMC peptides: their actions at the human MC-1 receptor and roles in the tanning response. Pigment Cell Res 13(Suppl 8):125–129
164. Busca R, Ballotti R (2000) Cyclic AMP a key messenger in the regulation of skin pigmentation. Pigment Cell Res 13(2):60–69
165. Raimondi S, Sera F, Gandini S et al (2008) MC1R variants, melanoma and red hair color phenotype: a meta-analysis. Int J Cancer 122(12):2753–2760

166. Valverde P, Healy E, Jackson I, Rees JL, Thody AJ (1995) Variants of the melanocyte-stimulating hormone receptor gene are associated with red hair and fair skin in humans. Nat Genet 11(3):328–330
167. Chatzinasiou F, Lill CM, Kypreou K et al (2011) Comprehensive field synopsis and systematic meta-analyses of genetic association studies in cutaneous melanoma. J Natl Cancer Inst 103(16):1227–1235
168. Palmer JS, Duffy DL, Box NF et al (2000) Melanocortin-1 receptor polymorphisms and risk of melanoma: is the association explained solely by pigmentation phenotype? Am J Hum Genet 66(1):176–186
169. Kennedy C, ter Huurne J, Berkhout M et al (2001) Melanocortin 1 receptor (MC1R) gene variants are associated with an increased risk for cutaneous melanoma which is largely independent of skin type and hair color. J Invest Dermatol 117(2):294–300
170. Bertolotto C, Lesueur F, Giuliano S et al (2011) A SUMOylation-defective MITF germline mutation predisposes to melanoma and renal carcinoma. Nature 480(7375):94–98
171. Fernandez LP, Milne RL, Pita G et al (2008) SLC45A2: a novel malignant melanoma-associated gene. Hum Mutat 29(9):1161–1167
172. Ibarrola-Villava M, Fernandez LP, Alonso S et al (2011) A customized pigmentation SNP array identifies a novel SNP associated with melanoma predisposition in the SLC45A2 gene. PLoS One 6(4):e19271
173. Ibarrola-Villava M, Hu HH, Guedj M et al (2012) MC1R, SLC45A2 and TYR genetic variants involved in melanoma susceptibility in southern European populations: results from a meta-analysis. Eur J Cancer 48(14):2183–2191
174. Brown KM, Macgregor S, Montgomery GW et al (2008) Common sequence variants on 20q11.22 confer melanoma susceptibility. Nat Genet 40(7):838–840
175. Gudbjartsson DF, Sulem P, Stacey SN et al (2008) ASIP and TYR pigmentation variants associate with cutaneous melanoma and basal cell carcinoma. Nat Genet 40(7):886–891
176. Bishop DT, Demenais F, Iles MM et al (2009) Genome-wide association study identifies three loci associated with melanoma risk. Nat Genet 41(8):920–925
177. Sturm RA, O'Sullivan BJ, Box NF et al (1995) Chromosomal structure of the human TYRP1 and TYRP2 loci and comparison of the tyrosinase-related protein gene family. Genomics 29(1):24–34
178. Yokoyama S, Woods SL, Boyle GM et al (2011) A novel recurrent mutation in MITF predisposes to familial and sporadic melanoma. Nature 480(7375):99–103
179. Sulem P, Gudbjartsson DF, Stacey SN et al (2008) Two newly identified genetic determinants of pigmentation in Europeans. Nat Genet 40(7):835–837
180. Song F, Qureshi AA, Giovannucci EL et al (2013) Risk of a second primary cancer after non-melanoma skin cancer in white men and women: a prospective cohort study. PLoS Med 10(4):e1001433
181. Green AC, O'Rourke MG (1985) Cutaneous malignant melanoma in association with other skin cancers. J Natl Cancer Inst 74(5):977–980
182. Marghoob AA, Slade J, Salopek TG, Kopf AW, Bart RS, Rigel DS (1995) Basal cell and squamous cell carcinomas are important risk factors for cutaneous malignant melanoma. Screening implications. Cancer 75(2 Suppl):707–714
183. Lindelof B, Sigurgeirsson B, Wallberg P, Eklund G (1991) Occurrence of other malignancies in 1973 patients with basal cell carcinoma. J Am Acad Dermatol 25(2 Pt 1):245–248
184. MacKie RM, Hauschild A, Eggermont AM (2009) Epidemiology of invasive cutaneous melanoma. Ann Oncol 20(Suppl 6):vi1–vi7
185. Ferrone CR, Ben Porat L, Panageas KS et al (2005) Clinicopathological features of and risk factors for multiple primary melanomas. JAMA 294(13):1647–1654
186. Caini S, Gandini S, Sera F et al (2009) Meta-analysis of risk factors for cutaneous melanoma according to anatomical site and clinico-pathological variant. Eur J Cancer 45(17): 3054–3063
187. Bevona C, Goggins W, Quinn T, Fullerton J, Tsao H (2003) Cutaneous melanomas associated with nevi. Arch Dermatol 139(12):1620–1624, discussion 1624

188. Marks R, Dorevitch AP, Mason G (1990) Do all melanomas come from "moles"? A study of the histological association between melanocytic naevi and melanoma. Australas J Dermatol 31(2):77–80

189. Kelly JW, Yeatman JM, Regalia C, Mason G, Henham AP (1997) A high incidence of melanoma found in patients with multiple dysplastic naevi by photographic surveillance. Med J Aust 167(4):191–194

190. Goodson AG, Grossman D (2009) Strategies for early melanoma detection: approaches to the patient with nevi. J Am Acad Dermatol 60(5):719–735, quiz 736–718

191. Goodson AG, Florell SR, Hyde M, Bowen GM, Grossman D (2010) Comparative analysis of total body and dermatoscopic photographic monitoring of nevi in similar patient populations at risk for cutaneous melanoma. Dermatol Surg 36(7):1087–1098

192. Olsen CM, Carroll HJ, Whiteman DC (2010) Estimating the attributable fraction for cancer: a meta-analysis of nevi and melanoma. Cancer Prev Res (Phila) 3(2):233–245

193. Vourc'h-Jourdain M, Martin L, Barbarot S (2013) Large congenital melanocytic nevi: therapeutic management and melanoma risk: a systematic review. J Am Acad Dermatol 68(3):493–498.e491–414

194. Kareus SA, Figueroa KP, Cannon-Albright LA, Pulst SM (2012) Shared predispositions of parkinsonism and cancer: a population-based pedigree-linked study. Arch Neurol 69(12):1572–1577

195. Leachman SA, Carucci J, Kohlmann W et al (2009) Selection criteria for genetic assessment of patients with familial melanoma. J Am Acad Dermatol 61(4):677.e671–614

196. Kohlmann W, Dunn K, Leachman S (2008) Role of genetic testing in hereditary melanoma. Expert Rev 3:639–643

197. Begg CB, Orlow I, Hummer AJ et al (2005) Lifetime risk of melanoma in CDKN2A mutation carriers in a population-based sample. J Natl Cancer Inst 97(20):1507–1515

198. Hansen CB, Wadge LM, Lowstuter K, Boucher K, Leachman SA (2004) Clinical germline genetic testing for melanoma. Lancet Oncol 5(5):314–319

199. Aspinwall LG, Taber JM, Leaf SL, Kohlmann W, Leachman SA (2013) Genetic testing for hereditary melanoma and pancreatic cancer: a longitudinal study of psychological outcome. Psychooncology 22(2):276–289

200. Aspinwall LG, Leaf SL, Kohlmann W, Dola ER, Leachman SA (2009) Patterns of photoprotection following CDKN2A/p16 genetic test reporting and counseling. J Am Acad Dermatol 60(5):745–757

201. Kasparian NA, Meiser B, Butow PN, Simpson JM, Mann GJ (2009) Genetic testing for melanoma risk: a prospective cohort study of uptake and outcomes among Australian families. Genet Med 11(4):265–278

202. Robson ME, Storm CD, Weitzel J, Wollins DS, Offit K (2010) American Society of Clinical Oncology policy statement update: genetic and genomic testing for cancer susceptibility. J Clin Oncol 28(5):893–901

203. Berliner JL, Fay AM, Cummings SA, Burnett B, Tillmanns T (2013) NSGC practice guideline: risk assessment and genetic counseling for hereditary breast and ovarian cancer. J Genet Couns 22(2):155–163

204. Aitken JF, Youl P, Green A, MacLennan R, Martin NG (1996) Accuracy of case-reported family history of melanoma in Queensland, Australia. Melanoma Res 6(4):313–317

205. Bataille V, de Vries E (2008) Melanoma—Part 1: epidemiology, risk factors, and prevention. BMJ 337:a2249

206. Lazovich D, Vogel RI, Berwick M, Weinstock MA, Warshaw EM, Anderson KE (2011) Melanoma risk in relation to use of sunscreen or other sun protection methods. Cancer Epidemiol Biomarkers Prev 20(12):2583–2593

207. Wolff T, Tai E, Miller T (2009) Screening for skin cancer: an update of the evidence for the U.S. Preventive Services Task Force. Ann Intern Med 150(3):194–198

208. Gimotty PA, Glanz K (2011) Sunscreen and melanoma: what is the evidence? J Clin Oncol 29(3):249–250

209. Lin JS, Eder M, Weinmann S (2011) Behavioral counseling to prevent skin cancer: a systematic review for the U.S. Preventive Services Task Force. Ann Intern Med 154(3):190–201
210. Bordeaux JS, Lu KQ, Cooper KD (2007) Melanoma: prevention and early detection. Semin Oncol 34(6):460–466
211. Austoker J (1994) Melanoma: prevention and early diagnosis. BMJ 308(6945):1682–1686
212. Rager EL, Bridgeford EP, Ollila DW (2005) Cutaneous melanoma: update on prevention, screening, diagnosis, and treatment. Am Fam Physician 72(2):269–276
213. Hamidi R, Peng D, Cockburn M (2010) Efficacy of skin self-examination for the early detection of melanoma. Int J Dermatol 49(2):126–134
214. Koh HK, Norton LA, Geller AC et al (1996) Evaluation of the American Academy of Dermatology's national skin cancer early detection and screening program. J Am Acad Dermatol 34(6):971–978

Chapter 6
The MAPK Pathway in Melanoma

Leomar Y. Ballester, Phyu P. Aung, and Chyi-Chia R. Lee

Abstract Dysregulation of the mitogen-activated protein kinase (MAPK) pathway has been associated with various neoplasms including melanomas. Common alterations in the MAPK pathway in melanomas include mutations in *BRAF, EGFR, KIT, RAS, MEK*, and *ERK*. The increased understanding of the biology and genetics of melanoma has generated interest in targeting the MAPK pathway for the treatment of melanoma. Vemurafenib, which targets the BRAF-V600E mutant protein, was the first FDA-approved drug for the treatment of patients with metastatic melanoma. In this chapter, we summarize the current understanding of the contributions of MAPK pathway alterations to melanoma development. We also discuss the association between mutations in particular genes and specific melanoma subtypes and the role of MAPK alterations in melanoma diagnosis. Therapeutic agents, in various stages of development, which target members of the MAPK pathway, are also discussed.

Keywords Mitogen-activated protein kinase pathway • MAPK • Targeted therapy • Melanoma • *BRAF* • *NRAS* • EGFR • KIT • *HRAS*

6.1   The MAPK Pathway

The mitogen-activated protein kinases (MAPK) pathway, also known as the Ras/Raf/MEK/ERK pathway, is a signaling cascade involved in transducing signals from the plasma membrane to the nucleus via consecutive phosphorylation events

L.Y. Ballester, MD, PhD (✉)
Department of Pathology and Genomic Medicine, Houston Methodist Hospital, Houston, TX, USA
e-mail: mreslyb@houstonmethodist.org

P.P. Aung, MD, PhD
Department of Pathology, The University of Texas, MD Anderson Cancer Center, Houston, TX, USA
e-mail: PAung@mdanderson.org

C.-C. R. Lee, MD, PhD (✉)
Laboratory of Pathology, National Cancer Institute, National Institutes of Health, Bethesda, MD, USA
e-mail: leechy@mail.nih.gov

© Springer Science+Business Media New York 2016
C.A. Torres-Cabala, J.L. Curry (eds.), *Genetics of Melanoma*, Cancer Genetics, DOI 10.1007/978-1-4939-3554-3_6

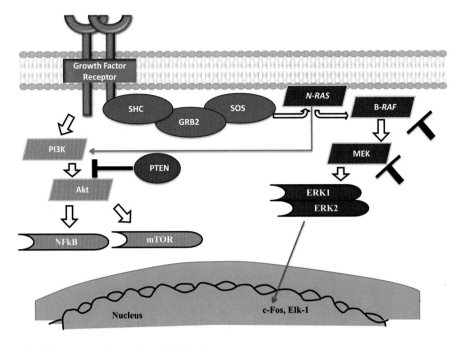

Fig. 6.1 Diagram of MAPK and PI3K pathways

(Fig. 6.1). The MAPK are a family of serine/threonine kinases that are involved in regulating cell growth, differentiation, and apoptosis [1]. The activity of the enzymes is regulated by a phosphorylation cascade initiated by the activation of a membrane receptor. The activation of the membrane receptor is the result of a conformational change in protein structure as a result of ligand binding. The ligand-induced confor-mational change promotes the interaction of the membrane receptor with an intracel-lular adaptor protein (i.e., Shc, GRB2, etc.). The adaptor protein, in turn, interacts with a guanine nucleotide exchange factor (i.e., SOS), which communicates the sig-nal to a small GTP-binding protein (i.e., RAS). Subsequently, RAS activates RAF (MAPKinase-kinase-kinase/MAPKKK), the first intracellular kinase in the cascade. RAF kinases are a family of serine/threonine kinases, including ARAF, BRAF and CRAF. Once activated, RAF phosphorylates the downstream kinase MEK (MAPKinase-kinase/MAPKK), which in turns activates the extracellular signal-reg-ulated kinase (ERK/MAPK). ERK can directly phosphorylate several transcription factors, regulating the expression of genes involved in cell growth and proliferation [2]. The complexity of this signaling pathway is highlighted by the existence of three RAS (HRAS, NRAS, KRAS), three RAF (ARAF, BRAF, CRAF), two MEK (MEK1 and MEK2), and two ERK isoforms (ERK1 and ERK2) (Table 6.1). Alterations at different points in this pathway can lead to uncontrolled cell growth and proliferation and contribute to the development of various cancers, including melanoma.

Table 6.1 Chromosomal location and molecular weight (MW) of key proteins in the MAPK pathway

	Chromosome	MW (Da)
EGFR (ERB1)	7p12	134,277
KIT (c-Kit)	4q11–q12	109,865
NRAS	1p13.2	21,229
HRAS	11p15.5	21,298
BRAF	7q34	84,437
MEK1 (MAP2K1)	15q22.1–q22.33	43,439
MEK2 (MAP2K2)	19p13.3	44,424
ERK1 (MAPK3)	16p11.2	43,136
ERK2 (MAPK1)	22q11.21	41,390

6.2 Common MAPK Alterations in Melanoma

Alterations at various points in the MAPK pathway have been associated with a variety of cancers [3]. Activating mutations in NRAS and BRAF occur in 15–30 and 60–70 % of melanomas, respectively [4] (Table 6.2). These alterations appear to be insufficient for the development of melanoma, considering that a number of benign nevi also carry mutations in the BRAF and NRAS genes. The additional genetic alterations, besides activating mutations in BRAF and NRAS, that are necessary for progression into melanoma, remain poorly understood.

The classification of melanomas according to specific genetic alterations will become important as more targeted therapies, designed against specific mutant proteins in selected pathways, become available. In addition to the well-known role of the MAPK pathway in growth and proliferation, it has been proposed that activation of the pathway also contributes to melanoma immune evasion, further contributing to cancer development [5]. This idea, in addition to contributing to our understanding of the mechanisms behind melanoma development, could have implications for immunotherapies that are currently under development for the treatment of melanoma.

6.3 EGFR

The epidermal growth factor receptor (EGFR), located in chromosome 7p12, is a 134 kDa protein member of the tyrosine kinase receptor family. Activation of EGFR leads to stimulation of the MAPK pathway and cell division. EGFR dysregulation has been shown to contribute to several cancers, and it has been studied as a potential therapeutic target for various malignancies [6]. EGFR is believed to be expressed at low-to-intermediate levels in melanoma cells [7]. Several studies have looked at EGFR mutations in melanoma; however, there is conflicting evidence regarding the contributions of EGFR alterations to melanoma development and its potential usefulness as a therapeutic target [8, 9].

Table 6.2 Common mutations in the MAPK pathway found in melanomas

Gene	Exon	DNA base change	AA change	Estimated frequency (%)
KIT	11	c.1727T>C	L576P	25
	11	c.1676T>C	V559A	20
	13	c.1924A>G	K642E	20
NRAS	2	c.182A>G	Q61R	35
	2	c.181C>A	Q61K	34
BRAF	15	c.1799T>A	V600E	80
	15	c.1798_1799delGTinsAA	V600K	5
MEK1	3	c.370C>T	P124S	a
	3	c.607G>A	E203K	a
MEK2	4	c.461C>T	S154F	a
	6	c.622G>A	E207L	a

Estimated frequency of specific amino acid changes as a percentage of melanomas with mutations in each particular gene
[a]Only a few cases reported
For a more comprehensive list of mutations in melanoma visit:
http://www.mycancergenome.org
http://cancer.sanger.ac.uk/cancergenome/projets/osmic/

6.4 KIT

The KIT gene, located in chromosome 4q12, encodes a 145 kDa membrane-associated receptor tyrosine kinase. KIT mutations have been reported in several cancers including melanomas. KIT mutations occur more frequently in acral and mucosal melanomas than in melanomas occurring at sites with intermittent sun exposure. A study looking at 102 primary melanomas from mucosa, acral skin, and the skin with and without chronic sun damage found KIT mutations in 39 % of mucosal, 36 % of acral, and 28 % of melanomas on the skin with chronic sun damage. However, no mutations were found in melanomas occurring in the skin without chronic sun damage [10]. The most common KIT mutations found in that study were K642E and L576P, both of which have also been reported in gastrointestinal stromal cell tumors (GIST) [11]. The reported frequency of KIT mutations in acral lentiginous melanoma (ALM) ranges between 10 and 15 % [12, 13].

In a study by Dika et al., 20 % of melanomas from the nail apparatus had mutations in the KIT gene including P551L (exon 11), V560D (exon 11), or D816N (exon 17) substitutions [14]. In contrast, only 4 % of sinonasal mucosal melanomas showed KIT mutations [12]. The majority of KIT mutations in acral lentiginous, mucosal, and nail apparatus melanoma are reported to occur in exon 11, with mutations occurring less frequently in exons 13 and 17 [12–14]. In contrast, no KIT mutations were identified in a study looking at 24 spindle cell melanomas [15]. Mutations in KIT have the potential of activating both the MAPK and PI3K pathways. In contrast, mutations affecting a protein downstream in the signaling cascade, such as BRAF, are less likely to activate the PI3K pathway (Fig. 6.1).

6.5 NRAS

Members of the RAS family are mutated in a number of tumors. The highest incidence of mutated RAS genes is found in tumors of the exocrine pancreas, colon carcinomas, and follicular and undifferentiated thyroid carcinomas [16]. NRAS is a 21 kDa protein, located in chromosome 1p13.2. It is a member of the small GTPase family of proteins, which also includes KRAS and HRAS. These are GTP-binding proteins with the intrinsic ability to hydrolyze GTP into GDP. The RAS protein becomes active upon GTP binding; the hydrolysis of GTP into GDP promotes the change into the inactive conformation. Mutations in RAS typically interfere with the ability of the protein to switch to the inactive conformation, leading to excessive RAS signaling. RAS proteins activate several pathways, and they serve as positive regulators of the MAPK pathway through activation of RAF.

Several studies have reported the presence of NRAS mutations in melanomas [12, 14, 17]. The percentage varies among melanoma subtypes, but about 15–20 % of all melanomas are believed to harbor a mutation in NRAS [18]. Although NRAS mutations occur at a low frequency in acquired nevi, they seem to be commonly present in congenital nevi (~80 %). This is in contrast to BRAF mutations, which are rare or absent in congenital nevi [19]. NRAS mutations also have been reported to occur more commonly in sun-exposed areas.

RAS proteins also have the ability to activate the PI3K/Akt pathway [20]. A study by Posch et al. showed that both the MEK/ERK and PI3K/mTor pathways were active in about half of melanoma samples harboring NRAS mutations [21]. In addition, a combination of MEK and PI3K pathway inhibitors showed greater growth inhibition of melanoma cells, than a MEK inhibitor alone. Increased phospho-Akt expression in melanoma has been associated with tumor progression and shorter survival [22].

It is interesting that the occurrence of BRAF and NRAS mutations in melanoma appear to be mutually exclusive events [23, 24]. This suggests that once the MAPK pathway becomes constitutively active by any particular mutation, the progression to melanoma depends on alterations in other proteins outside of the MAPK pathway (Table 6.1).

6.6 HRAS

HRAS is a 21 kDa GTPase involved in signal transduction in the MAPK pathway. The HRAS gene is located in chromosome 11p15.5. While NRAS mutations have been described in a subset of melanomas, HRAS mutations have been described in a subset of Spitz nevi [25–27]. The Spitz nevus is a melanocytic proliferation of epithelioid or spindled cells that occur more commonly in young patients. At times it can be difficult to distinguish Spitz nevi from Spitzoid melanoma. In a study looking at 170 Spitz lesions (93 Spitz nevi and 77 Spitz tumor of unknown malignant potential), it was found that 24 (14 %) lesions harbored an HRAS mutation. None of the patients with an HRAS mutation developed recurrences or metastases after a mean follow-up of 10.5 years. This has led various authors to conclude that the presence of an HRAS mutation in a Spitz lesion is an indicator of good prognosis [27, 28]. The idea is also supported by the fact that no HRAS mutations have been found in Spitzoid melanomas [29]. In contrast, 86 % of Spitzoid melanomas were found to have BRAF or NRAS mutations [26]. These data suggest that Spitzoid nevi and Spitzoid melanomas are genetically distinct lesions. It also suggests that incorporating genetic testing in the diagnosis of challenging Spitzoid lesions can be helpful. The most common *HRAS* mutations reported in Spitz nevi alter glutamine at position 61 (HRAS, Exon 3, c.182A>T : Q61L, c.182A>G : Q61R and c.181C>A : Q61K).

Sarin et al. published an interesting report on a single patient that provides a good example of progressive genetic alterations in Spitz nevi arising in association with a nevus spilus [25]. A 24-year-old patient presented with multiple pink papules arising in a large congenital pigmented patch. Histologic examination of two papules revealed Spitz nevi. The normal skin adjacent to the lesion, the pigmented patch, and the pink papules were genetically analyzed. The results showed the presence of HRAS mutation in cells from the pigmented patch and the Spitz nevi with adjacent normal skin having no HRAS mutations. In addition, the Spitz nevi showed increased copy number of chromosome 11p, where the HRAS gene is located. Amplification of chromosome 11p has been reported in Spitz nevi with a frequency of approximately 12 %, and HRAS mutations are detected at a higher frequency in cases with 11p amplification than in cases with normal copy numbers [30].

6.7   BRAF

Effectors or downstream targets of the RAS protein include ARAF, BRAF, and CRAF. The BRAF gene is an oncogene located in chromosome 7q34. It has 18 exons and encodes for an 84 kDa cytoplasmic serine/threonine kinase responsible for transducing mitogenic signals from the cell membrane to the nucleus. Several mutations in *BRAF* have been found in melanoma, the majority occurring within the P-loop and activation segments of the protein [31]. These mutations are thought to destabilize the inactive conformation, resulting in constitutive kinase activity leading to over activation of the pathway. The *BRAF-V600E* mutation, localized to exon 11, is the most common BRAF mutation found in melanomas [17, 32]. The V600E mutation introduces a conformational change in protein structure; the incorporation of glutamic acid acts as a phosphomimetic between the Thr598 and Ser601 phosphorylation sites, leading to constitutive activation of the protein with a substantial increase in the basal kinase activity [20]. The V600E mutation imparts a 480-fold increase in BRAF activity over the wild-type protein, which is associated with a 4.6-fold increase in ERK activity [31]. However, the increase in BRAF/ERK activity seems to be insufficient for melanoma development, given that BRAF mutations are also found in 86 % of benign nevi [33]. Additional alterations that are believed to contribute to melanoma progression remain to be identified.

A study with melanoma cell lines suggests that not only mutations that increased BRAF activity but also increased BRAF levels contribute to development of melanoma [34]. For example, cell lines with WT BRAF and NRAS showed higher levels of BRAF than cell lines with either of the genes mutated. It is also interesting that even when the MAPK pathway is constitutively active in uveal melanomas, these tumors typically do not have mutations in RAS or RAF genes [35], suggesting that other alterations can contribute to MAPK pathway activation in melanomas.

Similar rates of *BRAF* mutations are present in primary and metastatic melanomas, as well as in cultured malignant melanoma cell lines, suggesting that *BRAF* mutations occur before tumor dissemination and their incidence remains constant during tumor progression [36]. The frequency of BRAF mutations in melanoma varies among the four melanoma subtypes: the skin without chronic sun damage (59 %), acral skin (23 %), skin with chronic sun damage (11 %), and mucosal (11 %) [23, 37]. One study evaluating 16 cases of nail apparatus melanoma for *BRAF* mutations found that only one of the 16 cases had the *BRAF* mutation K601E [14]. The remaining 15 cases did not have a mutation in the *BRAF* gene. Another study looking at ALM in a cohort of Swedish patients found *BRAF* mutations in 17 % of cases, with KIT or *NRAS* mutations occurring in 15 % of cases, respectively [13]. In these series, *BRAF* mutations occur more commonly in women and in tumor located in the feet. Anatomical site was an independent predictor of survival, with tumors located in the hands having better prognosis than tumors located in the feet. One can speculate that the effect could be due to tumors in the upper extremities being discovered earlier than tumors in the lower extremities.

6.8 MEK

The mitogen-activated protein kinase (MEK) is a 43 kDa member of the MAPK pathway located in chromosome 15q22.1–q22.3. The RAF protein activates MEK, whose function is to activate ERK via phosphorylation. Mutations in *MEK1* (*MAP2K1*) and *MEK2* (*MAP2K2*) have been identified in melanomas at a frequency of 8 % (10/127 cases) according to one study [38]. The reported MEK1 mutations in order of frequency include P124S, E203L, F53L, and N382H. The mutations had a gain of function effect, leading to constitutive phosphorylation of ERK; however, E203L mutation was shown to have stronger effects on ERK phosphorylation compared to P124S. Two mutations in *MEK2* (S154F and E207L) were reported in the same study.

6.9 ERK

ERK1 (*MAPK3*, 41 kDa), located in chromosome 16p11.2, and *ERK2* (*MAPK1*, 43 kDa), located in chromosome 22q11.21, are protein kinases activated by MEK. Normal melanocytes do not have detectable ERK activity, but ERK's activity is increased in the majority of melanoma cell lines. The increase in ERK activity is often due to mutations in *BRAF* or *NRAS*. Upon activation, ERK can phosphorylate cytoplasmic targets and/or move to the nucleus where it can activate several transcription factors (Elk-1, Myc, CREB, Fos, etc.), which can bind the promoters of many genes [39]. Studies with melanoma cell lines have shown that reducing ERK expression by shRNA results in apoptosis, supporting the potential therapeutic effects of targeting ERK for the treatment of melanoma [40].

6.10   Targeting the MAPK Pathway for the Treatment of Melanoma

In the past, DNA alkylating agents, such as Dacarbazine, were the treatments of choice for metastatic melanoma. However, only a small (10–20 %) subset of patients responded, and it is questionable whether these drugs lead to any significant increase in life expectancy [41]. Considering the poor prognosis of patients with advanced metastatic melanomas, it is clear that more effective drugs are needed. Given the high incidence of MAPK pathway alterations in melanomas and other cancers, it is not surprising that several therapeutic strategies targeting specific proteins in the pathway have emerged. In 2011, the FDA approved the first drug directed against one of the proteins in the MAPK pathway, a BRAF inhibitor, for the treatment of metastatic melanoma, vemurafenib. Vemurafenib, which targets the BRAF protein with the V600E mutation, was the first drug to show a quantifiable increase in the life expectancy of patients with metastatic melanoma [42]. Subsequently, there has been an interest in drugs targeting other proteins in the pathway and combination strategies targeting multiple members of the pathway simultaneously.

6.10.1   Targeting KIT

Imatinib It is a potent kit inhibitor used in the treatment of chronic myelogenous leukemia and approved for the treatment of GIST. It is currently in clinical trials (trial# NCT00424515) for the treatment of metastatic melanoma originating from acral or mucosal sites (*KIT* mutations have been reported in melanomas from these sites).

6.10.2   Targeting RAS

Tipifarnib Addition of a farnesyl group to the RAS protein is important for its proper subcellular localization and function. The process of farnesylation is catalyzed by the enzyme farnesyl transferase. This enzyme is essential for the activation of RAS. Tipifarnib is an imidazole-containing methylquinoline, which is a selective inhibitor of farnesyl transferase [43]. Preclinical experiments with farnesyl transferase inhibitors have shown growth inhibition in 75 % of human tumor cell lines. A phase II clinical trial (NCT00060125) enrolled 14 patients with metastatic melanoma and looked at the effectiveness of tipifarnib (R115777) [44]. However, no clinical responses were observed in this trial, despite detecting 85–98 % inhibition of farnesyl transferase activity in tumor tissue biopsies. Another phase II clinical trial (NCT00281957) with 102 patients, comparing a combination of sorafenib and temsirolimus (an mTOR inhibitor) versus sorafenib and tipifarnib, failed to show significant activity in both arms of the study. The results of these trials put into question the usefulness of inhibiting farnesyl transferase in the treatment of melanoma.

6.10.3   Targeting BRAF

Vemurafenib   A BRAF inhibitor was the first drug approved in the US for the treatment of metastatic melanoma carrying a *BRAF* mutation. Various clinical trials have demonstrated the efficacy of vemurafenib in the treatment of advanced melanoma (NCT00949702, NCT01006980). A phase 3 randomized clinical trial with 675 patients with metastatic melanoma positive for the BRAF-V600E mutation showed higher response rates and increased overall survival with vemurafenib treatment [42]. Interestingly, whereas vemurafenib can inhibit the MAPK pathway, it has been shown to activate it in BRAF-WT cells. This effect might stimulate BRAF-WT melanoma cells and perhaps could contribute to the development of drug resistance. The development of drug resistance is a major problem limiting the effectiveness of vemurafenib, and some studies propose intermittent dosing as a mechanism to prevent the development of drug-resistant disease [45].

Sorafenib   An oral multi-kinase inhibitor that decreases activity of RAF, VEGFR 1-3, PDGFR, Flt-3, p38, c-kit, and FGFR-1. It has the ability of inhibiting tumor cell growth and angiogenesis [20, 43]. A phase II clinical trial evaluating sorafenib as a single agent in patients with advanced melanoma failed to show significant antitumor activity [46]. Similarly, a phase III clinical trial with 270 patients, evaluating the efficacy of sorafenib in combination with carboplatin and paclitaxel, showed that addition of sorafenib did not improve progression-free survival in patients with advanced melanoma [47]. It has been shown that sorafenib activates glycogen synthase kinase-3β (GSK-3β) in melanoma cell lines (129,130). Constitutive activation of this kinase correlates with a marked increase in basal levels of Bcl-2 and Bcl-x(L), inhibitors of apoptosis. Perhaps this effect contributes to reducing the antitumor efficacy of sorafenib [20].

Dabrafenib   A reversible, competitive inhibitor that inhibits *BRAF*-V600E activity. The results of various clinical trials (NCT00880321, NCT01227889, NCT01266967) have shown response rates of approximately 30–50 % and improvements in pro-gression-free survival in patients with metastatic melanoma harboring the V600E mutation.

Other compounds like RAF265 and XL281 are currently in clinical trials (NCT00304525, NCT00451880) for the treatment of melanoma [43].

6.10.4   Targeting MEK1/MEK2

Given that mutations in *c-KIT*, *NRAS*, and *BRAF* lead to activation of the pathway, it is sensible to hypothesize that inhibition of MEK could be an effective treatment for melanoma. Interestingly, a study by Solit et al. showed that the BRAF-V600E mutation was associated with enhanced sensitivity to MEK inhibitors, when com-pared to cells with either WT-*BRAF* or mutated *NRAS* [48]. The difference in sensi-tivity might be explained by the ability of mutant *NRAS* to activate the PI3K pathway in addition to the MAPK pathway. In contrast, the effects of mutant BRAF alter the MAPK pathway more selectively, making the cells more susceptible to MEK inhib-itors. Since the efficacy of MEK inhibitors is higher in melanomas with *BRAF* mutations than with *NRAS* mutations, it has been proposed the stratification of MEK inhibitor trials according to *BRAF* status. In fact, it appears that compounds with distinct mechanisms of inhibition are more effective in one melanoma versus another based on the presence of *BRAF* versus *NRAS* mutations [49]. This confirms the need to stratify MEK inhibitor trials according to the presence or absence of mutations in *BRAF*, *NRAS*, or *MEK*.

Several MEK inhibitors are being studied for the treatment of melanoma as sin-gle agent or in combination with BRAF inhibitors.

CI-1040   This was the first MEK inhibitor tested in clinical trials. However, efforts to move CI-1040 into the clinic were discontinued due to poor bioavailability and low antitumor activity [50, 51].

PD035901   This compound has improved pharmacologic properties, but an initial clinical trial (NCT00147550) was discontinued due to significant toxicity [52].

AZD6244   It is a very specific MEK1/MEK2 inhibitor that also has the ability to arrest cells in the G1 phase.

Trametinib   It is a selective MEK1 and MEK2 inhibitor. A clinical trial, with 322 patients with metastatic melanoma harboring the BRAF V600E or V600K mutation, compared trametinib versus chemotherapy. Patients treated with trametinib showed improved pro-gression-free and overall survival than patients treated with chemotherapy [53].

MEK162   It is a selective MEK1/MEK2 inhibitor. A phase II clinical trial with patients having *NRAS*- or *BRAF*-mutated advanced melanoma showed partial response in 20 % of patients in each group [54]. This is the first targeted therapy to show some activity in patients with *NRAS*-mutated melanoma.

References

1. Pearson G, Robinson F, Beers Gibson T et al (2001) Mitogen-activated protein (MAP) kinase pathways: regulation and physiological functions. Endocr Rev 22:153–183
2. McCubrey JA, Steelman LS, Chappell WH et al (2007) Roles of the Raf/MEK/ERK pathway in cell growth, malignant transformation and drug resistance. Biochim Biophys Acta 1773:1263–1284.
3. Dhillon AS, Hagan S, Rath O, Kolch W (2007) MAP kinase signalling pathways in cancer. Oncogene 26:3279–3290.
4. Gray-Schopfer VC, da Rocha DS (2005) The role of B-RAF in melanoma. Cancer Metastasis Rev 24:165–183
5. Sumimoto H, Imabayashi F, Iwata T, Kawakami Y (2006) The BRAF-MAPK signaling pathway is essential for cancer-immune evasion in human melanoma cells. J Exp Med 203:1651–1656.
6. Ciardiello F, Tortora G (2008) EGFR antagonists in cancer treatment. N Engl J Med 358: 1160–1174.
7. Ivanov VN, Hei TK (2004) Combined treatment with EGFR inhibitors and arsenite upregulated apoptosis in human EGFR-positive melanomas: a role of suppression of the PI3K-AKT pathway. Oncogene 24:616–626.
8. Boone B, Jacobs K, Ferdinande L et al (2011) EGFR in melanoma: clinical significance and potential therapeutic target. J Cutan Pathol 38:492–502.
9. Rákosy Z, Vízkeleti L, Ecsedi S et al (2007) EGFR gene copy number alterations in primary cutaneous malignant melanomas are associated with poor prognosis. Int J Cancer 121: 1729–1737.
10. Curtin JA, Busam K, Pinkel D, Bastian BC (2006) Somatic activation of KIT in distinct subtypes of melanoma. J Clin Oncol 24:4340–4346.
11. Heinrich MC, Corless CL, Demetri GD et al (2003) Kinase mutations and imatinib response in patients with metastatic gastrointestinal stromal tumor. J Clin Oncol 21:4342–4349.
12. Zebary A, Jangard M, Omholt K et al (2013) KIT, NRAS and BRAF mutations in sinonasal mucosal melanoma: a study of 56 cases. Br J Cancer 109:559–564.
13. Zebary A, Omholt K, Vassilaki I et al (2013) KIT, NRAS, BRAF and PTEN mutations in a sample of Swedish patients with acral lentiginous melanoma. J Dermatol Sci 72:284–289.
14. Dika E, Altimari A, Patrizi A et al (2013) KIT, NRAS, and BRAF mutations in nail apparatus melanoma. Pigment Cell Melanoma Res 26:758–760.
15. Kim J, Lazar AJ, Davies MA et al (2012) BRAF, NRAS and KIT sequencing analysis of spindle cell melanoma. J Cutan Pathol 39:821–825.
16. Bos JL (1989) ras oncogenes in human cancer: a review. Cancer Res 49:4682–4689
17. Davies H, Bignell GR, Cox C et al (2002) Mutations of the BRAF gene in human cancer. Nature 417:949–954.
18. Fedorenko IV, Gibney GT, Smalley KSM (2013) NRAS mutant melanoma: biological behavior and future strategies for therapeutic management. Oncogene 32:3009–3018.
19. Bauer J, Curtin JA, Pinkel D, Bastian BC (2006) Congenital melanocytic nevi frequently harbor NRAS mutations but no BRAF mutations. J Invest Dermatol 127:179–182.
20. Russo AE, Torrisi E, Bevelacqua Y et al (2009) Melanoma: molecular pathogenesis and emerging target therapies (review). Int J Oncol 34:1481–1489.
21. Posch C, Moslehi H, Feeney L et al (2013) Combined targeting of MEK and PI3K/mTOR effector pathways is necessary to effectively inhibit NRAS mutant melanoma in vitro and in vivo. Proc Natl Acad Sci USA 110:4015–4020.
22. Dhawan P, Singh AB, Ellis DL, Richmond A (2002) Constitutive activation of Akt/protein kinase B in melanoma leads to up-regulation of nuclear factor-kappaB and tumor progression. Cancer Res 62:7335–7342
23. Curtin JA, Fridlyand J, Kageshita T et al (2005) Distinct sets of genetic alterations in melanoma. N Engl J Med 353:2135–2147.

24. Lewis TB, Robison JE, Bastien R et al (2005) Molecular classification of melanoma using real-time quantitative reverse transcriptase-polymerase chain reaction. Cancer 104: 1678–1686.

25. Sarin KY, Sun BK, Bangs CD et al (2013) Activating HRAS mutation in agminated spitz nevi arising in a nevus spilus. JAMA Dermatol 149:1077–1081.

26. van Dijk MCRF, Bernsen MR, Ruiter DJ (2005) Analysis of mutations in B-RAF, N-RAS, and H-RAS genes in the differential diagnosis of Spitz nevus and spitzoid melanoma. Am J Surg Pathol 29:1145–1151

27. van Engen-van Grunsven ACH, van Dijk MCRF, Ruiter DJ et al (2010) HRAS-mutated spitz tumors: a subtype of Spitz tumors with distinct features. Am J Surg Pathol 34:1436–1441.

28. Da Forno PD, Pringle JH, Fletcher A et al (2009) BRAF, NRAS and HRAS mutations in spitzoid tumours and their possible pathogenetic significance. Br J Dermatol 161:364–372.

29. Takata M, Lin J, Takayanagi S et al (2007) Genetic and epigenetic alterations in the differential diagnosis of malignant melanoma and spitzoid lesion. Br J Dermatol 156:1287–1294.

30. Bastian BC, LeBoit PE, Pinkel D (2000) Mutations and copy number increase of HRAS in Spitz nevi with distinctive histopathological features. Am J Pathol 157:967–972.

31. Wan PTC, Garnett MJ, Roe SM et al (2004) Mechanism of activation of the RAF-ERK signaling pathway by oncogenic mutations of B-RAF. Cell 116:855–867.

32. Dhomen N, Marais R (2009) BRAF signaling and targeted therapies in melanoma. Hematol Oncol Clin North Am 23:529–545, ix.

33. Pollock PM, Harper UL, Hansen KS et al (2002) High frequency of BRAF mutations in nevi. Nat Genet 33:19–20.

34. Tanami H, Imoto I, Hirasawa A et al (2004) Involvement of overexpressed wild-type BRAF in the growth of malignant melanoma cell lines. Oncogene 23:8796–8804.

35. Zuidervaart W, van Nieuwpoort F, Stark M et al (2005) Activation of the MAPK pathway is a common event in uveal melanomas although it rarely occurs through mutation of BRAF or RAS. Br J Cancer 92:2032–2038.

36. Colombino M, Capone M, Lissia A et al (2012) BRAF/NRAS mutation frequencies among primary tumors and metastases in patients with melanoma. J Clin Oncol 30:2522–2529.

37. Blokx WAM, van Dijk MCRF, Ruiter DJ (2010) Molecular cytogenetics of cutaneous melanocytic lesions – diagnostic, prognostic and therapeutic aspects. Histopathology 56:121–132.

38. Nikolaev SI, Rimoldi D, Iseli C et al (2012) Exome sequencing identifies recurrent somatic MAP2K1 and MAP2K2 mutations in melanoma. Nat Genet 44:133–139.

39. Smalley K (2003) A pivotal role for ERK in the oncogenic behaviour of malignant melanoma? Int J Cancer 104:527–532.

40. Qin J, Xin H, Nickoloff BJ (2012) Specifically targeting ERK1 or ERK2 kills melanoma cells. J Transl Med 10:15.

41. Lui P, Cashin R, Machado M et al (2007) Treatments for metastatic melanoma: synthesis of evidence from randomized trials. Cancer Treat Rev 33:665–680.

42. Chapman PB, Hauschild A, Robert C et al (2011) Improved survival with vemurafenib in melanoma with BRAF V600E mutation. N Engl J Med 364:2507–2516.

43. Cheng Y, Zhang G, Li G (2013) Targeting MAPK pathway in melanoma therapy. Cancer Metastasis Rev 32:567–584.

44. Gajewski TF, Salama A (2012) Phase II study of the farnesyltransferase inhibitor R115777 in advanced melanoma (CALGB 500104). J Transl Med 10:246

45. Thakur Das M, Salangsang F, Landman AS et al (2013) Modelling vemurafenib resistance in melanoma reveals a strategy to forestall drug resistance. Nature 494:251–255.

46. Eisen T, Ahmad T, Flaherty KT et al (2006) Sorafenib in advanced melanoma: a phase II randomised discontinuation trial analysis. Br J Cancer 95:581–586.

47. Hauschild A, Agarwala SS, Trefzer U et al (2009) Results of a phase III, randomized, placebo-controlled study of sorafenib in combination with carboplatin and paclitaxel as second-line treatment in patients with unresectable stage III or stage IV melanoma. J Clin Oncol 27:2823–2830.

48. Solit DB, Garraway LA, Pratilas CA et al (2006) BRAF mutation predicts sensitivity to MEK inhibition. Nature 439:358–362.

49. Hatzivassiliou G, Haling JR, Chen H et al (2013) Mechanism of MEK inhibition determines efficacy in mutant KRAS- versus BRAF-driven cancers. Nature 501:232–236.
50. LoRusso PM, Adjei AA, Varterasian M et al (2005) Phase I and pharmacodynamic study of the oral MEK inhibitor CI-1040 in patients with advanced malignancies. J Clin Oncol 23:5281–5293.
51. Rinehart J, Rinehart J, Adjei AA et al (2004) Multicenter phase II study of the oral MEK inhibitor, CI-1040, in patients with advanced non-small-cell lung, breast, colon, and pancreatic cancer. J Clin Oncol 22:4456–4462
52. Boasberg PD, Redfern CH, Daniels GA et al (2011) Pilot study of PD-0325901 in previously treated patients with advanced melanoma, breast cancer, and colon cancer. Cancer Chemother Pharmacol 68:547–552.
53. Flaherty KT, Robert C, Hersey P et al (2012) Improved survival with MEK inhibition in BRAF-mutated melanoma. N Engl J Med 367:107–114.
54. Ascierto PA, Schadendorf D, Berking C et al (2013) MEK162 for patients with advanced melanoma harbouring NRAS or Val600 BRAF mutations: a non-randomised, open-label phase 2 study. Lancet Oncol 14:249–256.

Chapter 7
The PI3K-AKT Pathway in Melanoma

Alan E. Siroy, Michael A. Davies, and Alexander J. Lazar

Abstract Numerous signaling pathways are involved in the molecular pathogenesis of melanoma. Two of the most prominent pathways include the RAS-RAF-MEK-ERK pathway and the PI3K-AKT pathway. While targeted inhibition of BRAF/MEK have resulted in improved survival in patients with BRAF V600-mutated melanoma, therapeutic resistance is often the end result. The PI3K-AKT pathway plays a significant role in BRAF-/MEK-inhibitor resistance in melanoma patients and may represent a crucial target for combination therapy. This chapter will describe the components of the PI3K-AKT pathway, highlight their role in cellular physiology and melanoma pathogenesis, and examine their potential for molecular-targeted therapy.

Keywords Melanoma • PI3K • AKT • PTEN • mTOR • BRAF • NRAS • Molecular-targeted therapy • Therapeutic resistance • Immunotherapy

7.1 Introduction

Melanoma is an increasingly well-studied cancer in which a variety of signaling pathways critical to its pathogenesis have been elucidated. Although there are still pathologic mechanisms of melanoma that remain largely unknown, multiple genetic alterations in common molecular pathways have been found to contribute to the pathogenesis of melanoma [1]. The most common pathways that promote cellular growth, proliferation, and survival include the RAS-RAF-MEK-ERK pathway and the PI3K-AKT pathway, making their signaling components attractive targets for

A.E. Siroy • A.J. Lazar (✉)
Departments of Pathology & Translational Molecular Pathology, The University
of Texas MD Anderson Cancer Center, Houston, TX, USA
e-mail: AESiroy@mdanderson.org; alazar@mdanderson.org

M.A. Davies
Departments of Melanoma Medical Oncology & Systems Biology, The University
of Texas MD Anderson Cancer Center, Houston, TX, USA
e-mail: MDavies@mdanderson.org

© Springer Science+Business Media New York 2016
C.A. Torres-Cabala, J.L. Curry (eds.), *Genetics of Melanoma*, Cancer Genetics,
DOI 10.1007/978-1-4939-3554-3_7

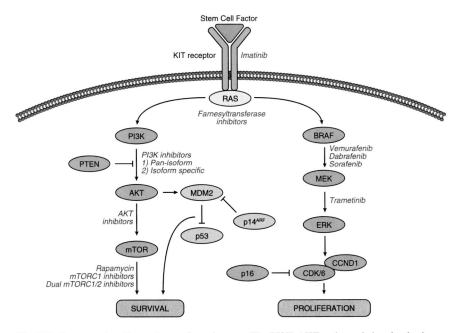

Fig. 7.1 Common signaling pathways in melanoma. The PI3K-AKT pathway is involved primarily in the regulation of cell survival, whereas the RAS-RAF-MEK-ERK regulates cellular proliferation. Potential therapeutic targets include components of the RAS-RAF-MEK-ERK and PI3K-AKT pathways as well as the receptor tyrosine kinases (prototyped here as the KIT receptor). Examples of therapeutic agents and their sites of action are shown in *red*

therapeutic agents (Fig. 7.1) [2]. Although the high frequency of *BRAF*- and *NRAS*-activating mutations in melanoma strongly support the role of the RAS-RAF-MEK-ERK pathway in the pathogenesis of melanoma [3, 4], numerous lines of evidence have shown that activation of this pathway alone is incomplete in establishing the pathogenicity of this disease [5, 6]. The PI3K-AKT pathway is an important regulator of normal cellular physiology and is observed to be activated with high frequency in many types of cancer [7, 8]. *PTEN* loss of function along with rare mutations in *PIK3CA* and *AKT* has been shown to activate the PI3K-AKT pathway specifically in melanoma [9–14]. Furthermore, multiple lines of evidence suggest that the PI3K-AKT pathway plays a significant role in BRAF-/MEK-inhibitor resistance [15–27]. Given the important role of this pathway in melanoma, this chapter will describe the components of the PI3K-AKT pathway, highlight their role in cellular physiology and melanoma pathogenesis, and examine their potential for molecular-targeted therapy.

7.2   PI3K-AKT Pathway: Normal Function in Cellular Physiology

The PI3K-AKT signaling pathway is broadly utilized by many cell types under normal physiologic conditions and depending on the cellular context is important in regulating cellular proliferation, survival, growth, protein synthesis, metabolism, and motility [28, 29]. PI3K, the main regulatory protein of the pathway, is a lipid kinase that consists of both a regulatory subunit (PIK3R, p85) and a catalytic subunit (PIK3C, p110), each of which includes multiple isoforms (i.e., PIK3CA, PIK3CB, PIK3CD, etc.) [30, 31]. Of note, PIK3CB has been demonstrated to be more involved with pathway activation, cell signaling, growth, and survival among the other isoforms of PIK3C, specifically in patients with *PTEN* loss of function [32, 33]. PI3K can be activated by receptor tyrosine kinases and activated RAS proteins (Fig. 7.2). As a result of this activation, phosphatidylinositols (PIPs) are phosphorylated by PI3K at their 3′ hydroxyl sites, producing phosphatidylinositol diphosphate (PIP_2) and phosphatidylinositol triphosphate (PIP_3). The resultant PIP_3 serves as a high-affinity binding ligand for PH-domain-containing AKT to be recruited to the cell membrane for phosphorylation at residues Ser473 and Thr308 by the mTORC2 complex and PDK1, respectively [29, 31]. Activated AKT inhibits the activity of the majority of its protein targets by phosphorylation, affecting cell growth, survival, and cell cycle entry [28]. Phosphorylation of FKHR-L1 by

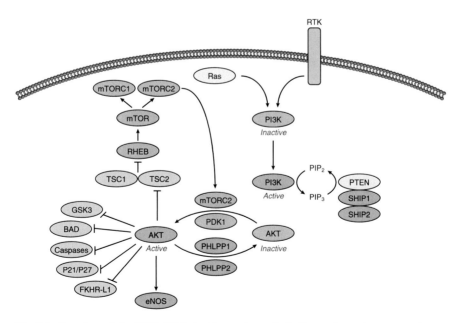

Fig. 7.2 Overview of the PI3K-AKT signaling pathway, including major activators, regulators, and effectors. *RTK* receptor tyrosine kinase

activated AKT promotes binding of the factor with 14-3-3 family of proteins, resulting in cytosolic retention and thus preventing transcription of Fas ligand genes responsible for apoptosis [34]. AKT similarly inhibits BAD protein from binding to Bcl-2 and Bcl-XL by coupling BAD with 14-3-3 proteins through phosphorylation, which inhibits apoptosis and increases cell survival [34]. The constitutively active protein kinase GSK3 is inhibited by phosphorylation by activated AKT, preventing its own inhibitory phosphorylation of cyclin D1, thus promoting cellular proliferation [28, 29]. AKT also phosphorylates and inhibits TSC2 which facilitates the activation of mTOR, a regulator of cell survival, growth, and metabolism [35, 36]. Along with the recruitment of AKT, PIP_3 has the ability to recruit and activate other PH-domain-containing proteins such as GDP-GTP exchange factors for Rac and ARF6, both of which are involved in remodeling the actin cytoskeleton for directional cellular motility [28]. Protein kinases of the Tec family are also activated by PIP_3, resulting in the regulation of cytosolic calcium concentrations and changes in gene expression [28].

Lipid phosphatases, such as the SH2-containing phosphatases (SHIP1 and SHIP2) and PTEN, downregulate the PI3K-AKT pathway by dephosphorylating PIP_3 which prevents both further recruitment and activation of PH-domain-containing proteins such as AKT, thus serving as a counterbalance to PI3K as critical regulators of AKT activity. SHIP1 and SHIP2 dephosphorylate the 5′ position of the PIP_3 inositol ring, whereas PTEN dephosphorylates the 3′-hydroxyl position of PIP_3, both producing PIP_2 [28]. Cancer makes use of existing physiologic cascades for its promotion and progression; we will now discuss how melanoma subverts the PI3K-AKT pathway to these ends.

7.3 PI3K-AKT Pathway Activation in Melanoma

A variety of mechanisms exist where the PI3K-AKT pathway is activated in melanoma. One of these mechanisms involves the loss of function of PTEN. As previously mentioned, PTEN is an important regulatory phosphatase of the PI3K-AKT pathway which decreases activity of the pathway through dephosphorylation of PIP_3. If PTEN expression or function is impaired, activation of the PI3K-AKT pathway results. Missense mutations, frameshift mutations, and/or deletions of the *PTEN* gene have been shown to produce loss of function of PTEN, resulting in inadequate or nonfunctional phosphatase activity of the resultant protein (Fig. 7.3) [9]. In addition to mutations and deletions, there is evidence that PTEN function can be lost due to epigenetic mechanisms (e.g., microRNAs, promoter methylation, etc.) [10, 11]. PTEN interactions with antagonizing exchange proteins such as P-REX2a have also been shown to epigenetically affect PTEN functionality through inhibition of phosphatase activity [37]. Loss of PTEN function has been shown to correlate with increased activity of AKT in multiple tumor types, and high levels of phosphorylated AKT have been specifically observed in cases of metastatic melanoma [38].

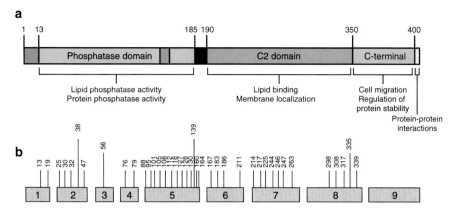

Fig. 7.3 PTEN protein and gene with associated mutations in melanoma. (**a**) PTEN protein and its major domains, including the phosphatase domain and the C2-domain. The phosphatase domain is responsible for lipid/protein phosphatase activity, whereas the C2 domain is primarily involved in lipid binding and membrane localization. (**b**) *PTEN* gene and associated mutations in melanoma. Boxes 1 through 9 represent the *PTEN* gene exons. The corresponding *vertical lines* with numbers represent the specific codons mutated in melanoma (Adapted from Aguissa-Toure AH, Li G (2012) Genetic alterations of PTEN in human melanoma. Cell Mol Life Sci 69 (9):1475–1491)

Genetic alterations of *PTEN* in melanomas are generally mutually exclusive with activating *NRAS* mutations due to their redundancy in activating the PI3K-AKT pathway (Fig. 7.1). However, a strong association does exist between loss of PTEN function and activating *BRAF* mutations likely due to the complimentary nature of activating both the PI3K-AKT and RAS-RAF-MEK-ERK pathways, respectively [39, 40]. Interestingly, preclinical studies involving genetically engineered mouse models have shown that loss of PTEN increases invasiveness and metastatic potential in both *BRAF*-mutant and *NRAS*-mutant melanomas, though the latter combination is infrequent in human melanoma [41, 42]. Dankort et al. noted that induction of the *BRAF* V600E mutation in the melanocytes of mice resulted merely in melanocytic hyperplasia [41]. However, with concurrent induction of PTEN loss, the combined activation of both RAS-RAF-MEK-ERK and PI3K-AKT pathways resulted in invasive/metastatic melanoma. Similarly, Nogueira et al. found that the addition of PTEN loss of function in mice with *RAS* mutation resulted in increased invasion and migration of melanoma cells [42]. Thus loss of PTEN function in preclinical models has provided evidence of pathway involvement in increased invasiveness and metastatic potential specifically in melanoma.

Although loss of PTEN is one of the more commonly studied mechanisms of PI3K-AKT activation, other events have also been shown to contribute to pathway activation in melanoma. Activating point mutations in *NRAS* occur in up to 20 % of melanomas, resulting in constitutive NRAS-mediated signaling and activation of multiple pathways, including PI3K-AKT [4]. Specific point mutations in the *PIK3CA* gene that encodes the catalytic subunit of PI3K tend to be quite rare in melanomas with a prevalence of 3–5 % [12, 13, 43]. Point mutations in *AKT1* and

AKT3 are also quite rare and have been detected in approximately 1 % and 1.5 % of melanomas, respectively [14, 30]. Similar to *NRAS*, activating mutations and amplifications of receptor tyrosine kinases (e.g., KIT, EGFR, HER2/neu, etc.) result in the activation of many different downstream pathways, including the PI3K-AKT and ERK pathways. Mutations and amplifications specific to *KIT* have been shown to frequently involve mucosal (20–30 %) and acral (10–15 %) melanomas as opposed to cutaneous melanomas (approximately 1 %) [44]. Somatic mutations of *ERBB4* have also been detected in approximately 19 % of melanomas, with the missense mutations resulting in increased kinase activity, though the significance of these mutations is uncertain and still debated [45].

Increased expression and activation of receptor tyrosine kinases may also occur epigenetically, resulting in PI3K-AKT pathway activation. Both PDGFRβ and IGF1R have been shown to be increased in expression and activation in melanoma cell lines with BRAF- and MEK-inhibitor resistance resulting from compensatory activation of the PI3K-AKT pathway [16, 17, 46]. Similarly, production of the protein hepatocyte growth factor (HGF) by non-transformed cells in the tumor microenvironment has been show to activate the PI3K-AKT pathway in melanoma cells, resulting in BRAF-inhibitor resistance in vitro [18, 19]. Expression of HGF in the stroma also correlated with decreased responsiveness to BRAF inhibitors in patients. Most recently, studies have found that the PI3K-AKT pathway can be activated during BRAF and MEK inhibition through upregulation of ERBB3 [20, 21]. When challenged with a BRAF inhibitor or MEK inhibitor, melanoma cell lines with *BRAF* V600 mutations were found to have hyper-phosphorylated ERBB3 receptors and increased phosphorylation of AKT [20]. BRAF inhibition also resulted in increased production of the ERBB3 ligand neuregulin, and antibodies to the heregulin isoform of neuregulin (anti-HRG) produced strong inhibition of phosphorylated ERBB3 and AKT. In another study, Abel et al. further noted that FOXD3 was produced by *BRAF*-mutant melanoma cells during BRAF or MEK inhibition and that this protein directly targets *ERBB3* for transcription resulting in increased ErbB3 protein production [21]. The study also found that BRAF/MEK inhibition enhances expression of *ERBB3* and enhances neuregulin/ErbB3 signaling to AKT through FOXD3 and that ERBB2 is required for neuregulin/ErbB3 signaling to occur.

Overall, the activation of the PI3K-AKT pathway in melanoma can occur through a variety of genetic and epigenetic mechanisms involving PTEN, NRAS, PIK3CA, AKT, and receptor tyrosine kinases. In this section, a few preclinical studies involving BRAF-/MEK-inhibitor resistance were mentioned to help illustrate various PI3K-AKT pathway activation mechanisms in melanoma. We will now examine further evidence of the role of the PI3K-AKT pathway in therapeutic resistance.

7.4   The PI3K-AKT Pathway and Therapeutic Resistance

Discovery of the genetic and epigenetic alterations that result in the constitutive activation of the RAS-RAF-MEK-ERK pathway in melanoma has led to treatments that focus on targeted therapies [3, 47, 48]. Three drugs targeting either the *BRAF*

V600 mutation (vemurafenib and dabrafenib) or MEK in the MAP kinase pathway (trametinib) have been approved by the FDA for the treatment of patients with metastatic melanoma. While these agents represent a marked advance in the treatment of this disease, their clinical benefit is limited by both de novo and acquired resistance [48–51].

There exist multiple lines of evidence to suggest that the PI3K-AKT pathway may play a significant role in BRAF-/MEK-inhibitor resistance. *BRAF*-mutant, PTEN-null human melanoma cell lines treated with BRAF and MEK inhibitors have demonstrated a reduction in MEK and ERK activity and cell growth inhibition [15, 22, 23]. Yet, when exposed to BRAF and MEK inhibition, the majority of PTEN-null melanoma cell lines undergo only cell cycle arrest with minimal cell death, whereas the PTEN-intact cell lines undergo apoptosis. In a study involving the analysis of melanoma tumor samples of patients treated in the phase II clinical trial of vemurafenib, immunohistochemical analysis revealed a modest association between PTEN expression and clinical response in which PTEN expression at baseline was found to be higher in treatment responders versus nonresponders [24]. Furthermore, patients with alterations in the *PTEN* gene who were treated with dabrafenib experienced shorter progression-free survival when compared to patients with intact PTEN [25]. These studies implicate a role for the PI3K-AKT pathway in de novo resistance through PTEN loss of function. There is growing evidence that the PI3K-AKT pathway may also be involved in acquired resistance to BRAF inhibition. Acquired resistance to BRAF inhibition through genetic loss of PTEN during treatment has been documented in a patient with intact PTEN prior to therapy induction [16]. Furthermore, studies involving exome sequencing of melanoma tumors from patients before treatment and after progression on BRAF inhibitors show mutations in a variety of genes of the PI3K-AKT pathway (e.g., *PTEN*, *PIK3CA*, *PIK3R*, etc.) present in progressive tumors [26, 27]. Shi et al. found that 22 % of progressive tumors contained PI3K-AKT pathway mutations in positive- and negative regulatory genes identified by whole exome sequencing analysis [26]. Furthermore, introduction of a number of these mutations into melanoma cell lines resulted in increased p-AKT levels and BRAF-inhibitor resistance. Another study involving whole exome sequencing of melanoma tumors in 45 patients who underwent vemurafenib or dabrafenib monotherapy also revealed mutations in PI3K-AKT pathway genes in 42 % of those with progressive disease, although experimental validation of these mutations confirming increased PI3K-AKT pathway activity or BRAF-inhibitor resistance was not performed in this study [27].

As mentioned in the previous section, increased expression and activation of receptor tyrosine kinases through genetic mechanisms (e.g., KIT, ERBB4) and epigenetic mechanisms (e.g., PDGFRβ, IGF1R, HGF, ERBB3) may also result in increased PI3K-AKT signaling [15–21, 44, 45]. Increased activation and expression of receptor tyrosine kinases may result in BRAF- and MEK-inhibitor resistance through compensatory activation of PI3K-AKT signaling. While in vitro experiments have shown that single-agent inhibition utilizing MEK inhibitors or PI3K-AKT pathway inhibitors alone failed to induce apoptosis in melanoma cells, concurrent inhibition of both the RAS-RAF-MEK-ERK and PI3K-AKT pathways produced marked cell death [16, 27, 46]. Therefore, while melanoma resistance to BRAF and MEK inhibition can occur through increased activation of the PI3K-AKT pathway to prevent apoptosis, additional targeting of the PI3K-AKT pathway may result in complete cell death for these resistant melanomas.

Along with molecular-targeted therapy, recent advances in understanding the relationship between melanoma and the immune system have resulted new treatment innovations with regard to immunotherapy. In addition to immunotherapeutic treatment involving exogenous cytokines interferon-α and interleukin-2 that have been used for years to treat melanoma patients with advanced disease [52–55], clinical trials involving anti-CTLA-4 blocking antibodies (e.g., ipilimumab, FDA approved), anti-PD-1 antibodies (e.g., pembrolizumab & nivolumab, both FDA approved, and combinations of these drugs) have resulted in promising results for patients with metastatic melanoma [56–59]. However, preclinical studies revealing PTEN as an immunologic regulator may provide early evidence of the PI3K-AKT pathway's role in potential resistance to immunotherapy. In a study involving PTEN-deficient melanoma cultures and melanoma cell lines, Dong et al. found that loss of PTEN resulted in the expression of immunosuppressive cytokines (IL-10, IL-6, and VEGF) and corresponded with melanoma samples lacking brisk host responses [60]. Furthermore, the study noted that PTEN was involved in the downregulation of the immunosuppressor PD-L1 in melanoma cells. Other data suggests that melanoma with loss of PTEN expression shows reduced levels of tumor infiltrating lymphocytes. This early data suggests that the PI3K-AKT pathway may play a potential role in resistance to immunotherapy in addition to its already proven role in BRAF-/MEK-inhibitor resistance in patients with *BRAF* V600-mutated melanoma.

7.5 PI3K-AKT-Targeted Therapies

The PI3K-AKT pathway contains multiple components that are potential targets for therapeutic agents. This is reflected by the multiple classes of inhibitors that are being developed and clinically tested against this pathway. The main classes of agents targeting components of the PI3K-AKT pathway include: single-target agents such as PI3K inhibitors, AKT inhibitors, and mTORC1 inhibitors and dual-target agents such as PI3K/mTOR inhibitors and mTORC1/mTORC2 inhibitors [61] (Table 7.1).

PI3K inhibitors include pan-isoform agents and isoform-specific agents. Several agents exist that target the different isoforms of the catalytic subunit of the PI3K enzyme [62]. As previously mentioned, these different isoforms of the PI3K catalytic subunit include p110α, p110β, and p110δ (i.e., PI3KCA, PI3KCB, and PI3KCD). Although p110α has been shown to mediate growth factor signaling from receptor tyrosine kinases, p110β has been demonstrated to be more involved with pathway activation, cell signaling, growth, and survival in cells with loss of PTEN [32, 33]. Thus, cancer cells with loss of PTEN appear to be more dependent on p110β rather than p110α, making p110β-selective inhibitors a rational strategy

Table 7.1 PI3K-AKT pathway inhibitors

	Category	Examples
Single-target agents	PI3K inhibitors	• BAY 80-6946 (Bayer, Morristown, New Jersey) • BKM120 (Novartis, Basel, Switzerland) • GDC-0941 (Genentech, San Francisco, California) • PX-866 (Oncothyreon, Seattle, Washington) • XL-147 (Exelixis, San Francisco, California) • ZSTK474 (Zenyaku Kogyo, Tokyo, Japan)
	PI3K isoform-specific inhibitors	• p110α-Specific: BYL719 (Novartis, Basel, Switzerland) • INK1117 (Intellikine, La Jolla, California) • p110C-Specific: AMG 319 (Amgen, Thousand Oaks, California) • CAL-101 (Calistoga, Seattle, Washington)
	AKT inhibitors	• GDC-0068 (Genentech, San Francisco, California) • GSK2110183 (GlaxoSmithKline, Middlesex, United Kingdom) • MK-2206 (Merck, Whitehouse Station, New Jersey) • Perifosine (Keryx, New York, New York)
	mTORC1 inhibitors	• Everolimus (Novartis, Basel, Switzerland) • Sirolimus (Pfizer, New York, New York) • Ridaforolimus (Merck, Whitehouse Station, New Jersey) • Temsirolimus (Pfizer, New York, New York)
Dual-target agents	Dual mTORC1/2 inhibitors	• AZD8055 (AstraZeneca, London, England) • OSI-027 (Astellas, Tokyo, Japan)
	Dual PI3K/mTOR inhibitors	• BEZ235, BGT226 (Novartis, Basel, Switzerland) • GDC-0980 (Genentech, San Francisco, California) • GSK2126458 (GlaxoSmithKline, Middlesex, United Kingdom) • PF-4691502, PF-5212384 (Pfizer, New York, New York) • SF-1126 (Semafore, Indianapolis, Indiana) • XL765 (Exelixis, San Francisco, California) • AKT inhibitors GDC-0068 (Genentech, San Francisco, California)

for melanoma patients with loss of PTEN. Clinical trials involving different p110β-selective inhibitors are currently ongoing. Interestingly, AKT inhibitors have been noted to be relatively selective for tumors with loss of PTEN [63, 64]. Although activating mutations of AKT in other cancers primarily involve the AKT1 isoform, evidence does show that mutations in the AKT3 gene are present in melanomas as well, albeit rarely [14]. A frequent switch from AKT1 to AKT3 expression has been demonstrated in metastatic melanomas, thus making AKT3-specific inhibitors preferential agents for patients with melanoma [65, 66]. Unfortunately, inhibitors of mTOR such as rapamycin and rapamycin analogs (rapalogs) have shown minimal activity in melanoma [67]. In explanation, recall that activation of mTOR occurs further downstream in the PI3K-AKT pathway

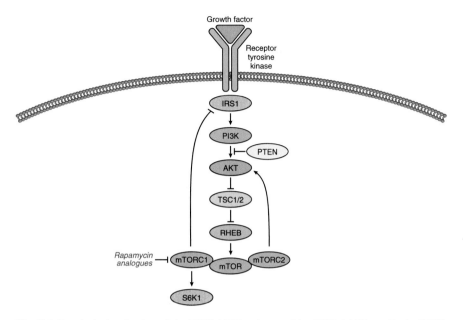

Fig. 7.4 Paradoxical activation of the PI3K-AKT pathway with mTOR inhibitors. In the PI3K-AKT pathway, mTORC1 negatively regulates IRS1 which subsequently decreases phosphorylation and activation of PI3K. Inhibition of mTORC1 by rapamycin analogs results in the disinhibition of IRS1 which allows for activation of PI3K and a subsequent increase in phosphorylated AKT, thus resulting in a "paradoxical" increase in AKT activity

through AKT-mediated inhibition of TSC2 and regulates cellular growth, survival, and metabolism [35, 36]. Although mTOR inhibitors have been shown to reach levels that significantly inhibit their target in vivo, further studies have shown that rapalogs paradoxically activate PI3K which may contribute to their lack of efficacy [68–70]. Rapalogs specifically inhibit the mTORC1 complex that activates P70-S6K1 (which is involved in activating protein translational machinery) and negatively regulates PI3K through a feedback loop mechanism (Fig. 7.4) [69]. It has been shown that mTORC1 inhibition results in the relief of the negative feedback loop and promotes activation of PI3K, AKT, and ERK [71, 72]. Since the mTORC2 complex is unaffected by rapalogs, it is able to phosphorylate and activate AKT [31]. Studies have shown that dual inhibition of mTORC1 and mTORC2 prevented activation of P70-S6K1 and AKT, thus more effectively inhibiting cancer cell growth and survival when compared to mTORC1 inhibition alone [73]. Similar to increased effectiveness of dual mTORC1/mTORC2 inhibitors over single mTORC1 inhibitor, dual PI3K/mTOR inhibitors have demonstrated broad and superior inhibition in melanoma cell lines when compared to single-agent PI3K or mTOR inhibitors alone [74, 75].

7.6 Challenges

Although the pharmacological development of a variety of PI3K-AKT pathway inhibitors continues to produce and test potential agents for targeted therapy, several significant challenges remain. One difficulty in the clinical application of these agents is the identification of appropriate pharmacodynamic markers that correlate with optimal PI3K-AKT pathway inhibition for effective clinical response [76]. For example, an analysis performed on a group of patients treated on the phase I trial of the BRAF-inhibitor vemurafenib showed that clinical effective responses were not achieved unless > 60 % of phosphorylated ERK (p-ERK) levels were inhibited [77]. In this case, p-ERK is a reasonably robust pharmacodynamic biomarker indicating the level of inhibition needed to be attained in order to achieve a clinically effective response. With regard to mTORC1 inhibitors, studies have shown marked inhibition of p-P70S6K and p-S6 levels in patients undergoing treatment with these agents [69, 78]. Currently, data available on the pharmacodynamics and biomarker assessment in patients treated with PI3K inhibitors and AKT inhibitors are limited [79]. Overall, single-agent PI3K and AKT inhibitors have only produced effective clinical responses at a very low frequency, complicating the validation of appropriate pharmacodynamics biomarkers based on preclinical data and models [30].

Another challenge to the effective clinical application of PI3K-AKT inhibitors is the presence of feedback loops and oncogenic cross talk. As previously mentioned, the mTORC1 complex negatively regulates PI3K through a feedback loop, and selective mTORC1 inhibition has been shown to promote the activation of PI3K, AKT, and ERK [71, 72]. This feedback loop involves the mTORC1 complex negatively regulating IRS-1 and subsequently PI3K (Fig. 7.4) [70, 80]. Thus, the application of mTORC1 inhibitors not only inhibits downstream signaling of mTORC1 but also inhibits the feedback loop that negatively regulates PI3K, thus promoting AKT activation through withdrawal of inhibition [69]. Single-agent PI3K and AKT inhibitors also result in the disruption of feedback loops that subsequently disinhibit FOXO transcription factors responsible for mediating the transcription of receptor tyrosine kinases, including HER3 and IGF1R [81–84]. The subsequent upregulation of these receptor tyrosine kinases results in "oncogenic cross talk" between the PI3K-AKT and the RAS-RAF-MEK-ERK pathways. Thus, the presence of feedback loops and oncogenic cross talk suggest that combination therapies employing multiple-targeted agents may be required to reach optimal inhibition and clinical effectiveness.

7.7 Summary

The molecular pathogenesis of melanoma is comprised of a variety of important signaling pathways, with two of the most prominent being the RAS-RAF-MEK-ERK pathway and the PI3K-AKT pathway. Although targeted therapy against the

RAS-RAF-MEK-ERK pathway through BRAF/MEK inhibition has improved survival in patients with BRAF V600-mutated melanoma, clinical efficacy is limited by therapeutic resistance. The PI3K-AKT pathway appears to play a significant role in BRAF-/MEK-inhibitor resistance in melanoma patients and could represent a crucial target for combination therapy. Continued pharmacological development of PI3K-AKT pathway inhibitors has resulted in a variety of agents that fall within several functional classes that include PI3K inhibitors, AKT inhibitors, mTORC1 inhibitors, PI3K/mTOR inhibitors, and mTORC1/mTORC2 inhibitors. Although these agents have the potential to target a variety of components of the PI3K-AKT pathway, numerous challenges remain, including the identification of pharmacodynamic biomarkers to assess clinical effective responses of these agents, overcoming feedback loops within the PI3K-AKT pathway, oncogenic cross talk between different pathways, and ultimately determining the optimal agents to prioritize for testing in melanoma patients. Further research in the clinical and molecular effects of PI3K-AKT pathway inhibition will contribute to the understanding of the pathogenesis of melanoma and hopefully improve patient outcomes. Multiple of these agents are now in clinical trial, usually in combination with other agents, and so we should learn much in the coming months and years.

References

1. Palmieri G, Capone M, Ascierto ML et al (2009) Main roads to melanoma. J Transl Med 7:86
2. Hocker TL, Singh MK, Tsao H (2008) Melanoma genetics and therapeutic approaches in the 21st century: moving from the benchside to the bedside. J Invest Dermatol 128(11):2575–2595
3. Davies H, Bignell GR, Cox C et al (2002) Mutations of the BRAF gene in human cancer. Nature 417(6892):949–954
4. Hocker T, Tsao H (2007) Ultraviolet radiation and melanoma: a systematic review and analysis of reported sequence variants. Hum Mutat 28(6):578–588
5. Pollock PM, Harper UL, Hansen KS et al (2003) High frequency of BRAF mutations in nevi. Nat Genet 33(1):19–20
6. Patton EE, Widlund HR, Kutok JL et al (2005) BRAF mutations are sufficient to promote nevi formation and cooperate with p53 in the genesis of melanoma. Curr Biol 15(3):249–254
7. Yuan TL, Cantley LC (2008) PI3K pathway alterations in cancer: variations on a theme. Oncogene 27(41):5497–5510
8. Vivanco I, Sawyers CL (2002) The phosphatidylinositol 3-Kinase AKT pathway in human cancer. Nat Rev Cancer 2(7):489–501
9. Aguissa-Toure AH, Li G (2012) Genetic alterations of PTEN in human melanoma. Cell Mol Life Sci 69(9):1475–1491
10. Mirmohammadsadegh A, Marini A, Nambiar S, Hassan M, Tannapfel A, Ruzicka T, Hengge UR (2006) Epigenetic silencing of the PTEN gene in melanoma. Cancer Res 66(13):6546–6552
11. Zhou XP, Gimm O, Hampel H, Niemann T, Walker MJ, Eng C (2000) Epigenetic PTEN silencing in malignant melanomas without PTEN mutation. Am J Pathol 157(4):1123–1128
12. Omholt K, Krockel D, Ringborg U, Hansson J (2006) Mutations of PIK3CA are rare in cutaneous melanoma. Melanoma Res 16(2):197–200

13. Curtin JA, Stark MS, Pinkel D, Hayward NK, Bastian BC (2006) PI3-kinase subunits are infrequent somatic targets in melanoma. J Invest Dermatol 126(7):1660–1663
14. Davies MA, Stemke-Hale K, Tellez C et al (2008) A novel AKT3 mutation in melanoma tumours and cell lines. Br J Cancer 99(8):1265–1268
15. Gopal YN, Deng W, Woodman SE, Komurov K, Ram P, Smith PD, Davies MA (2010) Basal and treatment-induced activation of AKT mediates resistance to cell death by AZD6244 (ARRY-142886) in Braf-mutant human cutaneous melanoma cells. Cancer Res 70(21):8736–8747
16. Villanueva J, Vultur A, Lee JT et al (2010) Acquired resistance to BRAF inhibitors mediated by a RAF kinase switch in melanoma can be overcome by cotargeting MEK and IGF-1R/PI3K. Cancer Cell 18(6):683–695
17. Shi H, Kong X, Ribas A, Lo RS (2011) Combinatorial treatments that overcome PDGFRbeta-driven resistance of melanoma cells to V600EB-RAF inhibition. Cancer Res 71(15):5067–5074
18. Straussman R, Morikawa T, Shee K et al (2012) Tumour micro-environment elicits innate resistance to RAF inhibitors through HGF secretion. Nature 487(7408):500–504
19. Wilson TR, Fridlyand J, Yan Y et al (2012) Widespread potential for growth-factor-driven resistance to anticancer kinase inhibitors. Nature 487(7408):505–509
20. Fattore L, Marra E, Pisanu ME et al (2013) Activation of an early feedback survival loop involving phospho-ErbB3 is a general response of melanoma cells to RAF/MEK inhibition and is abrogated by anti-ErbB3 antibodies. J Transl Med 11:180
21. Abel EV, Basile KJ, Kugel CH 3rd et al (2013) Melanoma adapts to RAF/MEK inhibitors through FOXD3-mediated upregulation of ERBB3. J Clin Invest 123(5):2155–2168
22. Paraiso KH, Xiang Y, Rebecca VW et al (2011) PTEN loss confers BRAF inhibitor resistance to melanoma cells through the suppression of BIM expression. Cancer Res 71(7):2750–2760
23. Xing F, Persaud Y, Pratilas CA et al (2012) Concurrent loss of the PTEN and RB1 tumor suppressors attenuates RAF dependence in melanomas harboring (V600E)BRAF. Oncogene 31(4):446–457
24. Trunzer K, Pavlick AC, Schuchter L et al (2013) Pharmacodynamic effects and mechanisms of resistance to vemurafenib in patients with metastatic melanoma. J Clin Oncol 31(14):1767–1774
25. Nathanson KL, Martin AM, Wubbenhorst B et al (2013) Tumor genetic analyses of patients with metastatic melanoma treated with the BRAF inhibitor Dabrafenib (GSK2118436). Clin Cancer Res 19:4868–4878
26. Shi H, Hugo W, Kong X et al (2014) Acquired resistance and clonal evolution in melanoma during BRAF inhibitor therapy. Cancer Discov 4(1):80–93
27. Van Allen EM, Wagle N, Sucker A et al (2014) The genetic landscape of clinical resistance to RAF inhibition in metastatic melanoma. Cancer Discov 4(1):94–109
28. Cantley LC (2002) The phosphoinositide 3-kinase pathway. Science 296(5573):1655–1657
29. Yap TA, Garrett MD, Walton MI, Raynaud F, de Bono JS, Workman P (2008) Targeting the PI3K-AKT-mTOR pathway: progress, pitfalls, and promises. Curr Opin Pharmacol 8(4):393–412
30. Davies MA (2012) The role of the PI3K-AKT pathway in melanoma. Cancer J 18(2):142–147
31. Davies MA, Gershenwald JE (2011) Targeted therapy for melanoma: a primer. Surg Oncol Clin N Am 20(1):165–180
32. Jia S, Liu Z, Zhang S et al (2008) Essential roles of PI(3)K-p110beta in cell growth, metabolism and tumorigenesis. Nature 454(7205):776–779
33. Wee S, Wiederschain D, Maira SM et al (2008) PTEN-deficient cancers depend on PIK3CB. Proc Natl Acad Sci USA 105(35):13057–13062
34. Brunet A, Datta SR, Greenberg ME (2001) Transcription-dependent and -independent control of neuronal survival by the PI3K-Akt signaling pathway. Curr Opin Neurobiol 11(3):297–305

35. Sarbassov DD, Ali SM, Sabatini DM (2005) Growing roles for the mTOR pathway. Curr Opin Cell Biol 17(6):596–603
36. Yecies JL, Manning BD (2011) mTOR links oncogenic signaling to tumor cell metabolism. J Mol Med (Berl) 89(3):221–228
37. Fine B, Hodakoski C, Koujak S et al (2009) Activation of the PI3K pathway in cancer through inhibition of PTEN by exchange factor P-REX2a. Science 325(5945):1261–1265
38. Davies MA, Stemke-Hale K, Lin E et al (2009) Integrated molecular and clinical analysis of AKT activation in metastatic melanoma. Clin Cancer Res 15(24):7538–7546
39. Tsao H, Goel V, Wu H, Yang G, Haluska FG (2004) Genetic interaction between NRAS and BRAF mutations and PTEN/MMAC1 inactivation in melanoma. J Invest Dermatol 122(2):337–341
40. Goel VK, Lazar AJ, Warneke CL, Redston MS, Haluska FG (2006) Examination of mutations in BRAF, NRAS, and PTEN in primary cutaneous melanoma. J Invest Dermatol 126(1):154–160
41. Dankort D, Curley DP, Cartlidge RA et al (2009) Braf(V600E) cooperates with Pten loss to induce metastatic melanoma. Nat Genet 41(5):544–552
42. Nogueira C, Kim KH, Sung H et al (2010) Cooperative interactions of PTEN deficiency and RAS activation in melanoma metastasis. Oncogene 29(47):6222–6232
43. Hodis E, Watson IR, Kryukov GV et al (2012) A landscape of driver mutations in melanoma. Cell 150(2):251–263
44. Woodman SE, Davies MA (2010) Targeting KIT in melanoma: a paradigm of molecular medicine and targeted therapeutics. Biochem Pharmacol 80(5):568–574
45. Prickett TD, Agrawal NS, Wei X et al (2009) Analysis of the tyrosine kinome in melanoma reveals recurrent mutations in ERBB4. Nat Genet 41(10):1127–1132
46. Nazarian R, Shi H, Wang Q et al (2010) Melanomas acquire resistance to B-RAF(V600E) inhibition by RTK or N-RAS upregulation. Nature 468(7326):973–977
47. Flaherty KT, Puzanov I, Kim KB et al (2010) Inhibition of mutated, activated BRAF in metastatic melanoma. N Engl J Med 363(9):809–819
48. Flaherty KT, Infante JR, Daud A et al (2012) Combined BRAF and MEK inhibition in melanoma with BRAF V600 mutations. N Engl J Med 367(18):1694–1703
49. Chapman PB, Hauschild A, Robert C et al (2011) Improved survival with vemurafenib in melanoma with BRAF V600E mutation. N Engl J Med 364(26):2507–2516
50. Sosman JA, Kim KB, Schuchter L et al (2012) Survival in BRAF V600-mutant advanced melanoma treated with vemurafenib. N Engl J Med 366(8):707–714
51. Hauschild A, Grob JJ, Demidov LV et al (2012) Dabrafenib in BRAF-mutated metastatic melanoma: a multicentre, open-label, phase 3 randomised controlled trial. Lancet 380(9839): 358–365
52. Lens MB, Dawes M (2002) Interferon alfa therapy for malignant melanoma: a systematic review of randomized controlled trials. J Clin Oncol 20(7):1818–1825
53. Mocellin S, Pasquali S, Rossi CR, Nitti D (2010) Interferon alpha adjuvant therapy in patients with high-risk melanoma: a systematic review and meta-analysis. J Natl Cancer Inst 102(7):493–501
54. Parkinson DR, Abrams JS, Wiernik PH et al (1990) Interleukin-2 therapy in patients with metastatic malignant melanoma: a phase II study. J Clin Oncol 8(10):1650–1656
55. Atkins MB, Lotze MT, Dutcher JP et al (1999) High-dose recombinant interleukin 2 therapy for patients with metastatic melanoma: analysis of 270 patients treated between 1985 and 1993. J Clin Oncol 17(7):2105–2116
56. Hodi FS, O'Day SJ, McDermott DF et al (2010) Improved survival with ipilimumab in patients with metastatic melanoma. N Engl J Med 363(8):711–723
57. Robert C, Thomas L, Bondarenko I et al (2011) Ipilimumab plus dacarbazine for previously untreated metastatic melanoma. N Engl J Med 364(26):2517–2526
58. Topalian SL, Hodi FS, Brahmer JR et al (2012) Safety, activity, and immune correlates of anti-PD-1 antibody in cancer. N Engl J Med 366(26):2443–2454

59. Brahmer JR, Tykodi SS, Chow LQ et al (2012) Safety and activity of anti-PD-L1 antibody in patients with advanced cancer. N Engl J Med 366(26):2455–2465
60. Dong Y, Richards JA, Gupta R et al (2013) PTEN functions as a melanoma tumor suppressor by promoting host immune response. Oncogene
61. Courtney KD, Corcoran RB, Engelman JA (2010) The PI3K pathway as drug target in human cancer. J Clin Oncol 28(6):1075–1083
62. Edgar KA, Wallin JJ, Berry M et al (2010) Isoform-specific phosphoinositide 3-kinase inhibitors exert distinct effects in solid tumors. Cancer Res 70(3):1164–1172
63. Lin J, Sampath D, Nannini MA et al (2013) Targeting activated Akt with GDC-0068, a novel selective Akt inhibitor that is efficacious in multiple tumor models. Clin Cancer Res 19(7):1760–1772
64. Vasudevan KM, Barbie DA, Davies MA et al (2009) AKT-independent signaling downstream of oncogenic PIK3CA mutations in human cancer. Cancer Cell 16(1):21–32
65. Robertson GP (2005) Functional and therapeutic significance of Akt deregulation in malignant melanoma. Cancer Metastasis Rev 24(2):273–285
66. Stahl JM, Sharma A, Cheung M et al (2004) Deregulated Akt3 activity promotes development of malignant melanoma. Cancer Res 64(19):7002–7010
67. Margolin K, Longmate J, Baratta T et al (2005) CCI-779 in metastatic melanoma: a phase II trial of the California Cancer Consortium. Cancer 104(5):1045–1048
68. Davies MA, Fox PS, Papadopoulos NE et al (2012) Phase I study of the combination of sorafenib and temsirolimus in patients with metastatic melanoma. Clin Cancer Res 18(4):1120–1128
69. Tabernero J, Rojo F, Calvo E et al (2008) Dose- and schedule-dependent inhibition of the mammalian target of rapamycin pathway with everolimus: a phase I tumor pharmacodynamic study in patients with advanced solid tumors. J Clin Oncol 26(10):1603–1610
70. O'Reilly KE, Rojo F, She QB et al (2006) mTOR inhibition induces upstream receptor tyrosine kinase signaling and activates Akt. Cancer Res 66(3):1500–1508
71. Carracedo A, Ma L, Teruya-Feldstein J et al (2008) Inhibition of mTORC1 leads to MAPK pathway activation through a PI3K-dependent feedback loop in human cancer. J Clin Invest 118(9):3065–3074
72. Soares HP, Ni Y, Kisfalvi K, Sinnett-Smith J, Rozengurt E (2013) Different patterns of Akt and ERK feedback activation in response to rapamycin, active-site mTOR inhibitors and metformin in pancreatic cancer cells. PLoS One 8(2):e57289
73. Chresta CM, Davies BR, Hickson I et al (2010) AZD8055 is a potent, selective, and orally bioavailable ATP-competitive mammalian target of rapamycin kinase inhibitor with in vitro and in vivo antitumor activity. Cancer Res 70(1):288–298
74. Deng W, Gopal YN, Scott A, Chen G, Woodman SE, Davies MA (2012) Role and therapeutic potential of PI3K-mTOR signaling in de novo resistance to BRAF inhibition. Pigment Cell Melanoma Res 25(2):248–258
75. Aziz SA, Jilaveanu LB, Zito C, Camp RL, Rimm DL, Conrad P, Kluger HM (2010) Vertical targeting of the phosphatidylinositol-3 kinase pathway as a strategy for treating melanoma. Clin Cancer Res 16(24):6029–6039
76. Andersen JN, Sathyanarayanan S, Di Bacco A et al (2010) Pathway-based identification of biomarkers for targeted therapeutics: personalized oncology with PI3K pathway inhibitors. Sci Transl Med 2(43):43ra55
77. Bollag G, Hirth P, Tsai J et al (2010) Clinical efficacy of a RAF inhibitor needs broad target blockade in BRAF-mutant melanoma. Nature 467(7315):596–599
78. Peralba JM, DeGraffenried L, Friedrichs W, Fulcher L, Grunwald V, Weiss G, Hidalgo M (2003) Pharmacodynamic evaluation of CCI-779, an Inhibitor of mTOR, in cancer patients. Clin Cancer Res 9(8):2887–2892
79. Yap TA, Yan L, Patnaik A et al (2011) First-in-man clinical trial of the oral pan-AKT inhibitor MK-2206 in patients with advanced solid tumors. J Clin Oncol 29(35):4688–4695
80. Shi Y, Yan H, Frost P, Gera J, Lichtenstein A (2005) Mammalian target of rapamycin inhibitors activate the AKT kinase in multiple myeloma cells by up-regulating the insulin-like growth

factor receptor/insulin receptor substrate-1/phosphatidylinositol 3-kinase cascade. Mol Cancer Ther 4(10):1533–1540

81. Chandarlapaty S, Sawai A, Scaltriti M et al (2011) AKT inhibition relieves feedback suppression of receptor tyrosine kinase expression and activity. Cancer Cell 19(1):58–71

82. Rodrik-Outmezguine VS, Chandarlapaty S, Pagano NC et al (2011) mTOR kinase inhibition causes feedback-dependent biphasic regulation of AKT signaling. Cancer Discov 1(3): 248–259

83. Chakrabarty A, Sanchez V, Kuba MG, Rinehart C, Arteaga CL (2012) Feedback upregulation of HER3 (ErbB3) expression and activity attenuates antitumor effect of PI3K inhibitors. Proc Natl Acad Sci USA 109(8):2718–2723

84. Serra V, Scaltriti M, Prudkin L et al (2011) PI3K inhibition results in enhanced HER signaling and acquired ERK dependency in HER2-overexpressing breast cancer. Oncogene 30(22): 2547–2557

Chapter 8
Biomarker Analysis of Gene-Mutated Protein Products by Immunohistochemistry in Melanoma

Carlos A. Torres-Cabala, Michael T. Tetzlaff, and Jonathan L. Curry

Abstract Melanoma has distinct yet highly interconnected genetic signaling network involved in cell proliferation, survival, and differentiation. Central to the molecular engine that drives melanoma are recurring activating *BRAF*, *NRAS*, *KIT*, and *GNAQ/GNA11* mutations in addition to a subset of tumors with functional loss of BAP1. The identification of these mutations in a subset of cutaneous melanomas has led to the development of novel mutation-specific-targeted therapies. Biomarker analysis, particularly with monoclonal anti-BRAF V600E has provided a highly sensitive and specific test for *BRAF V600E* mutation status, the most common mutation type in cutaneous melanoma. This chapter will examine the utility of biomarker expression by immunohistochemical methods in the evaluation of mutation status in melanoma and limitations to this testing method.

Keywords Biomarker • Gene mutation • Immunohistochemistry • Melanoma • BRAF • NRAS • KIT • GNAQ • GNA11 • BAP1

8.1 BRAF Mutation

BRAF belongs to RAF family of serine-threonine protein kinase in the MAPK cell signaling pathway and is one the three isoforms that include ARAF and CRAF [1]. BRAF activation triggers MAPK cell signaling pathway via phosphorylation of downstream targets MEK and ERK resulting in cell proliferation (Fig. 8.1). Compared to ARAF and CRAF, wild-type BRAF is constitutively activated thus

C.A. Torres-Cabala (✉) • J.L. Curry
Department of Pathology and Department of Dermatology, The University of Texas,
MD Anderson Cancer Center, Houston, TX, USA
e-mail: ctcabala@mdanderson.org; JLCurry@mdanderson.org

M.T. Tetzlaff
Department of Pathology, The University of Texas, MD Anderson Cancer Center,
Houston, TX, USA
e-mail: MTTetzlaff@mdanderson.org

© Springer Science+Business Media New York 2016
C.A. Torres-Cabala, J.L. Curry (eds.), *Genetics of Melanoma*, Cancer Genetics,
DOI 10.1007/978-1-4939-3554-3_8

Melanoma Genetic Signaling Network

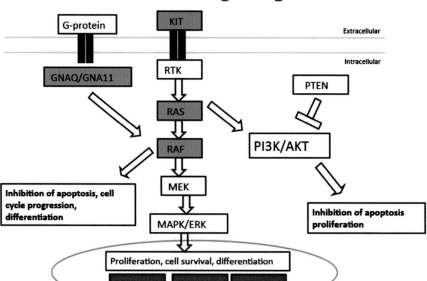

Fig. 8.1 Melanoma genetic signaling network. Most frequent genes mutated in melanoma involve growth-promoting signaling network with KIT, NRAS, BRAF, and GNAQ/GNA11 (*green boxes*) located extracellular and/or intracellular and growth inhibitory signaling network CDKN2A (p16) and BAP1 (*red boxes*) located in the nucleus. Melanoma has high degree of cross talk between the cell signaling pathways

more prone to mutation events than ARAF and CRAF isoforms [1]. A single DNA substitution point mutation thymine to adenine (T to A) that converts valine to glutamic acid at the 600 position of the amino acid (BRAF V600E) is the most frequent driver mutation in melanoma, occurring in ~75–90 % of patients with cutaneous melanoma [2–5]. *BRAF V600E* mutant melanomas that express the mutant protein exhibit greater than 400× more kinase activity wild-type BRAF [2, 6]. Not surprisingly, small molecule inhibitors (BRAFi) like vemurafenib that target BRAF V600E mutant protein demonstrated tremendous antitumor effect which translated into dramatic reduction of tumor burden and improved patient survival over standard chemotherapy [7].

The detection of BRAF V600E protein expression by monoclonal anti-BRAF V600E (clone VE1, Spring Bioscience, Pleasanton, CA) is a highly sensitive (97–100 %) and specific (97–100 %) biomarker in *BRAF V600E* mutation status of patients with melanoma [8–14]. In fact, the immunohistochemical (IHC) pattern of BRAF V600E protein expression and morphology of the melanoma cells significantly correlated with mutations status. Melanomas with epithelioid morphology (in contrast to spindle shape) that displayed a homogeneous expression pattern of BRAF V600E had a positive predictive value of ~98 % of harboring *BRAF V600E*

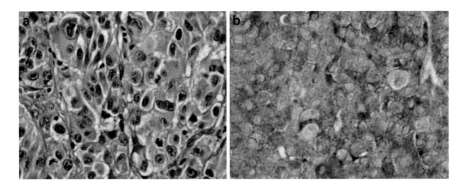

Fig. 8.2 (**a**) Metastatic melanoma with epithelioid cell morphology (hematoxylin and eosin, x400). (**b**) Tumor cells demonstrate strong and diffuse cytoplasmic immunohistochemical expression of BRAF V600E (anti-BRAF V600E with diaminobenzidine (DAB) and hematoxylin, x400)

mutation when tested by the next-generation sequencing (NGS) methods (Fig. 8.2) [14]. However, the inclusion of heterogeneous BRAF V600E protein expression as a positive test improved overall test sensitivity of this biomarker while lowering its test specificity. Since treatment of BRAFi to patients with BRAF non-600 mutations may enhance tumor growth, a lowered test specificity may have clinical implications [15]. In our practice, test specificity is clinically more critical, and in samples with heterogeneous or negative BRAF V600E IHC biomarker expression, we recommend correlation with DNA molecular analysis [14].

Molecular analysis of tumor DNA is con patient's sidered the gold standard in determining the mutation status of a patient's melanoma. However, on rare instances when biomarker test demonstrates unequivocal positivity for BRAF V600E IHC protein expression and there is a negative molecular test result, further investigation is warranted. We have experienced certain clinical situations in which expression of BRAF V600E biomarker was positive, while DNA molecular analysis was negative [16]. The discrepancy may be from tumor sampling particularly if only a focus of tumor is available in sections submitted for biomarker IHC expression and DNA analysis. Further investigation either by different molecular methods or testing alternative samples is advised.

The interpretation of BRAF V600E IHC expression in melanoma samples with notable melanin pigment can present a challenge. The presence of melanin pigment may obscure accurate visualization of the brown chromogen [3,3′-diaminobenzidine (DAB)] in the detection system and may be falsely interpreted as either "positive or negative." In these situations, we advise correlation with hematoxylin and eosin-stained slide and the use of Giemsa as the counterstain (melanin pigment will appear dark green, and positive IHC biomarker test result will remain brown) (Fig. 8.3). The use of red chromogen detection agent [3-amino-9-ethylcarbazole (AEC)] in selected cases is an alternative. Correlation with DNA analysis and results discussed with clinician will be essential.

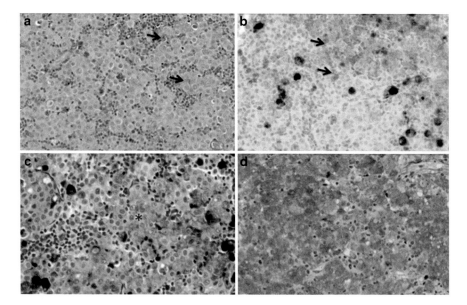

Fig. 8.3 (**a**) Melanoma with notable melanin pigment (*arrows*) (hematoxylin and eosin, x200). (**b**) Tumor cells may be misinterpreted as positive with anti-BRAF V600E immunohistochemical (IHC) stain when with diaminobenzidine (DAB) used as the detection system (Anti-BRAF V600E with diaminobenzidine (DAB) and hematoxylin, x200). (**c**) BRAF V600E IHC stain with DAB as the detection system and Giemsa as counterstain. Melanin pigment appears *dark green* not *brown* (*asterisk*); thus, tumor cells fail to express BRAF V600E (Anti-BRAF V600E with diaminobenzidine (DAB) and hematoxylin with Giemsa counterstain, x200). (**d**) *BRAF V600E* mutant melanoma. Tumor cells with immunohistochemical expression BRAF V600E will appear brown from DAB when counterstained with Giemsa (Anti-BRAF V600E with diaminobenzidine (DAB) and Giemsa counterstain, x200)

8.2 NRAS Mutation

NRAS belongs to the *RAS* oncogene family that also includes *HRAS* and *KRAS*. RAS activation recruits RAF which activates the MAPK cell signaling pathway promoting cell proliferation (Fig. 8.1). NRAS mutations occur in congenital melanocytic nevi and a 14–20 % of a subset of cutaneous melanoma [17–20]. Mutations in *NRAS* are activating mutations with Q61K and Q61R amino acid substitution commonly altered [5, 18].

The detection of NRAS Q61R protein expression by monoclonal anti-NRAS (Q61R) (clone SP174, Spring Bioscience, Pleasanton, CA) is a highly sensitive (~100 %) and specific (~100 %) IHC biomarker for *NRAS Q61R* mutation status [21, 22]. IHC expression of this biomarker appears to accurately identified melanomas that harbor the *NRAS Q61R* mutation. Further validation studies are in progress to examine the utility of this biomarker in melanoma.

8.3   KIT Mutation

KIT is the membrane tyrosine kinase receptor of the stem cell factor. The interaction between these two molecules is central for survival, proliferation, and differentiation of melanocytes [23]. In vitro studies initially demonstrated that, contrary to what happens in other tumors such as gastrointestinal stromal tumor (GIST) or mast cell leukemia where activating mutations in *KIT* induce malignant proliferation, melanoma cells should lose KIT in order to acquire proliferative advantage and become invasive [24]. In fact, observations of lack of expression of KIT in invasive and metastatic melanoma (in contrast to its detection in in situ melanoma) appeared to support this hypothesis [25]. However, it was subsequently noticed that some metastatic melanomas actually harbored mutations in *KIT* along with strong immunohistochemical expression of the protein [26, 27]. These findings were corroborated by array comparative genomic hybridization (aCGH) and mutation analysis studies [28] that identified a subset of mucosal, acral, and chronic sun-damaged-associated melanomas harboring activating mutations of *KIT*.

KIT can activate both the RAS-RAF-MEK-ERK and PI3K-AKT signaling pathways [29] (Fig. 8.1). Although activating mutations of *KIT* are rare in cutaneous melanomas in general, they are present in approximately 10–20 % of cases of acral lentiginous/mucosal and uveal melanomas [30–34]. The most frequent *KIT* mutations are found in exon 11 and exon 13 of the gene, located in 4q12. KIT L576P (exon 11) is the most common mutation identified in melanoma [32] (Fig. 8.4). This mutation promotes the dimerization and constitutive activation of KIT [28]. Identified mutations in exon 11 are V559A, V559G, and V560D, among others [32]. The K642E substitution in exon 13 affects the first tyrosine kinase domain of the protein. It appears that this mutation requires additional genetic alterations to be fully oncogenic. Indeed, a case carrying K642E mutation and a second mutation, N822I in exon 17, has been reported. Other mutations like D816V (exon 17), known to occur in acute myeloid leukemia and mastocytosis, have also been identified in melanoma [32]. D816V-mutated KIT has been reported to be insensitive to imatinib mesylate, as it occurs with D816H-mutated KIT in GIST [35] .

Fig. 8.4 The most common mutations of *KIT* in melanoma occur in exon 11. The mutation L576P, the most frequently encountered, derives from a point mutation in codon 576 that results in the substitution of leucine by proline

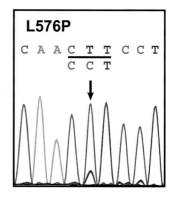

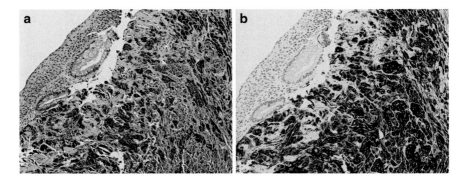

Fig. 8.5 Mucosal (anorectal) melanoma. (**a**) The tumor involves transitional squamous/glandular mucosa of the rectum. The tumor cells are heavily pigmented and numerous melanophages are present (hematoxylin and eosin, x100). (**b**) Immunohistochemical expression of KIT. Strong membranous and cytoplasmic expression is seen in this case. The tumor was demonstrated to harbor a mutation in *KIT*, V560D (Anti-KIT with diaminobenzidine (DAB) and hematoxylin, x100)

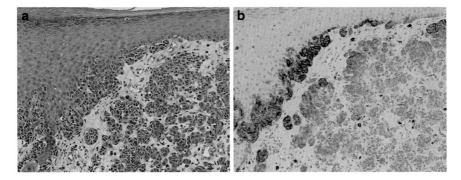

Fig. 8.6 Acral lentiginous melanoma. (**a**) The melanoma shows an in situ (lentiginous) component and invasion into the underlying dermis (hematoxylin and eosin, x200). (**b**) In this case, the in situ component of the tumor is diffusely and strongly positive for KIT by immunohistochemistry, whereas the invasive melanoma expresses the protein only focally (less than 10 % of the tumor cells). This melanoma was negative for mutations in *KIT* (Anti-KIT with diaminobenzidine (DAB) and hematoxylin, x200)

KIT can be detected by IHC using a polyclonal rabbit antibody (clone A4502, Dako Cytomation, Carpinteria, CA) in a high percentage of primary melanomas [36, 37]. Uveal and mucosal/acral lentiginous types are the most common KIT-positive melanomas (roughly between 40 and 80 %) [26, 32, 38, 39] (Fig. 8.5). Within the mucosal/acral lentiginous melanoma group, immunohistochemical detection of KIT appears to correlate with *KIT* mutation status as a strong negative predictor, since negative cases by IHC (less than 10 % of positive tumor cells) were not found to harbor any *KIT* mutations in a large study [32]. It appears that the in situ component of melanoma, regardless of mutation status, is almost always positive for KIT (Fig. 8.6), and metastases may show some decreased expression of the protein. The relatively high number of cases of melanoma that are negative for *KIT* mutation and show immunohistochemical expression of KIT may be explained by mechanisms other than gene mutation or amplification, such as epigenetic and autocrine/paracrine abnormalities [28]. Therefore, in contrast to the BRAF IHC stain, KIT IHC stain appears to be useful as a negative predictor of mutation and can be used to triage cases for molecular testing rather than as surrogate indicator for therapy with tyrosine kinase inhibitors. Nonetheless, isolated reports of cases showing partial response to imatinib mesylate in the absence of *KIT* mutation but strong expression of KIT by IHC [40] indicate that IHC detection of KIT per se may still play a role in the therapeutic decisions in some cases.

8.4   GNAQ/GNA11 Mutation

The *GNAQ* gene is located on chromosome 9q21. It encodes a heterotrimeric GTP-binding protein α-subunit that couples G-protein-coupled receptor signaling to the MAP kinase pathway [41] (Fig. 8.1). Mutations in the *GNAQ* gene at codon 209 of exon 5 (Q209L and Q209P) are found in uveal melanomas (around 50 %), primary melanocytic neoplasms of the central nervous system, and melanocytic nevi such as blue nevi and nevi of Ota [42, 43]. A case of mucosal melanoma harboring a *GNAQ* Q209L mutation has been reported [44].

Uveal melanomas that lack *GNAQ* mutation harbor mutations in a similar gene, *GNA11*, in up to 50 % [45]. In a series of uveal melanomas, mutations in *GNA11* were more frequent than mutations in *GNAQ* [46]. Most of these mutations are also mapped to exon 5 (Q209L), similar to *GNAQ*. It seems that *GNA11* Q209L mutations are more oncogenic and associated with a greater risk of distant metastasis than those involving *GNAQ* [47].

Immunohistochemical assays for GNAQ and GNA11 have been investigated in pancreatic and breast adenocarcinomas [48, 49]. To date, the correlation between IHC expression of GNAQ/GNA11 and *GNAQ/GNA11* mutation status in melanoma has not been reported.

8.5   BAP1 Mutation

BAP1 is a tumor suppressor gene mapped to 3p21.1 that encodes BRCA1-associated protein 1. BAP1 is a 90 kDa deubiquitinating enzyme located in the nucleus [50] (Fig. 8.1). BAP1 participates in several multiprotein complexes involved in repair of double-stranded DNA breaks, chromatin remodeling, cell cycle checkpoints, transcription, and apoptosis [50]. *BAP1* can be inactivated or lost as a result of a variety of mutations or deletions, which appear to be linked to specific functional abnormalities.

BAP1 mutations are associated with metastasizing uveal melanoma. It seems that while *GNAQ* mutations occur early in uveal melanoma and are not sufficient for malignant transformation, *BAP1* mutations occur later and coincide with the onset of metastasis [51]. In cutaneous melanocytic lesions, *BAP1* mutations were first described in the setting of an autosomal dominant syndrome associated with multiple clinically and morphologically distinct melanocytic neoplasms [52]. These BAP1-associated tumors ("BAPomas") show Spitzoid morphology and range from nevi to atypical proliferations with features of melanoma. This subset of Spitzoid tumors frequently displays *BRAF V600E* mutations [53].

Loss of BAP1 expression by IHC (clone C-4, Santa Cruz Biotechnology, CA) correlates well with biallelic inactivation of *BAP1* [53] (Fig. 8.7). In uveal melanoma, demonstration of loss of BAP1 by IHC correlates with poorer survival [54]. About 5 % of cutaneous melanomas appear to be lack expression of BAP1 by IHC [55]. It seems that desmoplastic melanoma is the subtype that more frequently loses expression of BAP1 and that this finding is independently associated with worse prognosis [55].

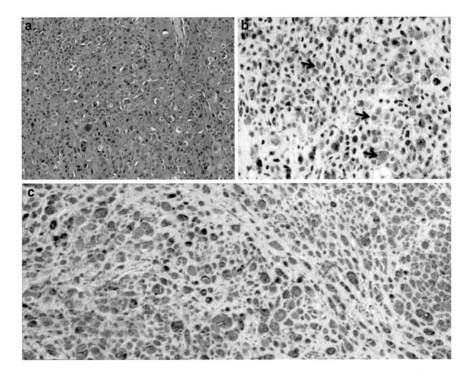

Fig. 8.7 BAP1-associated melanocytic tumor. (**a**) Epithelioid cells showing nuclear pleomorphism (Spitzoid features) are seen (hematoxylin and eosin, x200). (**b**) Loss of nuclear expression of BAP1 is detected by immunohistochemistry (*arrows*) (Anti-BAP1 with diaminobenzidine (DAB) and hematoxylin, x200). (**c**) The lesion demonstrates diffuse expression of BRAF V600E by immunohistochemistry, as it occurs in most of the BAP1-associated melanocytic lesions (Anti-BRAF V600E with diaminobenzidine (DAB) and hematoxylin, x200)

References

1. Mason CS, Springer CJ, Cooper RG, Superti-Furga G, Marshall CJ, Marais R (1999) Serine and tyrosine phosphorylations cooperate in Raf-1, but not B-Raf activation. EMBO J 18(8):2137–2148
2. Davies H, Bignell GR, Cox C et al (2002) Mutations of the BRAF gene in human cancer. Nature 417(6892):949–954
3. Xia J, Jia P, Hutchinson KE et al (2014) A meta-analysis of somatic mutations from next generation sequencing of 241 melanomas: a road map for the study of genes with potential clinical relevance. Mol Cancer Ther 13(7):1918–1928
4. Beadling C, Heinrich MC, Warrick A et al (2011) Multiplex mutation screening by mass spectrometry evaluation of 820 cases from a personalized cancer medicine registry. J Mol Diagn 13(5):504–513
5. Siroy AE, Boland GM, Milton DR et al (2015) Beyond BRAF(V600): clinical mutation panel testing by next-generation sequencing in advanced melanoma. J Invest Dermatol 135(2):508–515
6. Wan PT, Garnett MJ, Roe SM et al (2004) Mechanism of activation of the RAF-ERK signaling pathway by oncogenic mutations of B-RAF. Cell 116(6):855–867
7. Chapman PB, Hauschild A, Robert C et al (2011) Improved survival with vemurafenib in melanoma with BRAF V600E mutation. N Engl J Med 364(26):2507–2516
8. Marin C, Beauchet A, Capper D et al (2014) Detection of BRAF p.V600E mutations in melanoma by immunohistochemistry has a good interobserver reproducibility. Arch Pathol Lab Med 138(1):71–75
9. Capper D, Berghoff AS, Magerle M et al (2012) Immunohistochemical testing of BRAF V600E status in 1,120 tumor tissue samples of patients with brain metastases. Acta Neuropathol 123(2):223–233
10. Long GV, Wilmott JS, Capper D et al (2013) Immunohistochemistry is highly sensitive and specific for the detection of V600E BRAF mutation in melanoma. Am J Surg Pathol 37(1):61–65
11. Busam KJ, Hedvat C, Pulitzer M, von Deimling A, Jungbluth AA (2013) Immunohistochemical analysis of BRAF(V600E) expression of primary and metastatic melanoma and comparison with mutation status and melanocyte differentiation antigens of metastatic lesions. Am J Surg Pathol 37(3):413–420
12. Chen Q, Xia C, Deng Y et al (2014) Immunohistochemistry as a quick screening method for clinical detection of BRAF(V600E) mutation in melanoma patients. Tumour Biol 35(6):5727–5733
13. Feller JK, Yang S, Mahalingam M (2013) Immunohistochemistry with a mutation-specific monoclonal antibody as a screening tool for the BRAFV600E mutational status in primary cutaneous malignant melanoma. Mod Pathol 26(3):414–420
14. Tetzlaff MT, Pattanaprichakul P, Wargo J et al (2015) Utility of BRAF V600E immunohistochemistry expression pattern as a surrogate of BRAF mutation status in 154 patients with advanced melanoma. Hum Pathol 46(8):1101–1110
15. Kim DW, Nowroozi S, Kim K et al (2014) Clinical characteristics of patients with non-V600 BRAF mutant melanomas. J Clin Oncol 32(5s):suppl; abstr 9100
16. Jabbar KJ, Luthra R, Patel KP et al (2014) Comparison of next generation sequencing mutation profiling with BRAF and IDH1 mutation specific immunohistochemistry. Am J Surg Pathol 39(4):454–461
17. Ross AL, Sanchez MI, Grichnik JM (2011) Molecular nevogenesis. Dermatol Res Pract 2011:463184
18. Takata M, Saida T (2006) Genetic alterations in melanocytic tumors. J Dermatol Sci 43(1):1–10
19. Curtin JA, Fridlyand J, Kageshita T et al (2005) Distinct sets of genetic alterations in melanoma. N Engl J Med 353(20):2135–2147

20. Jakob JA, Bassett RL Jr, Ng CS et al (2012) NRAS mutation status is an independent prognostic factor in metastatic melanoma. Cancer 118(16):4014–4023
21. Ilie M, Long-Mira E, Funck-Brentano E et al (2015) Immunohistochemistry as a potential tool for routine detection of the NRAS Q61R mutation in patients with metastatic melanoma. J Am Acad Dermatol 72(5):786–793
22. Massi D, Simi L, Sensi E et al (2015) Immunohistochemistry is highly sensitive and specific for the detection of NRAS Q61R mutation in melanoma. Mod Pathol 28(4):487–497
23. Grichnik JM, Burch JA, Burchette J, Shea CR (1998) The SCF/KIT pathway plays a critical role in the control of normal human melanocyte homeostasis. J Invest Dermatol 111(2):233–238
24. Alexeev V, Yoon K (2006) Distinctive role of the cKit receptor tyrosine kinase signaling in mammalian melanocytes. J Invest Dermatol 126(5):1102–1110
25. Natali PG, Nicotra MR, Winkler AB, Cavaliere R, Bigotti A, Ullrich A (1992) Progression of human cutaneous melanoma is associated with loss of expression of c-kit proto-oncogene receptor. Int J Cancer 52(2):197–201
26. Guerriere-Kovach PM, Hunt EL, Patterson JW, Glembocki DJ, English JC 3rd, Wick MR (2004) Primary melanoma of the skin and cutaneous melanomatous metastases: comparative histologic features and immunophenotypes. Am J Clin Pathol 122(1):70–77
27. Willmore-Payne C, Holden JA, Tripp S, Layfield LJ (2005) Human malignant melanoma: detection of BRAF- and c-kit-activating mutations by high-resolution amplicon melting analysis. Hum Pathol 36(5):486–493
28. Curtin JA, Busam K, Pinkel D, Bastian BC (2006) Somatic activation of KIT in distinct subtypes of melanoma. J Clin Oncol 24(26):4340–4346
29. Glitza IC, Davies MA (2014) Genotyping of cutaneous melanoma. Chin Clin Oncol 3(3):27
30. Antonescu CR, Busam KJ, Francone TD et al (2007) L576P KIT mutation in anal melanomas correlates with KIT protein expression and is sensitive to specific kinase inhibition. Int J Cancer 121(2):257–264
31. Beadling C, Jacobson-Dunlop E, Hodi FS et al (2008) KIT gene mutations and copy number in melanoma subtypes. Clin Cancer Res 14(21):6821–6828
32. Torres-Cabala CA, Wang WL, Trent J et al (2009) Correlation between KIT expression and KIT mutation in melanoma: a study of 173 cases with emphasis on the acral-lentiginous/mucosal type. Mod Pathol 22(11):1446–1456
33. Kong Y, Si L, Zhu Y et al (2011) Large-scale analysis of KIT aberrations in Chinese patients with melanoma. Clin Cancer Res 17(7):1684–1691
34. Wallander ML, Layfield LJ, Emerson LL et al (2011) KIT mutations in ocular melanoma: frequency and anatomic distribution. Mod Pathol 24(8):1031–1035
35. Frost MJ, Ferrao PT, Hughes TP, Ashman LK (2002) Juxtamembrane mutant V560GKit is more sensitive to Imatinib (STI571) compared with wild-type c-kit whereas the kinase domain mutant D816VKit is resistant. Mol Cancer Ther 1(12):1115–1124
36. Potti A, Hille RC, Koch M (2003) Immunohistochemical determination of HER-2/neu overexpression in malignant melanoma reveals no prognostic value, while c-Kit (CD117) overexpression exhibits potential therapeutic implications. J Carcinog 2(1):8
37. Nazarian RM, Prieto VG, Elder DE, Duncan LM (2010) Melanoma biomarker expression in melanocytic tumor progression: a tissue microarray study. J Cutan Pathol 37(Suppl 1):41–47
38. Dai B, Cai X, Kong YY et al (2013) Analysis of KIT expression and gene mutation in human acral melanoma: with a comparison between primary tumors and corresponding metastases/recurrences. Hum Pathol 44(8):1472–1478
39. Santi R, Simi L, Fucci R et al (2015) KIT genetic alterations in anorectal melanomas. J Clin Pathol 68(2):130–134
40. Kim KB, Eton O, Davis DW et al (2008) Phase II trial of imatinib mesylate in patients with metastatic melanoma. Br J Cancer 99(5):734–740
41. Ross EM, Wilkie TM (2000) GTPase-activating proteins for heterotrimeric G proteins: regulators of G protein signaling (RGS) and RGS-like proteins. Annu Rev Biochem 69:795–827

42. Van Raamsdonk CD, Bezrookove V, Green G et al (2009) Frequent somatic mutations of GNAQ in uveal melanoma and blue naevi. Nature 457(7229):599–602
43. Kusters-Vandevelde HV, Klaasen A, Kusters B et al (2010) Activating mutations of the GNAQ gene: a frequent event in primary melanocytic neoplasms of the central nervous system. Acta Neuropathol 119(3):317–323
44. Kim CY, Kim DW, Kim K, Curry J, Torres-Cabala C, Patel S (2014) GNAQ mutation in a patient with metastatic mucosal melanoma. BMC Cancer 14:516
45. Van Raamsdonk CD, Griewank KG, Crosby MB et al (2010) Mutations in GNA11 in uveal melanoma. N Engl J Med 363(23):2191–2199
46. Griewank KG, van de Nes J, Schilling B et al (2014) Genetic and clinico-pathologic analysis of metastatic uveal melanoma. Mod Pathol 27(2):175–183
47. Patel M, Smyth E, Chapman PB et al (2011) Therapeutic implications of the emerging molecular biology of uveal melanoma. Clin Cancer Res 17(8):2087–2100
48. Mann KM, Ward JM, Yew CC et al (2012) Sleeping Beauty mutagenesis reveals cooperating mutations and pathways in pancreatic adenocarcinoma. Proc Natl Acad Sci USA 109(16):5934–5941
49. Asada K, Miyamoto K, Fukutomi T et al (2003) Reduced expression of GNA11 and silencing of MCT1 in human breast cancers. Oncology 64(4):380–388
50. Murali R, Wiesner T, Scolyer RA (2013) Tumours associated with BAP1 mutations. Pathology 45(2):116–126
51. Harbour JW, Onken MD, Roberson ED et al (2010) Frequent mutation of BAP1 in metastasizing uveal melanomas. Science 330(6009):1410–1413
52. Wiesner T, Obenauf AC, Murali R et al (2011) Germline mutations in BAP1 predispose to melanocytic tumors. Nat Genet 43(10):1018–1021
53. Wiesner T, Murali R, Fried I et al (2012) A distinct subset of atypical Spitz tumors is characterized by BRAF mutation and loss of BAP1 expression. Am J Surg Pathol 36(6):818–830
54. Shah AA, Bourne TD, Murali R (2013) BAP1 protein loss by immunohistochemistry: a potentially useful tool for prognostic prediction in patients with uveal melanoma. Pathology 45(7):651–656
55. Murali R, Wilmott JS, Jakrot V et al (2013) BAP1 expression in cutaneous melanoma: a pilot study. Pathology 45(6):606–609

Chapter 9
Molecular Platforms for Melanoma Mutation Analysis

Alaa A. Salim and Keyur Pravinchandra Patel

Abstract   Recurrent mutually exclusive somatic mutations including *BRAF*, *NRAS*, and *KIT* are among the most common genetic aberrations underlying pathogenesis of melanoma. Testing for these mutations can be useful in providing diagnostic, therapeutic, and prognostic information. Molecular diagnostic techniques for mutational analysis are becoming standard of care in melanoma as the detection of these mutations will contribute to the development of molecular classification of melanocytic tumors and guides through choosing the most appropriate therapy in the era of personalized medicine.

Keywords   Melanoma • Mutation analysis • Gene mutations • Prognosis • Targeted therapy • Personalized medicine • Sanger sequencing • Pyrosequencing • Sequenom • Next-generation sequencing • PCR • ASO-PCR

9.1   Introduction

9.1.1   Gene Mutations and Melanoma

Identification of somatic genetic aberrations in melanoma has led to better understanding of the biology of the disease which in turn led to better diagnosis, staging, and prognostication. This also facilitated molecular reclassification of melanoma in association with other pathological findings. For instance, acral, mucosal, ocular, chronic sun exposure and intermittent sun exposure melanomas have been proven to have a distinct genetic profile which reflects different susceptibility of different body parts to ultraviolet light [1]. Defining the molecular drivers of melanoma which regulate the tumor proliferation and survival opened the doors for discovery of targeted therapy that improved the disease control and the patient's overall

A.A. Salim, MD • K.P. Patel, MD, PhD (✉)
Department of Hematopathology, The University of Texas MD Anderson Cancer Center, Houston, TX, USA
e-mail: AAAlmohammedsali@mdanderson.org; KPPatel@mdanderson.org

© Springer Science+Business Media New York 2016   193
C.A. Torres-Cabala, J.L. Curry (eds.), *Genetics of Melanoma*, Cancer Genetics,
DOI 10.1007/978-1-4939-3554-3_9

survival rate. Molecular abnormalities in melanoma are mostly due to oncogenes related to the direct and indirect activation of the cell cycle regulatory proteins and signaling molecules including receptor tyrosine kinases (RTK) and the downstream mitogen-activated protein kinase (MAPK) *NRAS/BRAF/ERK* and phosphatidylinositol 3-kinase (PI3K)/*PTEN* pathways [2]. Common mutations include *BRAF*, *NRAS*, and *KIT* genes. *PTEN*, *GNAQ*, and *GNA11* gene mutations are less commonly involved.

BRAF activating mutation accounts for 65 % of melanomas with intermittent sun exposure. It most commonly affects codon 600 in exon 15 (V600E and less frequently, V600K, V600D, and V600R). *NRAS* activating mutation accounts for 20 % of melanomas with intermittent sun exposure and 15 % of melanomas arising in chronically sun-exposed skin. It most commonly affects residues in exon 1 (codon 12) or 2 (codon 60 and 61) of the gene [1]. *KIT* is a receptor tyrosine kinase that can activate several pathways, including MAPK, PI3K, and STAT3. Activating mutations are encountered in 15–20 % of melanomas involving acral, mucosal, and chronically sun-exposed sites. Most of these mutations are point mutations which occur in exons 11, 13, and 17 leading to in-frame amino acid substitution. *KIT* amplification at 4q12 locus has been reported in subset of cases [3]. *GNAQ* and *GNA11* activating mutations involve the hotspot residue on exon 5, which are mostly found in uveal melanomas, rarely on sun-damaged skin but not in acral or mucosal melanomas [4, 5]. All these mutations are mutually exclusive. In addition, large-scale genomic sequencing efforts have identified a distinct set of genes that are shown to be mutated at varying rate in melanoma [6].

9.1.2 Impact of Molecular Genetic Testing on Melanoma Care

Clinical utility of genetic mutations in melanoma can be categorized as diagnostic, prognostic, and predictive.

Diagnostic Mutational testing can help in subtyping of melanoma and therefore predicting the clinical behavior, e.g., *BRAF* mutations usually seen in younger age group (<55) and well known to be prevalent in cutaneous melanoma arising in intermittent sun-exposed skin like the trunk and proximal limbs from preexisting nevus with characteristic clinical and morphologic features [7]. *NRAS* mutations in some studies were shown to be more common in cutaneous melanoma arising in intermittent sun-exposed skin, nodular melanoma and lentigo maligna melanoma, while *KIT* mutations occur more frequently in acral, mucosal, and chronically sun-damaged sites like the head and neck and extremities. It can also help in identification of primary tumor sites in cases of metastatic melanoma of unknown primary.

Prognostic Characteristic mutations in the MAPK pathway are associated with poor prognosis. In a recent large series of melanoma comparing cases with *BRAF* and *NRAS* mutations to wild-type cases, patients with these mutations presented with higher-stage primary tumors [8].

Predictive Detection of *BRAF* mutations has significant therapeutic consequences. It has led to the development of selective *BRAF* inhibitors like vemurafenib and dabrafenib that induce tumor regression and improve the overall survival rate of patients with metastatic melanoma. Inhibitors of MEK a downstream mediator of RAS and RAF pathways were reported to be useful in *BRAF* mutations and possibly *NRAS* and *GNAQ/GNA11* mutations [9]. Although initial studies on unselected patients with advanced melanoma treated with imatinib showed minimal activity, tyrosine kinase inhibitors have a good clinical response in selected patients with activating *KIT* mutation [10, 11].

9.1.3 Mutation Analysis Platforms

A variety of molecular diagnostic strategies are available for gene mutation detection. The majority of these techniques require PCR-based amplification of the region of interest. Different detection strategies are applied based on the nature and location of the mutation within the gene. Mutations in melanoma which are limited to specific codons within the gene can be detected by direct pyrosequencing based on the detection of pyrophosphate released upon nucleotide incorporation, e.g., codon 600 mutations in *BRAF* and codons 12, 13, and 61 mutations in *NRAS*. *KIT* mutations including point mutations, deletions, and insertions involving exons 11, 13, and 17 are best detected by direct sequencing of DNA using Sanger sequencing.

The development of multiplex genotyping assays using single-nucleotide extension reactions such as Sequenom MassARRAY (Sequenom, San Diego, CA) allowed the detection of multiple mutations starting with a small amount of genomic DNA. The recent advent of massive parallel next-generation sequencing (NGS) platforms enabled the sequencing of large panels of genes involved in melanoma in a short period of time with less cost. Choosing the most appropriate test methodology depends on multiple factors such as the type of mutation, the frequency of mutation, anticipated test volume, sample type, sample volume, cost of technology, and preexistent instruments.

The vast majority of mutations in melanoma occur either at single-nucleotide level or small genetic alterations like insertions and deletions. Therefore, in this chapter we will discuss the most common testing methods used for detection of these mutations in a clinical setting which include Sanger sequencing, pyrosequencing, single-base primer extension MassARRAY (Sequenom), and NGS.

9.2   Sanger Sequencing

9.2.1   Principle of Sanger Sequencing

Sanger sequencing, considered as the gold standard method in DNA sequencing, is an enzymatic method works by chain termination approach. It is based on selective incorporation of chain-terminating dideoxynucleotide triphosphates (ddNTPs) by DNA polymerase during in vitro DNA replication. Four ddNTPs are used which lack the hydroxyl group required to connect with the next base to elongate the chain, and labeled with different colored fluorescent dyes, each with characteristic emission wavelength. In addition to the DNA template, the reaction contains primer, DNA polymerase, and dNTPs. The cycle sequencing reaction will result in DNA fragments of varying lengths differing by a single base that can be separated by capillary electrophoresis coupled with a laser detector which detects fluorescence from the four different dyes that are used to identify A, G, C, and T termination. The sequence then can be determined by correlating the color with a specific ddNTP.

Key steps in Sanger sequencing include:

1. First-round PCR to amplify the region of interest from the genomic DNA or cDNA, followed by cleanup of unincorporated nucleotides. An optional second-round nested PCR may help with increasing the amount of scant product or specificity of the analyzed product.
2. The next step, cycle sequencing (asymmetric PCR), generates chain-terminated fragments of various lengths. Generally speaking, bidirectional sequencing is preferred as it reduces the interpretation pitfalls resulting from sequencing artifacts.
3. Capillary electrophoresis (CE) is used to separate and read terminal base pair in sequencing products.
4. Analysis of the Sanger sequencing data includes primary analysis to check for dye incorporation, CE injection, and overall quality of sequence obtained using Sequencing Analysis software. Secondary analysis of sequencing traces, including trimming, assembly of forward and reverse strands, and comparison to normal gene template allows detection of mutations in the test sequence.

9.2.2   Result Reporting/Analytic Interpretation

For a high accuracy call, the identical insertion/deletion or point mutation must be present in both forward and reverse sequencing reaction (see Fig. 9.1). Depending on the gene protocol, mutations and equivocal mutations can be defaulted to or confirmed by alternate methodology (e.g., ASO-PCR or pyrosequencing) or repeated from the first PCR step. The final report includes each mutation, including the codon affected, nucleotide change, and the corresponding predicted amino acid change. Wherever possible, mutations and sequence variants are reported according to the HGVS/HUGO Gene Nomenclature.

Sanger   **Pyrosequencing**   **Sequenom**

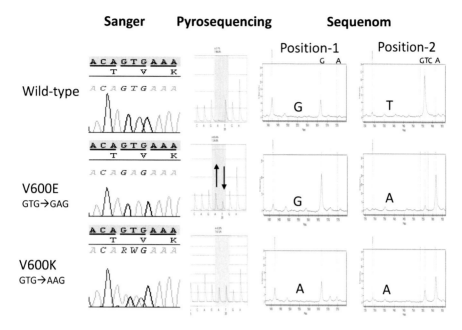

Fig. 9.1 Detection of *BRAF* V600 gene mutations on exon 15 by sequencing. *Upper panel*: wild-type sequence for amino acid valine (codon 600, GTG) shown by Sanger sequencing, *left*. The pyrogram shows wild-type sequence with three equal peaks (GTG), *middle*. Wild-type sequence by sequenom, *right*. *Middle panel*: the amino acid valine V600E point mutation, where a single-base substitution thymine>adenine (overlapping peaks) results in codon 600 mutation (GTG to GAG), changing the amino acid from valine to glutamic acid, detected by Sanger sequencing, *left*. On pyrosequencing, mutation is detected by increase in adenine peak and decrease in thymine peak, *middle*. Single-base mutation in codon 600 of *BRAF* gene (GTG>GAG) that would change the encoding amino acid from valine to glutamic acid (V600E) is detected by sequenom, *right*. *Lower panel*: the amino acid valine V600K point mutation, where two-base substitutions guanine>adenine and thymine>adenine result in codon 600 mutation (GTG to AAG), changing the amino acid from valine to lysine, detected by Sanger sequencing, *left*. In the *middle*, the mutation is seen on the pyrogram with increase in two adenine peaks and decrease in both guanine and thiamine peaks. On sequenom, two increasing adenine peaks and diminishing guanine and thymine peaks are indicative of two-base substitution (GTG>AAG) and V600E mutation, *right*

9.2.3   Limitations of Sanger Sequencing

1. For clinical purposes, the sensitivity of detection is approximately one mutated allele in a background of ten wild-type alleles. This translates into a minimum of one tumor cell with heterozygous mutation in a total of five cells without the mutation and hence the requirement for a minimum tumor percentage (20 %) in the sample tested. Samples with low tumor percentage may give a false-negative result with this assay.
2. Compared to other genotyping methods, Sanger sequencing is considered relatively more labor intensive, less sensitive, and lower throughput.

9.3 Pyrosequencing

9.3.1 Principle of Pyrosequencing

Pyrosequencing, also known as sequencing by synthesis, is a method that sequences a short strand of DNA using the target DNA template. It is based on the detection of released pyrophosphate during DNA synthesis. DNA sequence is determined by adding individual nucleotides at a time into an elongating strand of DNA in a predetermined order that results in natural release of pyrophosphate. This is followed by a cascade of enzymatic reactions which generate visible light proportional to the number of nucleotides incorporated. Measuring the light signals will identify the nucleotides added and then the sequence generated. In brief, a sequencing primer is hybridized with a single-strand target DNA generated by PCR and incubated with an enzyme cocktail (DNA polymerase, ATP sulfurylase, luciferase, and apyrase) and the substrates, adenosine 5′-phosphosulfate (APS) and luciferin. The first of four deoxynucleotide triphosphates (dNTP) is added to the reaction, and if it is complementary to the base in the DNA template, it will be incorporated to the single strand catalyzed by DNA polymerase. With each incorporation, pyrophosphate (PPi) is naturally released, and hence the term pyrosequencing, in a quantity equivalent to the amount of incorporated nucleotide. The released pyrophosphate is used in a sulfurylase reaction releasing ATP. The released ATP is used by luciferase in the conversion of luciferin to oxyluciferin. The reaction results in the emission of light which is proportional to the number of nucleotides incorporated. The light signals are recorded by a charge-coupled device camera in the form of peaks, known as pyrogram. If no nucleotide is incorporated, pyrophosphate will not be released and the unused nucleotide will be degraded by apyrase. As the process continues, the sequence of growing DNA strand can be determined from the magnitude of the peaks in the pyrogram as it is synthesized.

Major advantages of pyrosequencing include higher sensitivity (10–20 %) in mutation detection compared to Sanger sequencing (5–10 %), flexibility of the assay design, amenability to degraded/low-quality source DNA, low cost, and short-time procedure.

Key steps in pyrosequencing include:

1. First-round PCR to amplify the region of interest from genomic DNA or cDNA.
2. Pyrosequencing of the amplified PCR product using a sequencing primer. Due to the constraints on placement of sequencing primers, the pyrosequencing assays intend to be unidirectional. Clinical analyses are typically performed in duplicates.
3. Analysis of pyrograms including comparison with reference wild-type and mutant sequences.

9.3.2 Results Reporting/Analytical Interpretation of Pyrosequencing

– Pyrosequencing results (pyrograms) are essentially graphs of light intensity versus time.
– Each test sample pyrogram is compared against the negative control. If no differences in peak heights are observed, the sample is reported as negative for mutation. If there is a difference in a peak height, or an additional peak appears, the mutation is determined and reported.
– Mutations will be indicated as additional peaks to the wild type or alterations in the height of wild-type peaks with relation to a reference peak (see Fig. 9.1).

The sensitivity of detection is approximately 10 % mutation-containing cells present in the sample.

9.3.3 Limitations of Pyrosequencing

1. Short sequence read length (30 bases long) although with improved chemistry, it can be capable of read lengths between 400 and 500 bp
2. Low resolution with long repeats of the same nucleotides

9.4 Single-Base Primer Extension MassARRAY (Sequenom)

9.4.1 Principle of Single-Base Primer Extension MassARRAY (Sequenom)

The MassARRAY platform is used to for genotyping genetic variations such as single-nucleotide polymorphisms (SNPs), insertion/deletions, and mutations. Available gene panels like MelaCarta v1.0 can be used to assess mutation status of 72 hotspot regions of 20 oncogenes and tumor suppressors in melanoma: *AKT1, BRAF, CDK4, CXCR4, CTTNB1, ERBB4, EPHA10, EPHB6, GNA11, GNAQ, KIT, KRAS, MEK, MET, NEK10, NRAS, PDGFRA, PIK3CA, PTK2B,* and *ROR2.*

Briefly, the MassARRAY system is based on multiplex PCR followed by a single-base primer extension reaction. The primer extension products are analyzed using Matrix-assisted laser desorption/ionization time-of-flight mass spectrometry or MALDI-TOF MS. During MALDI-TOF MS, a matrix is used to protect the biomolecule (DNA) from being destroyed by direct laser beam and to facilitate vaporization and ionization. The biomolecule is ionized via laser pulses. Molecules are separated according to mass to charge ratio. The ionized molecules "fly" through the vacuum tube toward the detector. Low-mass molecules reach the detector first.

The time of flight is converted to a spectrogram that graphs mass verses intensity. Mass-modified terminator nucleotides incorporated during the single-base extension are used to distinguish different genotypes.

9.4.2 Result Reporting/Analytic Interpretation

Spectra of each assays in a well is compared against the negative control for all patients. Calls made by the Typer Software are based on the height of each peak. Manual calls are made based on extra peaks lining up with individual nucleotides (see Fig. 9.1).

The sensitivity of this assay for detection of a mutation, as established during assay validation, is 1 in 10 mutation-bearing cells in the population. Final report includes the results of the mutational analysis for the gene, codon involved, and the amino acid change.

9.4.3 Limitations of Single-Base Primer Extension MassARRAY (Sequenom)

1. The sensitivity of detecting a point mutation by PCR-based single-base extension assay on the MassARRAY platform is approximately one mutated cell in ten cells without the mutation. Therefore, samples in which the tumor is present in small numbers compared to nonneoplastic cells may give a false-negative result with this assay. The presence of mutations outside the tested codons cannot be excluded.
2. Multiplexing capability in between the conventional sequencing platforms and recent NGS platforms.

9.5 Next-Generation Sequencing

9.5.1 Principle of Next-Generation Sequencing

The discovery of NGS technology has increased the throughput of DNA sequencing and tremendously decreased the time and cost associated with comprehensive genome analysis. It represents a major departure from traditional Sanger sequencing technique by allowing whole-genome and whole-exome sequencing along with the flexibility of multiplexing and screening specific panels of genes for mutations. Advantages of NGS technologies include the ability to screen multiple genes with limited starting material compared to conventional sequencing platforms that require relatively larger DNA quantities. In addition, its compatibile with real-life melanoma specimens, such as formalin-fixed, paraffin-embedded (FFPE) or fine-needle aspiration (FNA) biopsy specimens with potentially fragmented and cross-linked DNA. Currently, several NGS platforms and panels are available for sequencing of target genomic regions. Majority of the commercially available NGS panels for oncologic testing include *BRAF*, *NRAS*, and *KIT* genes. The coverage is either focused on the frequently mutated regions (hotspots) or entire coding sequence of the gene to detect point mutations, deletions, and insertions. Commercially available platforms used include Ion Torrent Personal Genome Machine (IT-PGM; Life Technologies, Carlsbad, CA) and Illumina (the GAII; Illumina, San Diego, CA).

Different NGS technologies may employ different techniques but all have the following common steps:

1. *DNA library preparation*. It involves preparation of DNA template, which needs to be sequenced. In the case of whole genome, this would be fragmented and size-selected genomic DNA. In the case of targeted regions, areas of interest would be clonally PCR amplified to generate a DNA library which will be used as templates for sequencing. The DNA to be sequenced (fragmented, if whole genome, or the targeted amplicon library prepared by multiplexed PCR amplification reaction) is ligated to adaptors. Special adaptors with specific barcodes sequence can be ligated to amplicon library prepared to facilitate simultaneous sequencing of several samples each identified by a specific DNA barcode.

2. *Sequencing and data acquisition*. The DNA sample to be sequenced is used as a template and sequenced. Monitoring the sequence of incorporated nucleotides in real time is used to obtain the sequence information of the template being sequenced. This is also referred to as "sequencing by synthesis." During Ion Torrent sequencing (Ion PGM, Ion Proton), four nucleotides are flowed in a predetermined order. The pH change resulting from the release of hydrogen ion during nucleotide incorporation is measured to determine the nucleotide sequence. In comparison, Illumina sequencing platforms (MiSeq, HiSeq, NextSeq) utilize laser and optics to detect incorporation of a fluorescently labeled nucleotide during each synthesis cycle.

3. *Sequence alignment and data analysis*. This constitutes a very important step, where the sequence information collected is aligned to the respective reference sequence which helps to determine the quality of the sequencing and also detect the presence of sequence alterations by comparing test sequence against the wild-type sequences. This process is computationally intensive and requires specialized aligner and variant caller softwares.

9.5.2 Result Reporting/Analytic Interpretation

Each sequence variant identified for the sample is visualized in a genome browser such as integrative genomic viewer (IGV) and is decided by several criteria which include variant frequency of 10 % or more, adequate sequencing coverage (250×), presence of the variant in both forward and reverse reads, and comparable variant

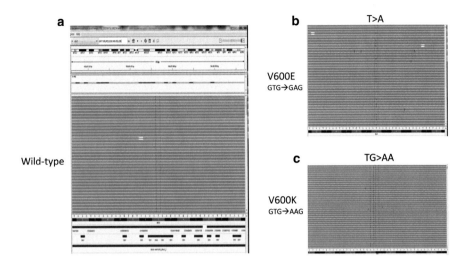

Fig. 9.2 Detection of *BRAF* V600E mutation on exon 15 by next-generation sequencing. In the *upper panel*, IGV shows wild-type *BRAF* V600 sequence (GTG). In the *lower panel*, IGV shows V600E point mutation with single-base substitution thymine > T (adenine in reverse direction), in both forward (*red*) and reverse (*blue*) reads changing the base sequence (GTG > GAG) and the amino acid from valine to glutamic acid

frequency in reads of both directions (see Fig. 9.2). Since NGS analysis assesses a wider genomic region, mutations can be found in any of the covered region. Also, a variety of sequencing artifacts may be detected. Statistical analysis of the available data allows filtering of nonspecific calls.

9.5.3 Limitations of Next-Generation Sequencing

1. The possibility of any detected mutation being a germline mutation cannot be ruled out unless a germline sample is tested.
2. At homopolymer stretch, nonlinear correlation between signal generated and the number of nucleotides incorporated leads to erroneous mutation calls in some NGS platforms.
3. Certain mutations like deletions and insertions could be missed by the variant caller software unless specifically optimized. This necessitates manual review of the sequence and read alignment of the gene of interest in IGV.

9.6 Summary

In summary, mutational analysis in melanoma is currently considered a standard of care since the diagnosis of the disease, providing prognostic information and guiding therapeutic decisions heavily rely on the mutational status of the disease. The critical role of these molecular markers in driving the advancement of melanoma research can't be overemphasized. In this chapter, we have discussed different molecular diagnostic procedures used in detection of gene mutations commonly seen in melanoma taking in consideration the advantages, technical difficulties, and limitations of each procedure which will have a great impact on choosing the most appropriate testing platform.

References

1. Curtin JA, Fridlyand J, Kageshita T et al (2005) Distinct sets of genetic alterations in melanoma. N Engl J Med 353(20):2135–2147
2. Tubbs RR, Stoler MH (2009) Cell and tissue based molecular pathology. Churchill Livingstone, Philadelphia
3. Curtin JA, Busam K, Pinkel D, Bastian BC (2006) Somatic activation of KIT in distinct subtypes of melanoma. J Clin Oncol 24:4340–4346
4. Van Raamsdonk CD, Bezrookove V, Green G et al (2009) Frequent somatic mutations of GNAQ in uveal melanoma and blue naevi. Nature 457:599–602
5. Van Raamsdonk CD, Griewank KG, Crosby MB et al (2010) Mutations in GNA11 in uveal melanoma. N Engl J Med 363:2191–2199
6. Xia J, Jia P, Hutchinson KE et al (2014) A meta-analysis of somatic mutations from next generation sequencing of 241 melanomas: a road map for the study of genes with potential clinical relevance. Mol Cancer Ther 13(7):1918–1928
7. Viros A, Fridlyand J, Bauer J et al (2008) Improving melanoma classification by integrating genetic and morphologic features. PLoS Med 5:e120
8. Thomas NE, Edmiston SN, Alexander A et al (2015) Association between NRAS and BRAF mutational status and melanoma-specific survival among patients with higher-risk primary melanoma. JAMA Oncol 1(3):359–368
9. Solit DB, Garraway LA, Pratilas CA et al (2006) BRAF mutation predicts sensitivity to MEK inhibition. Nature 439(7074):358–362
10. Hodi FS, Friedlander P, Corless CL et al (2008) Major response to imatinib mesylate in KIT-mutated melanoma. J Clin Oncol 26:2046–2051
11. Lutzky J, Bauer J, Bastian BC (2008) Dose-dependent, complete response to imatinib of a metastatic mucosal melanoma with a K642E KIT mutation. Pigment Cell Melanoma Res 21:492–493

Part IV
Melanoma Therapeutics

Chapter 10
Immunotherapy in Melanoma

Van A. Trinh, Yeorim Ahn, and Wen-Jen Hwu

Abstract Clinical and laboratory observations suggest that host immunity may influence the course of melanoma progression, rationalizing the investigation of immunotherapeutic approaches in this disease. Areas of active investigation have included the use of recombinant cytokines, either alone or in combination with other biologic response modifiers, cancer vaccines, gene therapy, adoptive immunotherapy, or monoclonal antibodies. Although cytokine therapies of interferon alpha (IFN) and interleukin-2 (IL-2) are effective in only a small percentage of patients, the results can be quite dramatic and durable.

Resistance to immunotherapy has been documented to result from a number of immunoevasive maneuvers used by cancer cells. The most effective defense mounted by cancer cells is accomplished through hijacking the host's complex check and balance system governing peripheral tolerance—the mechanism operated by numerous immune checkpoint molecules to prevent autoimmune attacks on normal tissues. The strategy of using monoclonal antibodies to block the inhibitory immune checkpoint receptors of cytotoxic T-lymphocyte antigen-4 (CTLA-4), programmed cell death-1 (PD-1), and programmed cell death ligand-1 (PD-L1) has been shown to restore effective host immunity against melanoma.

This chapter will focus on the use of cytokines and immune checkpoint-targeted antibodies in the management of patients with advanced melanoma.

Keywords Melanoma • Immunotherapy • Ipilimumab • Nivolumab • Lambrolizumab • Pembrolizumab • Tumor immunity barrier • Immune checkpoint-targeted therapy • Monoclonal antibody • Biologic response modifiers • CTLA-4 • PD-1/PD-L1 pathway • Anti-CTLA-4 antibody • Anti-PD-1 antibody • Anti-PD-L1 antibody

V.A. Trinh, PharmD • W.-J. Hwu, MD, PhD (✉)
Department of Melanoma Medical Oncology, The University of Texas MD Anderson Cancer Center, Houston, TX, USA
e-mail: wenjhwu@mdanderson.org

Y. Ahn, MD
Ritz Dermatology Clinic, Seoul, South Korea

© Springer Science+Business Media New York 2016
C.A. Torres-Cabala, J.L. Curry (eds.), *Genetics of Melanoma*, Cancer Genetics,
DOI 10.1007/978-1-4939-3554-3_10

10.1   Introduction

Melanoma has traditionally been recognized as the prototypical immunogenic cancer among human malignancies. Spontaneous tumor regression observed in all stages of melanoma [1] and increased prevalence of the disease in the immunosuppressed population [2] are direct and indirect evidence of immune surveillance of melanoma. Over the past 20 years, significant insights into the complex interaction between host immunity and human cancer have contributed valuable immunologic interventions, from the classic cytokines to the novel immune checkpoint-targeted agents, to the therapeutic repertoire for malignant melanoma. In this chapter, we will briefly discuss the cytokine therapy, i.e., interferon alpha (IFN) and interleukin-2 (IL-2), used in current melanoma treatment schema and examine in depth the recent breakthroughs with the monoclonal antibodies (mAbs) directing at immune checkpoint molecules such as cytotoxic T-lymphocyte antigen-4 (CTLA-4) and programmed cell death-1 (PD-1).

10.2   The Cytokines

10.2.1   Interferon Alpha

Upon binding to the cell-surface receptors IFNAR1 and IFNAR2, IFN produces pleiotropic biological activities by inducing the transcription of hundreds of genes via the JAK-STAT and other signaling pathways [3]. The mechanism of its antitumor effect is not completely understood, but is thought to be the cumulative results of cytostatic, antiangiogenic, and immunostimulatory activities. The immunomodulating effect of IFN is broad, including induction of cytokines, upregulation of major histocompatibility antigen expression, enhancement of the phagocytic activity of natural killer (NK) cells and macrophages, and augmentation of the specific cytotoxicity of lymphocytes against tumor cells [4].

Despite much controversy, IFN remains the widely recognized adjuvant therapy for patients with resected melanoma at high risk of disease relapse. Patients with stage IIC and stage III disease have a relapse rate of 50 % or higher and a 5-year mortality rate of 40–60 % despite definitive surgical resection [5]. Numerous adjuvant trials utilizing IFN at different dosing schedules in various risk groups have been carried out (Table 10.1) [6–12]. The high-dose regimen of IFN alfa-2b, administered at 20 million units/m^2 daily intravenously (IV) five times a week for 4 weeks (induction phase) followed by 10 million units/m^2 subcutaneously (SC) three times weekly for 48 weeks (maintenance phase), has consistently demonstrated relapse-free survival (RFS) benefit with an inconsistent impact on overall survival (OS).

Pegylated IFN alfa-2b (PEG-IFN) is a derivative of recombinant IFN, containing polyethylene glycol covalently linked to IFN. PEG-IFN has similar spectrum of biological activity as IFN; however, its plasma half-life increased by tenfold, allowing for weekly administration [13]. Adjuvant PEG-IFN has been evaluated in

Table 10.1 Select adjuvant IFN trials [1, 4, 6–12]

Study	IFN dose and schedule	Impact on survival	Patient population (n)
High-dose IFN			
ECOG 1684	Arm 1: 20 MU/m²/day IV × 5 days per week × 4 weeks, then 10 MU/m²/day SC TIW × 48 weeks Arm 2: observation	RFS: increased ($p=0.002$) OS: increased ($p=0.02$)	II–III ($n=287$)
ECOG 1690	Arm 1: 20 MU/m²/day IV × 5 days per week × 4 weeks, then 10 MU/m²/day SC TIW × 48 weeks Arm 2: 3 MU SC TIW × 2 years Arm 3: observation	Arm 1 vs. arm 3: RFS: increased ($p=0.03$) OS: NS	II–III ($n=642$)
Low-dose IFN			
ECOG 1690	As above	Arm 2 vs. arm 3: RFS and OS: NS	II–III ($n=642$)
EORTC 18871	Arm 1: 1 MU SC QOD × 1 year Arm 2: IFN-γ Arm 3: Iscador M (mistletoe extract) Arm 4: observation	Arm 1 vs. arm 4: RFS and OS: NS	II–III ($n=830$)
Intermediate-dose IFN			
EORTC 18952	Arm 1: 10 MU SC × 5 days per week × 4 weeks, then 10 MU SC TIW × 12 months Arm 2: 10 MU SC × 5 days per week × 4 weeks, then 5 MU SC TIW × 24 months Arm 3: observation	DMFI and OS: NS	II–III (1388)
Nordic collaborative	Arm 1: 10 MU SC × 5 days per week × 4 weeks, then 10 MU SC TIW × 12 months Arm 2: 10 MU SC × 5 days per week × 4 weeks, then 10 MU SC TIW × 24 months Arm 3: observation	Arm 1 + 2 vs. arm 3: *RFS: increased ($p=0.03$)* OS: NS Arm 1 vs. arm 3: RFS: increased ($p=0.034$) OS: NS	II–III ($n=855$)
Pegylated IFN			
EORTC 18991	Arm 1: 6 mcg/kg/week SC × 8 weeks, then 3 mcg/kg/week SC × up to 5 years Arm 2: observation	RFS: increased ($p=0.01$) DMFS and OS: NS	III ($n=1256$)
Other dosing or duration			
Hellenic cooperative	Arm 1: 15 MU/m²/day IV × 5 days per week × 4 weeks, then 10 MU SC TIW × 48 weeks Arm 2: 15 MU/m²/day IV × 5 days per week × 4 weeks	RFS and OS: NS	II–III ($n=364$)
E1697	Arm 1: 20 MU/m²/day IV × 5 days per week × 4 weeks Arm 2: observation	RFS and OS: NS	II–III (1150)

RFS relapse-free survival, *OS* overall survival, *DMFI* distant metastases free interval, *NS* not statistically significant

patients with stage III melanoma in a large randomized controlled trial conducted by the European Organisation for Research and Treatment of Cancer (EORTC) [14]. In this trial (EORTC 18991), 1256 patients with resected stage III disease were randomly assigned to PEG-IFN or observation and stratified by known prognostic factors, such as nodal tumor burden (microscopic versus macroscopic), number of involved lymph nodes, Breslow thickness, and ulceration status of the primary lesion. The dose of PEG-IFN was 6 mcg/kg of body weight SC weekly for the first 8 weeks (induction phase) followed by 3 mcg/kg once a week for up to 5 years (maintenance phase). The results indicate a statistically significant prolongation of RFS for all patients and a decreased risk of distant metastasis in patients with microscopic lymph node involvement and ulcerated primary tumor. There was no significant OS benefit for PEG-IFN-treated patients.

Two meta-analyses pooling data from 13 or 14 randomized controlled trials between 1990 and 2008 have ascertained a statistically significant improvement in both RFS and OS favoring adjuvant IFN even though the impact on OS is small [15, 16]. Factoring in the cost and serious toxicities associated with high-dose IFN or PEG-IFN, the challenge is to uncover predictive factors to identify patients who will benefit from adjuvant IFN. Manifestation of autoimmunity, either clinical or serological, was found to correlate with favorable survival outcome from adjuvant IFN in the phase III study conducted by the Hellenic Oncology Group [17]. This association has not been substantiated in other trials and needs further exploration in prospective studies [18]. Ulceration of the primary lesion has also been suggested to signify a subset of patients who derive the most benefit from adjuvant IFN [15, 19]. This observation is being investigated in the ongoing EORTC 18081 trial prospectively evaluating adjuvant PEG-IFN in patients with stage II ulcerated primary melanoma.

10.2.2 Interleukin-2

The antitumor activity of IL-2 is believed to be immune based; however, the exact mechanism is unclear. Upon binding to the high-affinity IL-2 receptor expressed on immune cells, IL-2 induces a cytokine cascade comprising various interferons, interleukins, and tumor necrosis factors. These cytokines further stimulate the proliferation and differentiation of B and T cells, monocytes, macrophages, and NK cells, inducing both specific and nonspecific antitumor cytotoxicity [20].

High-dose IL-2, administered at 600,000 IU/kg IV every 8 h for up to a maximum of 14 doses per cycle, was approved by the US Food and Drug Administration (FDA) for the treatment of advanced melanoma based on durable disease control observed in a small group of patients in phase II studies. Pooled analysis of eight clinical trials evaluating high-dose IL-2 between 1985 and 1993 demonstrated an overall response rate (ORR) of 16 %, with long-term remission of 5 years or more occurring in about 4 % of responders [21]. However, high-dose IL-2 has a substantial toxicity profile, limiting its clinical utility to those patients with good performance status and without preexisting cardiopulmonary comorbidities. Safe administration of high-dose IL-2 should take place in intensive care units with the supervision of an experienced oncology team.

10.3   Immune Checkpoint-Targeted Therapy

Over the past two decades, improved understanding of the interactions among the immune system, the tumor, and its associated microenvironment has unearthed several molecular targets for immunotherapy. Generally, a pathogen- or tumor antigen-specific T-cell activation within the secondary lymphoid tissues requires two signals [22]. The first signal occurs when a T-cell receptor (TCR) recognizes and binds to tumor-associated antigen presented in association with major histocompatibility complex by antigen-presenting cells (APCs). By itself, this interaction is usually not meaningful and results in an anergic state unless a costimulatory signal (second signal) is provided by the binding of the CD28 cell-surface antigen on T cells to the B7-1 (CD80) or B7-2 (CD86) receptors on APCs. Both signals are required for the activation, differentiation, and proliferation of antigen-specific T cells, which then migrate to the source of antigens in the periphery to elicit effector function. T-cell-mediated immunity is tightly regulated by a check and balance system involving many stimulatory and inhibitory molecules (Fig. 10.1) [23]. These immune checkpoints work in concert to modulate the duration and amplitude of antigen-specific immune responses to safeguard the body against pathogenic invasion and tumor formation while maintaining self-tolerance.

10.3.1   CTLA-4 Blocking Monoclonal Antibodies

Immediately following T-cell activation, the expression of CTLA-4, an inhibitory checkpoint molecule that competes with CD28 for binding to B7, is upregulated on the T-cell surface. CTLA-4-B7 ligation interrupts the costimulatory signal, blunting

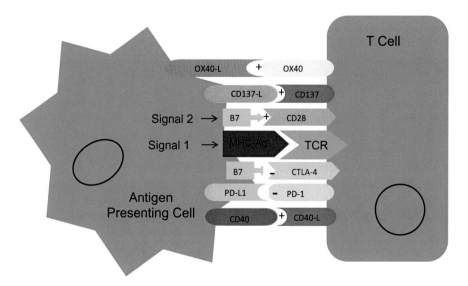

Fig. 10.1   Complex interactions to regulate T-cell activation at the immune synapse

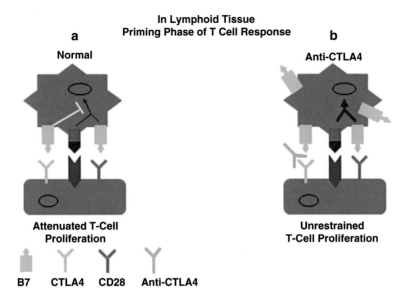

**In Lymphoid Tissue
Priming Phase of T Cell Response**

a Normal   **b** Anti-CTLA4

Attenuated T-Cell
Proliferation

Unrestrained
T-Cell Proliferation

B7   CTLA4   CD28   Anti-CTLA4

Fig. 10.2 Mechanism of action of anti-CTLA-4 in lymphoid tissue priming phase of T-cell response. (**a**) Normally, CTLA4 is upregulated following T-cell activation. CTLA4 competes with CD28 for B7 ligation, putting a brake on T-cell activation. (**b**) Ipilimumab interrupts CTLA4-B7 ligation, releasing the brake

T-cell response [24]. Thus, targeting CTLA-4 with a blocking mAb has been shown to significantly enhance antitumor immunity in preclinical studies (Fig. 10.2) [25]. In the last decade, two fully human anti-CTLA4 mAbs, ipilimumab (Bristol-Myers Squibb) and tremelimumab (Pfizer), have been developed and evaluated in clinical trials.

10.3.1.1 Ipilimumab

The efficacy and safety of ipilimumab in patients with advanced melanoma were demonstrated in two large randomized phase III trials. In the first study (MDX010-20), 676 previously treated patients with unresectable stage III or IV melanoma were randomized 3:1:1 to ipilimumab, 3 mg/kg IV every 3 weeks (Q3W) for four doses, with the melanoma peptide vaccine gp100 ($n=403$), ipilimumab with gp100 placebo ($n=137$), or gp100 vaccine with ipilimumab placebo ($n=136$) [26]. At a median follow-up of approximately 20 months, median OS was 10.0 [95 % confidence interval (CI) 8.5–11.5], 10.1 (95 % CI 8.0–13.8), or 6.4 months (95 % CI 5.5–8.7) for patients treated with the combination, ipilimumab alone, or gp100 alone, respectively. The OS advantage favoring both ipilimumab-containing regimens was statistically significant. The ORR was 10.9 % (95 % CI 6.3–17.4) in the ipilimumab-alone group. Ipilimumab's side effect profile mostly comprised immune-related adverse events (irAEs), with grade 3 or 4 incidents observed in 10–15 % of patients. There were eight treatment-related deaths in the combination group, of which five were associated with irAEs (four from colitis and one from Guillain–Barre syndrome). Two out of four deaths were secondary to irAEs in the ipilimumab-alone group (one from colitis and one from liver failure) [26].

In the second phase III study (CA184-024), 502 previously untreated patients with advanced melanoma were randomly assigned with dacarbazine (DTIC) plus ipilimumab ($n = 250$) or DTIC plus ipilimumab placebo ($n = 252$). The dosing schedule of ipilimumab was 10 mg/kg Q3W for four doses followed by a maintenance phase. The addition of ipilimumab to DTIC significantly improved OS compared to DTIC alone [11.2 vs. 9.1 months, hazard ratio (HR) $= 0.72$, $p < 0.001$] [27]. Most of the toxicities of the combination were irAEs; however, the presentation of irAEs was slightly different than in previous clinical reports for ipilimumab, with higher rates of elevated liver function tests and lower rates of gastrointestinal (GI) complications and endocrinopathies. No treatment-related mortality was observed in the combination arm [27].

Tumor responses to ipilimumab were durable. In the pooled analysis of survival data of 1861 ipilimumab-treated patients in eight phase 2, two phase 3, and two retrospective observational studies, the median OS was 11.4 months (95 % CI 10.7–12.1), with a 3-year OS rate of 22 % (95 % CI 20–24). When including 2985 patients in the ipilimumab expanded access program (EAP), the median OS was 9.5 months (95 % CI 9.0–10.0) and 3-year OS rate was 21 % (95 % CI 20–22). It should be noted that patients in the EAP were more likely to carry unfavorable prognostic factors, such as poor performance status, active brain metastases, and non-cutaneous primaries. The plateau in the OS curve, emerging at 3 years and extending to 10 years, was independent of prior systemic therapies or ipilimumab dosing schedules [28].

Attempts to identify biomarkers to predict whether patients would respond to CTLA-4 blockade or develop life-threatening irAEs have accompanied the clinical development of ipilimumab [29]. So far, various immunologic parameters, such as absolute lymphocyte count value at week 7 post therapy initiation [30], antibody and CD8$^+$ T-cell responses to the cancer testis antigen NY-ESO-1 [31], or pretreatment intratumoral regulatory T-cell population [32], have been shown to correlate with ipilimumab's clinical benefit; however, the associations were inconsistent across trials and will need further exploration in prospective studies.

Considering the OS benefit and safety profile of ipilimumab from the aforementioned phase III trials, the FDA and European Medicines Agency approved ipilimumab for patients with unresectable or metastatic melanoma. The current approved dosing schedule for ipilimumab is 3 mg/kg Q3W for four doses or up to 16 weeks from the first dose, whichever comes first [33, 34]. To determine whether a higher dose of ipilimumab further extends survival, a randomized phase III trial comparing 3 mg/kg to 10 mg/kg of ipilimumab is underway in patients with advanced melanoma. Maintenance ipilimumab was utilized in a number of clinical trials but has not been systematically evaluated.

In the previously mentioned MDX010-20 study, 31 patients with tumor response or stable disease to previous ipilimumab were given reinduction therapy upon disease progression. Most patients were able to receive all four doses in the first reinduction cycle, five completed the second retreatment series, and one concluded the whole third round. Reinduction ipilimumab were able to restore disease control in approximately 70 % of patients with best ORR approaching 40 % [26, 35]. No new safety concerns were observed with reinduction therapy. The development of irAEs during the induction cycle did not increase the risk of toxicities of reinduction series.

Traditionally, the World Health Organization (WHO) or Response Evaluation Criteria in Solid Tumors (RECIST) criteria are used to evaluate clinical responses to cytotoxic chemotherapy. Through ipilimumab development, it has become increasingly clear that these criteria are not well suited to assess response to immunotherapy because immunotherapy can induce significant inflammatory reaction [36]. Thus, tumor size may increase before eventual regression. Since antitumor immunity takes time to fully develop, response can occur after the emergence of new lesions. Wolchok and colleagues have proposed the so-called immune-related response criteria (irRC) for response assessment in patients treated with immunotherapy [37]. The irRC permit the inclusion of new lesions in the total measurable disease burden. Progressive disease must be confirmed twice, at least 4 weeks apart, provided that patients do not have rapid clinical deterioration. This approach was able to identify an additional 10 % of patients who eventually benefit from ipilimumab but would otherwise be categorized as nonresponders with WHO or RECIST criteria. However, irRC may also overestimate response to therapy and lead to unnecessary prolongation of potentially toxic treatment [38]. The irRC are currently being prospectively validated in clinical trials investigating immune checkpoint inhibitors.

The utility of ipilimumab is being expanded into the adjuvant setting. In EORTC 18071, ipilimumab is compared against placebo in 951 patients with resected stage III melanoma [39]. The administration schedule of ipilimumab was 10 mg/kg Q3W for four doses, then every 12 weeks for 3 years. The study population was at particularly high risk for disease relapse: 36 % with stage IIIC, 44 % with stage IIIB, and 20 % with stage IIIA (N1a disease must have at least one metastatic focus of greater than 1 mm in diameter). At a median follow-up of 2.74 years, adjuvant ipilimumab significantly prolonged RFS compared with placebo, with median RFS of 26.1 and 17.1 months, respectively (HR=0.75, 95 % CI 0.64–0.90; $p=0.0013$). Compared with the experience of ipilimumab in metastatic disease, the severity of toxicities appeared more substantial with adjuvant ipilimumab, causing treatment discontinuation in 49 % of patients and limiting the median number of doses per patient to four. Five patients (1.1 %) died of irAEs, three from colitis, one from myocarditis, and one from Guillain–Barre syndrome. EORTC 18071 remain blinded for distant metastasis-free survival and OS.

Another ongoing phase III adjuvant study, E1609, examines the efficacy of postoperative ipilimumab at 3 or 10 mg/kg for four induction doses followed by four maintenance doses every 12 weeks versus standard adjuvant high-dose interferon for 1 year (NCT01274338). This study will supplement EORTC 18071 in defining the role of ipilimumab, especially at the dose recommended by regulatory agencies worldwide, in preventing disease recurrence in patients with resected high-risk melanoma. At present, the FDA is reviewing supplemental label indication of ipilimumab as adjuvant therapy in patients with resected, high-risk melanoma.

Ipilimumab monotherapy has also been evaluated in patients with active untreated brain metastases in a multicenter phase II study [40]. The antitumor activity of ipilimumab was similar at intra- and extracranial sites. Among the 51 patients who did not require corticosteroid for symptoms of brain metastases, eight achieved partial response and four had stable disease in the brain. However, intracranial disease control appeared inferior in the steroid-dependent group ($n = 21$), with one complete response and one stable disease. This encouraging result has led to the NIBIT-M1 trial, evaluating ipilimumab plus fotemustine, a nitrosourea able to cross the blood–brain barrier, in 20 patients with asymptomatic brain metastases [41]. Most patients had 2–3 intracranial lesions; a third of them had received prior local therapy including stereotactic radiosurgery or whole brain radiation. Eight patients achieved an objective response and two had disease stabilization in the brain. The result of this trial is being confirmed in the ongoing phase III NIBIT-M2 trial, in which the combination is compared with fotemustine alone in patients with melanoma brain metastases.

The most common adverse events associated with ipilimumab are irAEs, reflecting its mechanism of action [33, 42]. At 3 mg/kg dose, irAEs affect approximately 60 % of patients; 10–15 % of these are grade 3 or 4 in severity. The gastrointestinal (GI) tract and skin are most frequently affected while hepatic, endocrine, and neurologic events are less common. Typically, irAEs occur during the 12-week induction period, although rarely they can develop several months after the last dose of ipilimumab. Dermatologic toxicities tend to occur early, usually after the first dose. The median onset of GI and hepatic events is between the sixth and seventh weeks, followed by endocrinopathies at 9–11 weeks after treatment initiation [42].

Generally, irAEs are mild to moderate in severity; however, high-grade irAEs have been observed in 15 % of patients. To ensure patient safety, ipilimumab is approved with a Risk Evaluation and Mitigation Strategy (REMS) to advise patients about the risks of irAEs and to assist clinicians in the evaluation and management of irAEs [43]. Although high-grade irAEs can be life-threatening, they can be controlled through patients' early reporting and immediate initiation of appropriate therapy. Treatment algorithms have been developed to guide irAE management. Besides symptom-directed measures, the cornerstone of these guidelines is high-dose systemic steroid (1–2 mg/kg/day of prednisone or equivalent). Interestingly, evidence to date suggests corticosteroid administration for irAEs does not appear to affect tumor response to ipilimumab [44, 45].

The management strategies for specific irAEs are summarized in Table 10.2 [43]. Time to resolution is dependent on the affected organ system. Dermatologic, GI, and liver immune-related toxicities improve in 2–4 weeks; however, endocrinopathies take a long time to resolve and in some cases are irreversible. Once symptoms improve, it is critical to taper off steroid slowly over 4–6 weeks to avoid

Table 10.2 Recommended management of irAEs [43, 46]

Site	Signs and symptoms	Management

GI	Assess patients for changes in bowel habits and for the following signs and symptoms: diarrhea, abdominal pain, blood or mucus in stool with or without fever, peritoneal signs consistent with bowel perforation and ileus	Initiate workup to rule out infectious etiologies
		Mild (grade 1): <4 stools/day over baseline
		• Symptomatic management: dietary modifications and antidiarrheals
		Moderate (grade 2): 4–6 stools/day over baseline, abdominal pain, blood, or mucus in stool
		• Withhold immunotherapy and administer antidiarrheals
		• For symptoms that persist for more than 1 week
		  – Start systemic corticosteroids (0.5–1 mg/kg/day of prednisone or equivalent)
		  – Taper steroid down slowly over 4 or 6 weeks upon improvement to mild severity or resolution
		  – Resume immunotherapy if symptoms improve to at least mild severity and steroid dose is 7.5 mg prednisone equivalent or less
		  – If symptoms worsen, treat as below
		Severe or life-threatening (grade 3 or 4): >7 stools/day over baseline, signs consistent with perforation, ileus, fever
		• Permanently discontinue immunotherapy
		• Rule out bowel perforation
		• If perforation is present, do not administer corticosteroids
		• If no perforation
		  – Start systemic corticosteroids at 1–2 mg/kg/day of prednisone or equivalent
		  – Taper steroid down slowly over 4 or 6 weeks upon improvement to mild severity or resolution
		• If persistent symptoms
		  – Continue to evaluate for perforation or peritonitis
		  – Consider infliximab and/or other immunosuppressants

(continued)

Table 10.2 (continued)

Site	Signs and symptoms	Management
Skin	Evaluate patients for signs and symptoms of pruritus or rash	*Mild (grade 1)*: mild or localized itching, rash covering <10 % of skin surface • Symptomatic management: topical moisturizers, oatmeal baths, or antipruritics *Moderate (grade 2)*: intense or generalized itching, skin changes from scratching, rash involving 10–30 % of skin surface • Withhold immunotherapy • For symptoms that persist for more than 1 week: – Start high-potency topical steroids or systemic corticosteroids (0.5 mg/kg/day of prednisone or equivalent) – Taper steroid down slowly over 4 or 6 weeks upon improvement to mild severity or resolution – Resume immunotherapy if symptoms improve to mild severity and steroid dose is 7.5 mg prednisone equivalent or less *Severe or life-threatening (grade 3 or 4)*: Stevens–Johnson syndrome, toxic epidermal necrolysis, or rash complicated by full thickness dermal ulceration or necrotic, bullous, or hemorrhagic manifestations • Permanently discontinue immunotherapy • Start systemic corticosteroids at 1–2 mg/kg/day of prednisone or equivalent • Taper steroid down slowly over 4 or 6 weeks when improvement to mild severity or resolution

(continued)

Table 10.2 (continued)

Site	Signs and symptoms	Management
Liver	Evaluate LFTs and assess for signs and symptoms of hepatitis before each infusion. Elevations in LFTs (e.g., AST, ALT) and/or total bilirubin may occur in absence of clinical symptoms	Initiate workup to rule out infectious or malignant etiologies Increase frequency of LFT monitoring until resolution *Mild (grade 1)*: AST or ALT ≤2.5 times ULN and/or total bilirubin ≤1.5 times ULN • Monitor *Moderate*: AST or ALT >2.5 times to ≤5 times ULN and/or total bilirubin elevation >1.5 times but ≤3 times ULN • Withhold immunotherapy • Resume immunotherapy if LFTs ≤ 2.5 × ULN or return to baseline and bilirubin ≤ 1.5 × ULN or return to baseline *Severe or life-threatening (grade 3 or 4)*: AST or ALT >5 times ULN; and/or total bilirubin >3 times ULN • Permanently discontinue immunotherapy • Start systemic corticosteroids at 1–2 mg/kg/day of prednisone or equivalent • Taper steroid down slowly over 4 or 6 weeks upon sustained improvement or return to baseline • For persistent symptoms: consider other immunosuppressants
Hypophysitis	Evaluate signs and symptoms such as fatigue, headache, changes in mental status, abdominal pain, unusual bowel habits, hypotension, abnormal thyroid function tests, and/or serum chemistries	Initiate workup to rule out brain or meningeal metastases or other underlying etiologies *Moderate to life-threatening* • Evaluate endocrine function • Consider radiographic pituitary gland imaging • Withhold immunotherapy in symptomatic patients • Initiate appropriate hormone replacement therapy • Start systemic corticosteroids at 1–2 mg/kg/day of prednisone or equivalent • Resume immunotherapy if patient stable and symptoms resolve or return to baseline, patient is stable on hormone replacement therapy, and steroid dose is 7.5 mg prednisone equivalent or less

(continued)

Table 10.2 (continued)

Site	Signs and symptoms	Management
Neurologic	Advise patient to report changes in muscle weakness, numbness, or other sensory alterations. Unless alternative etiology identified, signs and symptoms of neuropathy should be considered immune mediated	*Mild (grade 1)*: asymptomatic; loss of deep tendon reflexes or paresthesia *Moderate (grade 2)*: symptoms clinically detectable without impact on ADLs • Withhold immunotherapy • Initiate appropriate medical interventions • Resume immunotherapy when symptoms resolve or return to baseline *Severe or life-threatening (grade 3 or 4)*: severe symptoms with impact on ADLs or life-threatening • Permanently discontinue immunotherapy • Institute appropriate medical interventions • Consider systemic corticosteroids at 1–2 mg/kg/day of prednisone or equivalent
Ocular	Assess patients for uveitis, iritis, or episcleritis	• Administer corticosteroid eye drops • Permanently discontinue immunotherapy for immune-mediated ocular disease that is unresponsive to local immunosuppressive therapy
Pulmonary	Advise patient to report changes in coughing and breathing status Assess chest imaging	*Mild (grade 1)*: asymptomatic; radiographic changes only • Monitor every 2–3 days *Moderate (grade 2)*: mild to moderate symptoms, worsens from baseline • Monitor daily • Withhold immunotherapy • Start systemic corticosteroids at 1–2 mg/kg/day of prednisone or equivalent • Consider pulmonary consult for bronchoscopy and/or lung biopsy • Taper steroid down slowly over 4 or 6 weeks upon sustained improvement or return to baseline • Resume immunotherapy if benefit outweighs risk *Severe or life-threatening (grade 3 or 4)*: severe symptoms; hypoxia; life-threatening • Permanently discontinue immunotherapy • Monitor daily • Start systemic corticosteroids at 1–2 mg/kg/day of prednisone or equivalent • Consider pulmonary consult for bronchoscopy and/or lung biopsy • Taper steroid down slowly over 4 or 6 weeks upon sustained improvement or return to baseline • For persistent symptoms: add other immunosuppressants

Table 10.2 (continued)

Site	Signs and symptoms	Management
Nephritis	Evaluate creatinine before each infusion	Initiate workup to rule out other etiologies
		Increase frequency of creatinine monitoring until resolution
		Mild (grade 1): Cr >ULN and baseline but ≤1.5 times baseline
		• Monitor Cr weekly
		Moderate (grade 2): Cr >1.5 times to ≤6 times ULN or >1.5 times baseline
		• Withhold immunotherapy
		• Monitor Cr every 2–3 days
		• Start systemic corticosteroids (0.5–1 mg/kg/day of prednisone or equivalent)
		• Taper steroid down slowly over 4 or 6 weeks upon sustained improvement or return to baseline
		• Resume immunotherapy
		Severe or life-threatening (grade 3 or 4): Cr >6 times ULN
		• Permanently discontinue immunotherapy
		• Monitor Cr daily
		• Start systemic corticosteroids at 1–2 mg/kg/day of prednisone or equivalent
		• Consult nephrology
		• Consider renal biopsy

ADL activities of daily living, *ALT* alanine aminotransferase, *AST* aspartate aminotransferase, *Cr* creatinine, *GI* gastrointestinal, *LFTs* liver function tests, *ULN* upper limit of normal

relapse [42, 43]. Ipilimumab rechallenge can be considered in patients with grade 1 or 2 irAEs once symptoms resolved to grade 0–1. Generally, ipilimumab should be permanently discontinued in patients experiencing grade 3 or 4 irAEs.

10.3.1.2 Tremelimumab

Tremelimumab is a fully human anti-CTLA-4 IgG2 mAb with a half-life of 19.6 days [47]. The randomized dose-finding phase II study comparing tremelimumab at either 10 mg/kg monthly or 15 mg/kg every 3 months (Q3M) demonstrated similar efficacy with either schedule; however, the Q3M administration appeared better tolerated and more convenient to patients [47]. Thus, 15 mg/kg Q3M was selected for subsequent trials. At this dose, tremelimumab produced an ORR of 6.6 %, comparable to that of ipilimumab, in patients with advanced refractory or relapsed melanoma [48]. Responses to tremelimumab were also durable. The toxicities, consisting of irAEs, mirror the safety profile of ipilimumab.

Tremelimumab was further evaluated in a large phase III study, in which 655 previously untreated patients with advanced melanoma were randomly assigned at 1:1 ratio to receive tremelimumab or conventional chemotherapy, either temozolomide or DTIC [49]. In this trial, tremelimumab was dosed at 15 mg/kg IV Q3M, temozolomide at 200 mg/m^2 orally daily for 5 days every 28 days, and DTIC at 1 g/m^2 IV Q3W. The primary end point of this study was OS; the secondary end points included ORR, duration of response (DOR), progression-free survival (PFS) at 6 months, and adverse events. At the planned second interim analysis, the median OS for the tremelimumab group was 11.8 months compared to 10.7 months for the chemotherapy arm (HR = 0.96; $p = 0.73$). The secondary end points of ORR and 6-month PFS did not differ between the two arms. Diarrhea, pruritus, and rash were the most common toxicities of tremelimumab. Considering the results, the data and safety monitoring board recommended early discontinuation of the trial. Tremelimumab administered at 15 mg/kg Q3M failed to yield superior OS benefit over conventional chemotherapy as the first-line therapy for patients with advanced melanoma. However, a post hoc analysis of salvage therapy in approximately 60 % of the study population revealed that 16 % of the patients in the chemotherapy arm received ipilimumab on a compassionate use basis subsequently. This unintended crossover might have compromised the benefit of tremelimumab [49].

10.3.2 PD-1, PD-1 Ligand 1 (PD-L1), and PD-1 Ligand 2 (PD-L2) Blocking Monoclonal Antibodies

PD-1 receptor, expressed on activated T and B cells, NK cells, and monocytes, is another important negative regulator of the immune system. PD-1 ligand 1, (PD-L1 or B7-H1) and PD-1 ligand 2 (PD-L2 or B7-DC) are two known natural ligands of PD-1. PD-L1 is widely expressed on hematopoietic cells and normal tissues whereas PD-L2 expression is restricted to myeloid cells and few non-hematopoietic tissues [50, 51]. Engagement of PD-1 to PD-L1 inhibits T-cell effector function, ultimately inducing T-cell exhaustion and deletion; however, the biology of PD-1-to-PD-L2 ligation is currently unclear and requires further investigation. The PD-1–PD-L1 pathway plays a critical role in fine-tuning host immunity to thwart pathogenic invasion while preserving self-tolerance. Intriguingly, this protective mechanism can be hijacked by cancer cells to evade immunosurveillance. Indeed, upregulation of PD-L1 and to a lesser extent PD-L2 expression has been demonstrated in many human tumor systems. Moreover, interrupting the binding of PD-1 to its ligands has been shown to induce tumor regression in animal models [52, 53]. These discoveries fuel rapid clinical development of mAbs against the PD-1–PD-L1 pathway as immunotherapeutic strategies for various human cancers (Fig. 10.3).

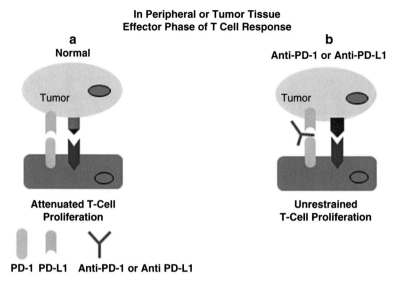

In Peripheral or Tumor Tissue
Effector Phase of T Cell Response

a
Normal

Tumor

Attenuated T-Cell
Proliferation

b
Anti-PD-1 or Anti-PD-L1

Tumor

Unrestrained
T-Cell Proliferation

PD-1 PD-L1   Anti-PD-1 or Anti PD-L1

Fig. 10.3 Mechanism of action of anti-PD-1 or anti-PD-L-1 in peripheral or tumor tissue effector phase of T-cell response. (**a**) PD-L1 is upregulated on peripheral tissue following T-cell activation, dampening immune response upon binding to PD-1 on T cell. Tumor cells evade host immunity by expressing PD-L1. (**b**) Anti-PD-1 or anti-PD-L1 interrupts PD-1-PD-L1 ligation, restoring anti-tumor immunity

10.3.2.1 PD-1 Blocking Monoclonal Antibodies

Nivolumab (Bristol-Myers Squibb)

Nivolumab (BMS 936558, MDX-1106) is a fully human IgG4 mAb that directly antagonizes the PD-1 receptor. Based on the preliminary single-dose safety and efficacy data from a pilot study in 39 patients with treatment-refractory cancers [54], a large phase I trial was conducted to further explore the activity and tolerability of multidose nivolumab [55]. In this study, 296 previously treated patients with advanced cancers of various tumor types, a third of them with melanoma, received nivolumab 0.1–10 mg/kg IV every 2 weeks (Q2W) for up to 2 years. Patients with prior therapies with T-cell-modulating mAbs, including anti-CTLA4, anti-PD-1, or anti-PD-L1, were excluded.

Long-term follow-up data in 107 patients with advanced melanoma revealed an ORR of 31 % (95 % CI 22.3–40.5), a median PFS of 3.7 months (95 % CI 1.9–9.1) and a median OS of 16.8 months (95 % CI 12.5–31.6). The antitumor activity of nivolumab appeared rapid and durable, with half of the responses observed at the first restaging evaluation (8 weeks after treatment initiation) and a median DOR of 2 years. Maximum tolerated dose (MTD) was not reached within the dose range evaluated. The 3 mg/kg dose level yielded numerically superior results (ORR: 41 %, median PFS: 9.7 months, median OS: 20.3 months), thus was chosen for subsequent studies [56].

Nivolumab was well tolerated, with 5 % of patients discontinuing treatment due to toxicities. Common side effects included fatigue, diarrhea, rash, pruritus, appetite loss, and nausea. Grade 3 or 4 adverse events occurred in 14 % of patients. Immune-based toxicities, mostly manageable and reversible with treatment interruption and glucocorticoids, were seen in 6 % of patients. Nivolumab-induced pneumonitis affected 12 (4 %) patients and was the cause of death in 3 (1 %) individuals [56].

CheckMate 037

The safety and efficacy of nivolumab as second-line therapy for advanced melanoma was evaluated in CheckMate 037, a randomized, open-label phase III trial. In this study, patients with advanced melanoma whose disease progressed after ipilimumab and, if *BRAF V600* mutation positive, a *BRAF* inhibitor were assigned 2:1 to nivolumab 3 mg/kg Q2W (*n* = 272) or investigator's choice of chemotherapy (ICC) (*n* = 133). The options of ICC were DTIC or carboplatin–paclitaxel Q3W. The co-primary end points were OS for the entire study population and non-comparative ORR (RECIST 1.1) in the first 120 nivolumab-treated patients with at least a 24-week follow-up [57].

At a median follow-up of 8.4 months, ORR was 31.7 % (95 % CI 23.5–40.8) in the 120 nivolumab-treated patients and 10.6 % (95 % CI 3.5–23.1) in the 47 ICC-treated participants. The favorable effect of nivolumab on ORR was independent of *BRAF* mutation status. Nivolumab appeared to induce more rapid onset of response than ICC, with median time to response of 2.1 and 3.5 months, respectively. Median DOR was not reached in the nivolumab arm, as compared with 3.5 months in the ICC group. PFS and OS data were not yet mature.

Overall, 9 % and 31 % of patients receiving nivolumab and ICC had grade 3–4 treatment-related adverse events, respectively. Common high-grade toxicities were elevated lipase, transaminitis, fatigue, and anemia with nivolumab and myelosuppression with ICC. High-grade irAEs, comprising rash, diarrhea/colitis, hepatitis, and nephritis, occurred in 3 % of nivolumab-treated patients. Approximately 2 % of nivolumab-treated patients experienced low-grade immune-mediated pneumonitis. Toxicities led to treatment discontinuation in 3 % and 7 % of the nivolumab and ICC groups, respectively. Treatment-related mortalities were not observed in either arm [57].

CheckMate 066

This is an international, randomized, double-blind phase III trial conducted outside of the USA, where ipilimumab had not been commercially available. Previously untreated patients with *BRAF* wild-type advanced melanoma were randomly assigned 1:1 to nivolumab 3 mg/kg Q2W plus a DTIC-matched placebo Q3W (*n* = 210) or DTIC 1 g/m2 Q3W plus a nivolumab-matched placebo Q2W (*n* = 208). The primary end point was OS, and secondary end points included investigator-assessed PFS and ORR [58].

Nivolumab significantly prolonged OS compared with DTIC. At a median follow-up of 8.9 months in the nivolumab group and 6.8 months in the DTIC group, median OS was not reached in the nivolumab group versus 10.8 months in the DTIC group (HR=0.42, 99.79 % CI 0.25–0.73; $p<0.001$). Nivolumab also significantly improved PFS, with median PFS of 5.1 and 2.2 months in the nivolumab and DTIC groups, respectively (HR=0.43, 95 % CI 0.34–0.56; $p<0.001$). ORR was 40 % in the nivolumab group compared with 13.9 % in the DTIC group (odds ratio=4.06; $p<0.001$). Median time to response was 2.1 months in either arm. Median DOR was not reached in the nivolumab group versus 6.0 months (95 % CI 3.0-not reached) in the DTIC group.

Grade 3–4 treatment-related toxicities occurred more frequently in the dacarbazine group (17.6 vs. 11.7 %), leading to a higher rate of treatment discontinuation due to adverse events (11.7 vs. 6.8 %). Grade 3–4 irAEs occurred in 6 % of nivolumab-treated patients, with high-grade rash/pruritus, diarrhea/colitis, and transaminitis each affecting 1.5 % of patients. There were three cases of low-grade immune-mediated pneumonitis with nivolumab therapy. Treatment-related mortality was not observed in either group [58].

CheckMate 067

Because ipilimumab is the current standard frontline treatment for patients with *BRAF* wild-type AM in the USA, the CheckMate 067, a randomized, double-blind, phase III trial, was conducted to compare the safety and efficacy of upfront nivolumab, either as monotherapy or in combination with ipilimumab, against ipilimumab alone in treatment-naïve patients with advanced melanoma. Patients were randomized 1:1:1 to nivolumab 3 mg/kg Q2W plus ipilimumab-matched placebo ($n=316$), nivolumab 1 mg/kg with ipilimumab 3 mg/kg Q3W for four doses, followed by nivolumab 3 mg/kg Q2W ($n=314$), or ipilimumab 3 mg/kg Q3W for four doses plus nivolumab-matched placebo ($n=315$) [59]. The co-primary end points were PFS and OS, and secondary end points included ORR, safety, and PD-L1 as predictive biomarker for efficacy.

At a median follow-up of approximately 12 months, median PFS were 11.5, 6.9, and 2.9 months in the groups treated with the combination, nivolumab, and ipilimumab, respectively. The PFS advantage favoring both nivolumab-containing regimens was statistically significant. ORR was also significantly higher with the combination (57.6 %) or nivolumab monotherapy (43.7 %) versus ipilimumab monotherapy (19.0 %). Although the study was not designed to compare nivolumab monotherapy with the combination, combined checkpoint blockade produced numerically superior PFS, particularly in the PD-L1-negative subgroup [59].

The incidence and nature of treatment-related adverse events associated with single-agent nivolumab or ipilimumab were similar to prior experience. However, the combination was more toxic. Grade 3–4 treatment-related adverse events affected 55.0 % of patients and led to treatment discontinuation in one-third of the study population. Common grade 3–4 irAEs were diarrhea/colitis and elevated liver enzymes. Most toxicities were manageable and reversible with standard irAE management guidelines. There was no treatment-related death in the combination arm [59].

Pembrolizumab (Merck Sharp and Dohme)

KEYNOTE-001

Pembrolizumab (lambrolizumab, MK-3475) is a humanized anti-PD-1 IgG4 mAb. KEYNOTE-001, the largest phase I trial in oncology, examined the safety profile, antitumor activity, and dose–response relationship of pembrolizumab in 655 patients with advanced melanoma, of whom 342 were ipilimumab treated. There were no significant differences in terms of efficacy and toxicity among three dose levels: 10 mg/kg IV Q2W, 10 mg/kg Q3W, or 2 mg/kg Q3W [55]. At a median follow-up of 21 months, an ORR of 33 % (95 % CI 30–37), median PFS of 4.4 months (95 % CI 3.1–5.5), and median OS of 22.8 months (95 % CI 19.8–28.7) were observed across all dose levels. Better results were seen in the ipilimumab-naïve subgroup, with ORR of 45.1 %, median PFS of 13.8 months and median OS of 31.1 months [60].

Drug-related adverse events, mostly low grade, were observed in 83 % of patients. Frequent adverse effects comprised fatigue, rash, pruritus, and diarrhea. Grade 3 or 4 toxicities occurred to 14 % of patients and led to treatment discontinuation in 4 % of the study population. High-grade irAEs were infrequent and reversible with appropriate management. Pembrolizumab-induced pneumonitis, mostly of grade 1 or 2, affected 3 % of patients. Treatment-related mortality was not observed [61].

KEYNOTE-002

KEYNOTE-002, a randomized phase II trial involving 540 patients with advanced melanoma whose disease progressed after ipilimumab and, if *BRAF V600* mutation positive, a *BRAF* inhibitor, evaluated the efficacy of second-line pembrolizumab against ICC [62]. Patients were randomized 1:1:1 to pembrolizumab 2 mg/kg Q3W ($n = 180$) or 10 mg/kg Q3W ($n = 181$) or ICC ($n = 179$). Chemotherapy options were DTIC, temozolomide, carboplatin, paclitaxel, or carboplatin–paclitaxel combination. At a median follow-up of 10 months, half of the ICC-treated patients had crossed over to the pembrolizumab arms. The PFS rates at 6 months were 34 % (95 % CI: 27–41) and 38 % (95 % CI: 31–45) in the pembrolizumab 2 mg/kg and 10 mg/kg groups, respectively, versus 16 % (95 % CI: 10–22) in the chemotherapy arm ($p < 0.0001$ for both comparisons). The ORRs were 21 % and 25 % in the pembrolizumab 2 mg/kg and 10 mg/kg groups, respectively, as compared with 4 % in the chemotherapy arm ($p < 0.0001$ for both comparisons). Median times to response were 13, 15, and 13 weeks in the pembrolizumab 2 mg/kg, 10 mg/kg, and ICC group, respectively. Median DOR was 37 weeks in the chemotherapy group, whereas it has not been reached in either pembrolizumab arm. OS results were not yet mature.

The rate of treatment-related grade 3–4 toxicities was higher in the chemotherapy group compared with either pembrolizumab arm (26 vs. 11 % and 14 %). The most common serious adverse effects of pembrolizumab were diarrhea (1 %) and pneumonitis (1 %). Toxicities led to treatment discontinuation in 3 %, 7 %, and 6 % of patients treated with pembrolizumab 2 mg/kg, 10 mg/kg, and ICC, respectively. Treatment-related deaths were not observed [62].

KEYNOTE-006

This randomized, open-label phase III trial compared three treatment arms, pembrolizumab 10 mg/kg Q2W or Q3W for up to 2 years, or ipilimumab 3 mg/kg Q3W for four doses, in 834 advanced melanoma patients who were treatment-naïve or had received one prior systemic treatment (exclude anti-CTLA-4 and anti-PD-1) [63]. Pembrolizumab produced statistically significant and clinically meaningful improvement in the co-primary end points of PFS and OS as compared to ipilimumab. At the first interim analysis, median PFS were 5.5 (95 % CI 3.4–6.9) and 4.1 months (95 % CI 2.9–6.9) in the pembrolizumab 2 mg/kg and 10 mg/kg groups, respectively, as compared with 2.8 months (95 % CI 2.8–2.9) in the ipilimumab arm. At the second interim analysis, the 1-year OS rates were 74.1 %, 68.4 %, and 58.2 % in the patients treated with pembrolizumab 2 mg/kg, 10 mg/kg, and ipilimumab, respectively. The OS advantage favoring the pembrolizumab arms are statistically significant. The ORRs were 33.7 % and 32.9 % in the pembrolizumab 2 mg/kg and 10 mg/kg groups, respectively, as compared with 11.9 % in the ipilimumab arm. Median time to response was approximately 85 days, and median DOR was not reached in any of the treatment group.

The rate of treatment-related grade 3–4 toxicities was higher with ipilimumab than pembrolizumab (19.9 vs. 13.3 % and 10.1 %). The most common serious adverse effects of pembrolizumab were colitis (1.4 and 2.5 %) and hepatitis (1.1 and 1.8 %). Toxicities led to treatment discontinuation in 4 %, 6.9 %, and 9.4 % of patients treated with pembrolizumab 2 mg/kg, 10 mg/kg, and ipilimumab, respectively. Treatment-related deaths were not observed in either pembrolizumab arms, whereas one patient in the ipilimumab group died from complications of immune-related diarrhea/colitis [63].

Considering the favorable efficacy and safety profiles of pembrolizumab and nivolumab, the FDA approved their use for the management of patients with advanced melanoma who have progressed on ipilimumab and, if *BRAF* V600 mutation positive, a *BRAF* inhibitor [46, 64]. Supplemental label indication as frontline therapy for advanced melanoma is expected in the near future. The clinical utility of anti-PD-1 antibodies will continue to expand to other settings, including adjuvant therapy for resected high-risk melanoma or treatment of melanoma brain metastases.

Pidilizumab (CureTech/Teva)

Pidilizumab (CT-011) is a humanized anti-PD-1 IgG1 mAb. A phase I trial in 17 patients with advanced hematologic malignancies was conducted to examine the tolerability of single-dose pidilizumab at escalating doses ranging from 0.2 to 6 mg/kg [65]. MTD was not reached within this dose range. Pidilizumab administration was without serious adverse events, infusion-related reactions, or irAEs. Its safety and efficacy profile were subsequently evaluated in 100 patients with metastatic melanoma in a multicenter, randomized phase II study. Patients were randomly assigned to pidilizumab 1.5 or 6 mg/kg IV Q2W for up to 54 weeks and stratified by prior ipilimumab exposure. An ORR of 6 %, median PFS of 1.9 months, and 1-year OS rate of 64.5 % were observed. Pidilizumab was well tolerated, with the most common toxicities being fatigue (31 %) and diarrhea (16 %). Serious adverse events, including appendicitis, arthritis, hepatitis, and pneumonitis, were reported in 4 % of patients. Two percent of patients discontinued treatment due to treatment-related toxicities. Treatment-related mortality was not observed [66].

10.3.2.2 Anti-PD-L1 Blocking Antibodies

BMS-936559 (Bristol-Myers Squibb)

BMS-936559 is a fully human anti-PD-L1 IgG4 mAb that blocks the engagement of PD-1-L1 to PD-1 and CD-80. To date, BMS-936559 has been evaluated in a large phase I dose-finding study enrolling 207 previously treated patients with advanced malignancies of various types [67]. Of note, prior therapy with a T-cell modulating mAb (e.g., anti-CTLA4, anti-PD-1, or anti-PD-L1) was not allowed. BMS-936559 was administered at escalating dosing levels, 0.3, 1, 3, and 10 mg/kg, IV Q2W for up to 2 years. The median duration of therapy was 12 weeks. MTD was not defined within the evaluated dose range.

Objective responses were documented in patients with NSCLC, melanoma, RCC, and ovarian cancer at doses of 1 mg/kg or higher. Of 52 evaluable patients with advanced melanoma, three individuals achieved complete response, while six others had partial tumor reduction, resulting in an ORR of 17 %. Five of those nine responses were durable, lasting more than 1 year. Additionally, 27 % of patients had stable disease that sustained for at least 24 weeks. The PFS rate at 24 weeks was 42 % [67].

Treatment-related adverse events were reported in 61 % of patients, commonly manifesting as fatigue, infusion reaction, diarrhea, arthralgia, rash, nausea, pruritus, and headache. The quality and quantity of toxic effects were similar across all dose levels, except for infusion reaction which typically occurred at 10 mg/kg dose level. Immune-related side effects, mostly of grade 1 or 2, affected 39 % of patients. Grade 3 or 4 side effects were infrequent; 6 % of patients discontinued treatment because of toxicities related to BMS-936559. Interestingly, treatment-associated pneumonitis was not reported in this study [67].

Above safety and efficacy data provided proof of concept that BMS-936559, an anti-PD-L1 mAb, could also induce durable tumor regression in patients with advanced melanoma or select solid tumors, justifying further development of this agent.

Atezolizumab (Genentech)

Atezolizumab (MPDL3280A, RG7446) is a fully human anti-PD-L1 IgG1 mAb engineered to avoid antibody-dependent cellular cytotoxicity. Early results of a large phase I dose-finding study in previously treated patients with advanced malignancies of various types were presented at the 2013 ASCO meeting [68]. MPDL3280A was administered IV every 3 weeks at doses ranging from 0.01 to 20 mg/kg. By the data cutoff date, 171 and 122 patients were evaluable for safety and efficacy, respectively. MTD was not yet identified. The median duration of therapy was 127 days. Grade 3 or 4 adverse events, regardless of attribution, were reported in 39 % of patients. Immune-related toxicities included hepatitis, rash, and colitis. High-grade pneumonitis was not observed. Objective responses were documented in patients with NSCLC, melanoma, RCC, colorectal carcinoma, and gastric cancer, with a response rate of 29 % in those with advanced melanoma. MPDL3280A is currently being developed in multiple phase I or II studies as monotherapy or in combination with other agents in patients with advanced solid tumors. Of interest is a phase I dose escalation trial examining the safety and preliminary efficacy of MPDL3280A and vemurafenib, a selective *BRAF* inhibitor, in previously untreated patients with *BRAFV600* mutant metastatic melanoma.

MEDI4736 (MedImmune)

MEDI4736 is another fully human mAb targeting PDL-1 ligand. It is currently being evaluated in a multicenter, first-in-human, phase I study in patients with advanced solid tumors, including melanoma [51].

10.3.2.3 Anti-PD-L2 Monoclonal Antibody

AMP-224 (Amplimmune/GlaxoSmithKline)

AMP-224 is a recombinant protein fusing the extracellular domain of PD-L2 to the Fc-portion of IgG1, potentially blocking the PD-1-to-PD-L2 ligation. A first-in-human phase I study of AMP-224 in patients with refractory cancer is underway [51].

In general, the anti-PD-1 and anti-PD-L1mAbs have more robust antitumor activity and more favorable safety profile than ipilimumab; however, new irAEs emerge with the administration of agents targeting the PD-1–PD-L1–PD-L2 pathway: pneumonitis with the anti-PD-1 and infusion-related reaction with the anti-PD-L1. Clinical investigations of the anti-PD-1 or anti-PD-L1 also attempted to correlate clinical response with PD-L1 expression in pretreatment tumor samples; however, the association between disease regression and positive PD-L1 expression in tumor tissues has been inconsistent across trials. The role of PD-L1 expression in tumor tissues as a biomarker predictive of clinical response to the mAbs directing at the PD-1–PD-L1–PD-L2 pathway continues to be an area of active research.

10.3.3 Other Immune Checkpoint-Targeted Agents

In addition to the costimulatory signal provided by the binding of CD28 on T cells to B7-1 (CD80) or B7-2 (CD86) on APCs, engagement of other costimulatory molecules are required at the immune synapse to promote survival and proliferation of the activated T cells and to generate memory T cells [69, 70]. CD40, 4-1-BB, or OX40 are the most studied immune-potentiating molecules to date.

10.3.3.1 CD40-Targeting Monoclonal Antibodies

CD40, a member of the tumor necrosis factor (TNF) receptor superfamily, is expressed on APCs like dendritic cells, B cells, and monocytes. CD40 can also be found on non-immune cells and is overexpressed in approximately 50 % of carcinomas and melanomas and nearly 100 % of hematological B-cell malignancies. Its natural ligand, CD-40 L or CD154, is expressed on the surface of activated T-helper cells. Upon ligand binding, CD40 enhances antigen presentation, strengthens macrophages' antitumor cytotoxicity, and boosts antigen-specific antibody production [70–72]. Cross-linking of CD40 on cancer cells yields variable outcome depending on tumor types. Activation of CD40 on tumor cells of melanomas, certain carcinomas, and select B-cell lymphomas can result in direct tumor killing [73–75]. On the contrary, CD40 ligation on low-grade B-cell malignancies may actually stimulate tumor growth [76]. Many mAbs directing at CD40 have entered clinical trials, demonstrating promising activity in melanoma and other hematologic and solid tumors. Among them, CP-870893 is the agent at more advanced stage of clinical development [70, 72].

CP-870893 (Pfizer) is a fully human CD40 agonist IgG2 mAb. The first-in-human phase I dose-finding trial evaluated the safety profile of single-dose CP-870893 up to 0.3 mg/kg in 29 patients with advanced solid tumors [77]. The MTD was established at 0.2 mg/kg. Four partial responses, all in patients with melanoma, were observed at doses of 0.2 or 0.3 mg/kg. One response was durable, lasting at least 14 months. CP-870893 was generally tolerated, with the most common adverse event being low-grade cytokine release syndrome (CRS). CRS appeared dose proportional, occurred shortly after infusion ended, and paralleled with TNFα and IL-6 surges. Typical manifestation of CRS included fever, chills, muscle aches, back pain, nausea, and vomiting. Premedications with acetaminophen and H-1 antagonists did not seem to prevent the syndrome. Autoimmune-like side effects were not documented. Transient decrease in peripheral lymphocytes, monocytes, and platelets and elevation of hepatic enzymes happened within 24–48 h and resolved by day 8 after dose administration. Venous thromboembolism developed in one patient and has been occasionally reported in other studies involving CP-870893; this procoagulant state has been linked to its action on activated platelets and endothelial vascular cells [78].

A subsequent phase I trial evaluated repeat dosing of CP-870893 at 0.05–0.25 mg/kg/dose weekly in 27 patients with advanced malignancies [79]. The MTD was again determined at 0.2 mg/kg. No objective responses were seen; stable diseases were achieved in 26 % of patients. Suboptimal activity of weekly CP-870893 may result from the detrimental effect of chronic CD40 activation which may lead to eventual deletion of tumor antigen-specific T cells [79]. Therefore, subsequent studies of CP-870893 utilize every 3- or 4-week schedule. This mAb, combined with tremelimumab, is currently being tested in a phase I trial involving patients with advanced melanoma. Clinical development is also ongoing in patients with advanced solid tumors, mostly in combination with chemotherapy.

10.3.3.2 CD137 (4-1-BB) Targeting Monoclonal Antibody

CD137 or 4-1-BB is an inducible cell-surface receptor that modulates T-cell costimulatory responses and enhances the activity of T cells and natural killer cells [70, 80]. A monoclonal antibody with CD137 agonistic activity, urelumab, or BMS-663513 (Bristol-Myers Squibb) has been tested in clinical trials, exhibiting antitumor effects in some patients with advanced melanoma [81]. However, the phase II study in patients with refractory melanoma was halted in May 2009 due to unusually high incidence of grade 4 hepatitis [82]. Trial with urelumab has recently been resumed using a lower-dose regimen.

10.3.3.3 OX40 Targeting Monoclonal Antibody

OX40 or CD134, another member of the TNF receptor superfamily, is an inducible costimulatory molecule mainly expressed on activated T cells. The only known ligand of OX40 is OX40-L, expressed on activated APCs. OX40 ligation also promotes survival and proliferation of the activated T cells and expands the pool of memory T cells. Humanized OX40 agonist mAb is being developed for future clinical trials in human subjects [80].

In general, activating mAbs targeting stimulatory immune checkpoints can produce immune-mediated antitumor response in patients with melanoma; however, their clinical activity as single agent does not appear as impressive as that of inhibitory checkpoint blocking mAbs. Thus, combinatorial approach will be the platform to advance the clinical development of these agents.

10.3.4 Combinations with Immune Checkpoint-Targeted Agents

Theoretically, rapid antigen release from apoptotic tumor cells after radiotherapy, chemotherapy, or selective *BRAF* inhibitor can effectively prime antigen-specific cytotoxic T lymphocytes. Supporting this hypothesis is the observation of abscopal effect, an event in which local radiotherapy causes tumor regression at a distant site, in a patient who subsequently achieved global tumor response when radiotherapy was added to ipilimumab upon disease progression [83]. Therefore, there is a strong interest in combining novel immune checkpoint inhibitors with other treatment modalities. At present, most of the data are with ipilimumab-based combinations. Several trials are ongoing to examine ipilimumab with concomitant radiotherapy in patients with metastatic melanoma with or without brain metastases. Current data have shown that ipilimumab generated at least additive antitumor effect when combined with DTIC at the expense of higher incidence of hepatic irAEs [27]. Studies combining ipilimumab with other chemotherapy or biochemotherapy are ongoing.

Given the dramatic responses observed with therapies that target the mitogen-activated protein kinase pathway in patients with *BRAFV600E*-positive melanoma, a phase I dose-finding study was conducted to explore the safety of concurrent ipilimumab and vemurafenib, an oral selective *BRAF* inhibitor [84]. The first six-patient cohort received both drugs at full dose concomitantly after 1-month vemurafenib lead-in. Within 5 weeks after the first dose of ipilimumab, four out of six patients developed grade 3 transaminitis. A reduced dose of vemurafenib was used for the second cohort. Despite this modification, grade 2 or 3 elevation in liver function tests was again observed within 3 weeks from the first ipilimumab administration in three out of four patients. The additive hepatotoxicity seen with concurrent administration of these two agents led to the discontinuation of the trial.

Dabrafenib, another selective *BRAF* inhibitor, plus or minus trametinib, a MEK inhibitor, has been investigated in combination with ipilimumab in a phase I study in patients with *BRAF*V600 mutant advanced melanoma. Preliminary safety data were presented at the 2014 ASCO Annual Meeting [85]. The doublet regimen, in which both ipilimumab and dabrafenib were administered at full dose, was well tolerated ($n=8$). Common adverse events, primarily of grade 1 or 2, were chills, fatigue, hand-foot syndrome, pyrexia, and maculopapular rash. Transient grade 3 transaminitis was documented in one out of eight patients after the second dose of ipilimumab and resolved after a week of high-dose steroid. The doublet arm is in the expansion phase. The triplet regimen began with ipilimumab at full dose with dabrafenib 100 mg twice daily and trametinib 1 mg daily ($n=7$). Early-onset high-grade colitis and intestinal perforation were seen in two out of seven patients, leading to the discontinuation of the triplet arm [85].

Ipilimumab or tremelimumab has also been combined with other biologics such as sargramostim, bevacizumab, vaccines, cytokines, or immune checkpoint-targeted antibodies. Of note is the result of a phase I/II study combining ipilimumab with high-dose IL-2 [86]. Three patients each received ipilimumab at 0.1, 0.3, 1, and 2 mg/g/dose; 24 patients had ipilimumab at full dose. The first dose of ipilimumab was given without IL-2. All subsequent doses of ipilimumab were followed by high-dose IL2 within 24 h. At a median follow-up duration of 84 months, the ORR was 25 %, with unprecedented complete response rate of 17 %. All CRs are durable, from 76 to 89+ months. The median OS was 16 months and a 5-year OS rate of 25 %. The combination was well tolerated, with 17 % grade 3 or 4 irAEs. Patients received up to six cycles of the combination.

Even more remarkable is the clinical activity of combined checkpoint blockade as demonstrated in the CheckMate 067 [59]. However, concurrent administration of ipilimumab and nivolumab is quite toxic. Whether the higher ORR and improved PFS observed with the combination will translate into an OS advantage and whether this improvement in OS justifies the increased toxicities remain to be seen.

After 20 years of dormancy, the field of immuno-oncology has awakened with groundbreaking scientific advances and innovative therapeutic strategies. A new family of mAbs that tamper with key regulators of the immune system to augment antitumor immunity has entered clinical trials. Pioneered by ipilimumab, these novel immunotherapeutic agents offer oncologists endless potential to unleash the immune system to attack and destroy cancers, bringing within reach the prospect of durable remission to patients with advanced melanoma. While clinicians are embracing these new treatment strategies, special attentions should be directed at agent-specific immune-related toxicities and their respective management. Companion gene expression and immunologic profiling, also an area of active research, will help improve the therapeutic indices and personalize the utilities of these agents in the near future.

References

1. Kalialis LV, Drzewiecki KT, Klyver H (2009) Spontaneous regression of metastases from melanoma: review of the literature. Melanoma Res 19:275–282
2. Kubica AW, Brewer JD (2012) Melanoma in immunosuppressed patients. Mayo Clin Proc 87:991–1003
3. Platanias LC (2005) Mechanisms of type-I- and type-II-interferon-mediated signalling. Nat Rev Immunol 5:375–386
4. Jonasch E, Haluska FG (2001) Interferon in oncological practice: review of interferon biology, clinical applications, and toxicities. Oncologist 6:34–55
5. Balch CM, Soong SJ, Atkins MD et al (2004) An evidence-based staging system for cutaneous melanoma. CA Cancer J Clin 54:131–149
6. Kirkwood JM, Strawderman MH, Ernstoff MS et al (1996) Interferon alfa-2b adjuvant therapy of high-risk resected cutaneous melanoma: the eastern cooperative oncology group trial EST 1684. J Clin Oncol 14:7–17
7. Kirkwood JM, Ibrahim JG, Sondak VK et al (2000) High- and low-dose interferon alfa-2b in high-risk melanoma: first analysis of intergroup trial E1690/S9111/C9190. J Clin Oncol 18:2444–2458
8. Kleeberg UR, Suciu S, Brocker EB et al (2004) Final results of the EORTC 18871/DKG 80-1 randomised phase III trial. rIFN-alpha2b versus rIFN-gamma versus ISCADOR M versus observation after surgery in melanoma patients with either high-risk primary (thickness >3 mm) or regional lymph node metastasis. Eur J Cancer 40:390–402
9. Eggermont AM, Suciu S, Mackie R et al (2005) Post-surgery adjuvant therapy with intermediate doses of interferon alfa 2b versus observation in patients with stage IIb/III melanoma (EORTC 18952): randomised controlled trial. Lancet 366:1189–1196
10. Hansson J, Aamdal S, Bastholt L et al (2011) Two different duration of adjuvant therapy with intermediate-dose interferon alfa-2b in patients with high-risk melanoma (Nordic IFN trial): a randomised phase III trial. Lancet Oncol 12:144–152

11. Pectasides D, Dafni U, Bafaloukos D et al (2009) Randomized phase III study of 1 month versus 1 year of adjuvant high-dose interferon alfa-2b in patients with resected high-risk melanoma. J Clin Oncol 27:939–944
12. Agarwala SS, Lee SJ, Flaherty LE et al (2011) Randomized phase III study of high-dose interferon alfa-2b (HDI) for 4 weeks induction only in patients with intermediate- and high-risk melanoma (intergroup trial E 1697). J Clin Oncol 29:Abstract 8505
13. Merck Sharp and Dohme Corp. (2012) Sylatron™ US prescribing information. http://www.sylatron.com/peginterferon/sylatron/hcp/index.jsp. Accessed 28 Jun 2013
14. Eggermont AM, Suciu S, Testori A et al (2012) Long-term results of the randomized phase III trial EORTC 18991 of adjuvant therapy with pegylated interferon alfa-2b versus observation in resected stage III melanoma. J Clin Oncol 30:3810–3818
15. Wheatley K, Ives N, Eggermont AMM et al (2007) Interferon-α as adjuvant therapy for melanoma: an individual patient meta-analysis of randomised trials. J Clin Oncol 25:Abstract 8526
16. Mocelin S, Pasquali S, Rossi CR et al (2010) Interferon alpha adjuvant therapy in patients with high-risk melanoma: a systematic review and meta-analysis. J Natl Cancer Inst 102:492–501
17. Gogas H, Ioannovich J, Dafni U et al (2006) Prognostic significance of autoimmunity during treatment of melanoma with interferon. N Engl J Med 354:709–718
18. Krauze MT, Tarhini A, Gogas H et al (2011) Prognostic significance of autoimmunity during treatment of melanoma with interferon. Semin Immunopathol 33:385–391
19. Eggermont AM, Suciu S, Testori A et al (2012) Ulceration and stage are predictive of interferon efficacy in melanoma: results of the phase III adjuvant trials EORTC 18952 and EORTC 18991. Eur J Cancer 48:218–225
20. Prometheus Laboratories Inc. (2012) Proleukin® US prescribing information. http://www.proleukin.com. Accessed 28 Jun 2013
21. Atkins MB, Lotze MT, Dutcher JP et al (1999) High-dose recombinant interleukin-2 therapy for patients with metastatic melanoma: analysis of 270 patients treated between 1985 and 1993. J Clin Oncol 17:2105–2116
22. Rudd CE, Taylor A, Schneider H (2009) CD28 and CTLA-4 coreceptor expression and signal transduction. Immunol Rev 229:12–26
23. Pardoll DM (2012) The blockade of immune checkpoints in cancer immunotherapy. Nat Rev Cancer 12:252–264
24. Graziani G, Tentori L, Navarra P (2012) Ipilimumab: a novel immunostimulatory monoclonal antibody for the treatment of cancer. Pharmacol Res 65:9–22
25. Leach DR, Krummel MF, Allison JP (1996) Enhancement of antitumor immunity by CTLA-4 blockade. Science 271:1734–1736
26. Hodi FS, O'Day SJ, McDermott DF et al (2010) Improved survival with ipilimumab in patients with metastatic melanoma. N Engl J Med 363:711–723
27. Robert C, Thomas L, Bondarenko I et al (2011) Ipilimumab plus dacarbazine for previously untreated metastatic melanoma. N Engl J Med 364:2517–2526
28. Schadendorf D, Hodi FS, Robert C et al (2015) Pooled analysis of long-term survival data from phase II and phase III trials of ipilimumab in unresectable or metastatic melanoma. J Clin Oncol 33(17):1889–1994
29. Callahan MK, Wolchok JD, Allison JP (2010) Anti-CTLA-4 antibody therapy: immune monitoring during clinical development of a novel immunotherapy. Semin Oncol 37:473–484
30. Ku GY, Yuan J, Page DB et al (2010) Single-institution experience with ipilimumab in advanced melanoma patients in the compassionate use setting: lymphocyte count after 2 doses correlates with survival. Cancer 116(7):1767–1775
31. Yuan J, Adamow M, Ginsberg BA et al (2011) Integrated NY-ESO-1 antibody and CD8+ T-cell responses correlate with clinical benefit in advanced melanoma patients treated with ipilimumab. Proc Natl Acad Sci USA 108:16723–16728
32. Hamid O, Schmidt H, Nissan A et al (2011) A prospective phase II trial exploring the association between tumor microenvironment biomarkers and clinical activity of ipilimumab in advanced melanoma. J Transl Med 9:204
33. Bristol-Myers Squibb (2013) Yervoy™ US prescribing information. http://packageinserts.bms.com/pi/pi_yervoy.pdf. Accessed 28 Jun 2013

34. Datapharm Communications Limited (2013) YERVOY™ (ipilimumab) summary of product characteristics. http://www.medicines.org.uk/emc/medicine/24779. Accessed 29 Jun 2013
35. Robert C, Schadendorf D, Messina M et al (2013) Efficacy and safety of retreatment with ipilimumab in patients with pretreated advanced melanoma who progressed after initially achieving disease control. Clin Cancer Res 19:2232–2239
36. Bronstein Y, Ng CS, Hwu P et al (2011) Radiologic manifestations of immune-related adverse events in patients with metastatic melanoma undergoing anti-CTLA-4 antibody therapy. AJR Am J Roentgenol 197:W992–W1000
37. Wolchok JD, Hoos A, O'Day S et al (2009) Guidelines for the evaluation of immune therapy in solid tumors: immune-related response criteria. Clin Cancer Res 15:7412–7420
38. Ribas A, Chmielowski B, Glaspy JA (2009) Do we need a different set of response assessment criteria for tumor immunotherapy? Clin Cancer Res 15:7116–7118
39. Eggermont AM, Chiarion-Sileni V, Grob JJ et al (2015) Adjuvant ipilimumab versus placebo after complete resection of high-risk stage III melanoma (EORTC 18071): a randomised, double-blind, phase 3 trial. Lancet Oncol 16(5):522–530
40. Margolin K, Ernstoff MS, Hamid O et al (2012) Ipilimumab in patients with melanoma and brain metastases: an open-label, phase 2 trial. Lancet Oncol 13:459–465
41. Di Giacomo AM, Ascierto PA, Pilla L et al (2012) Ipilimumab and fotemustine in patients with advanced melanoma (NIBIT-M1): an open-label, single-arm phase 2 trial. Lancet Oncol 13:879–886
42. Kähler KC, Hauschild A (2011) Treatment and side effect management of CTLA-4 antibody therapy in metastatic melanoma. J Dtsch Dermatol Ges 9:277–286
43. Bristol-Myers Squibb (2013) Yervoy™ US prescribing information: risk evaluation and mitigation strategy. http://www.yervoy.com/hcp/rems.aspx. Accessed 29 Aug 2015
44. Amin A, de Pril V, Hamid O et al (2009) Evaluation of the effect of systemic corticosteroids for the treatment of immune-related adverse events (irAEs) on the development or maintenance of ipilimumab clinical activity. J Clin Oncol 27:Abstract 9037
45. Horvat TZ, Adel NG, Dang TO et al (2015) Immune-related adverse events, need for systemic immunosuppression, and effects on survival and time to treatment failure in patients with melanoma treated with ipilimumab at memorial Sloan Kettering cancer center. J Clin Oncol 33:3193–3198
46. Bristol-Myers Squibb (2015) Opdivo® Prescribing information. http://packageinserts.bms.com/pi/pi_opdivo.pdf. Accessed 1 Sept 2015
47. Camacho LH, Antonia S, Sosman J et al (2009) Phase I/II trial of tremelimumab in patients with metastatic melanoma. J Clin Oncol 27:1075–1081
48. Kirkwood JM, Lorigan P, Hersey P et al (2010) Phase II trial of tremelimumab (CP-675,206) in patients with advanced refractory or relapsed melanoma. Clin Cancer Res 16:1042–1048
49. Ribas A, Kefford R, Marshall MA et al (2013) Phase III randomized clinical trial comparing tremelimumab with standard-of-care chemotherapy in patients with advanced melanoma. J Clin Oncol 31:616–622
50. Flies DB, Sandler BJ, Sznol M et al (2011) Blockade of the B7-H1/PD-1 pathway for cancer immunotherapy. Yale J Biol Med 84:409–421
51. Sznol M, Chen L (2013) Antagonist antibodies to PD-1 and B7-H1 (PD-L1) in the treatment of advanced human cancer. Clin Cancer Res 19:1021–1034
52. Okudaira K, Hokari R, Tsuzuki Y et al (2009) Blockade of B7-H1 or B7-DC induces an anti-tumor effect in a mouse pancreatic cancer model. Int J Oncol 35:741–749
53. Zhou Q, Xiao H, Liu Y et al (2010) Blockade of programmed death-1 pathway rescues the effector function of tumor-infiltrating T cells and enhances the antitumor efficacy of lentivector immunization. J Immunol 185:5082–5092
54. Brahmer JR, Drake CG, Wollner I et al (2010) Phase I study of single-agent anti-programmed death-1 (MDX-1106) in refractory solid tumors: safety, clinical activity, pharmacodynamics, and immunologic correlates. J Clin Oncol 28:3167–3175
55. Topalian SL, Hodi FS, Brahmer JR et al (2012) Safety, activity, and immune correlates of anti-PD-1 antibody in cancer. N Engl J Med 366:2443–2454

56. Topalian SL, Sznol M, Mcdermott DF et al (2014) Survival, durable tumor remission, and long-term safety in patients with advanced melanoma receiving nivolumab. J Clin Oncol 32(10):1020–1030

57. Weber JS, D'Angelo SP, Minor D et al (2015) Nivolumab versus chemotherapy in patients with advanced melanoma who progressed after anti-CTLA-4 treatment (CheckMate 037): a randomised, controlled, open-label, phase 3 trial. Lancet Oncol 16(4):375–384

58. Robert C, Long GV, Brady B et al (2015) Nivolumab in previously untreated melanoma without BRAF mutation. N Engl J Med 372(4):320–330

59. Larkin J, Chiarion-Sileni V, Gonzalez R et al (2015) Combined nivolumab and ipilimumab or monotherapy in untreated melanoma. N Engl J Med 373(1):23–34

60. Daud A, Ribas A, Robert C (2015) Long-term efficacy of pembrolizumab in a pooled analysis of 655 patients with advanced melanoma enrolled in KEYNOTE-001. J Clin Oncol 33:Abstract 9005

61. Hamid O, Robert C, Daud A et al (2013) Safety and tumor responses with lambrolizumab (anti-PD-1) in melanoma. N Engl J Med 369(2):134–144

62. Ribas A, Puzanov I, Dummer R et al (2015) Pembrolizumab versus investigator-choice chemotherapy for ipilimumab-refractory melanoma (KEYNOTE-002): a randomised, controlled, phase 2 trial. Lancet Oncol 16(8):908–918

63. Robert C, Schachter J, Long GV et al (2015) Pembrolizumab versus ipilimumab in advanced melanoma. N Engl J Med 372(26):2521–2532

64. Merck Sharp and Dohme (2014) Keytruda® prescribing information. http://www.merck.com/product/usa/pi_circulars/k/keytruda/keytruda_pi.pdf. Accessed 1 Sept 2015

65. Berger R, Rotem-Yehudar R, Slama G et al (2008) Phase I safety and pharmacokinetic study of CT-011, a humanized antibody interacting with PD-1, in patients with advanced hematologic malignancies. Clin Cancer Res 14:3044–3051

66. Atkins MB, Kudchadkar RR, Sznol M et al (2014) Phase 2, multicenter, safety and efficacy study of pidilizumab in patients with metastatic melanoma. J Clin Oncol 32:Abstract 9001

67. Brahmer JR, Tykodi SS, Chow LQ et al (2012) Safety and activity of anti-PD-L1 antibody in patients with advanced cancer. N Engl J Med 366:2455–2465

68. Herbst RS, Gordon MS, Fine GD et al (2013) A study of MPDL3280A, an engineered PD-L1 antibody in patients with locally advanced or metastatic tumors. J Clin Oncol 31:Abstract 3000

69. Gilboa E (2004) The promise of cancer vaccines. Nat Rev Cancer 4:401–411

70. Melero I, Grimaldi AM, Perez-Gracia JL et al (2013) Clinical development of immunostimulatory monoclonal antibodies and opportunities for combination. Clin Cancer Res 19:997–1008

71. Fonsatti E, Maio M, Altomonte M et al (2010) Biology and clinical applications of CD40 in cancer treatment. Semin Oncol 37:517–523

72. Vonderheide RH, Glennie MJ (2013) Agonistic CD40 antibodies and cancer therapy. Clin Cancer Res 19:1035–1043

73. von Leoprechting A, van der Bruggen P, Pahl HL et al (1999) Stimulation of CD40 on immunogenic human malignant melanomas augments their cytotoxic T lymphocyte-mediated lysis and induces apoptosis. Cancer Res 59:1287–1294

74. Ghamande S, Hylander BL, Oflazoglu E et al (2001) Recombinant CD40 ligand therapy has significant antitumor effects on CD40-positive ovarian tumor xenografts grown in SCID mice and demonstrates an augmented effect with cisplatin. Cancer Res 61:7556–7562

75. Funakoshi S, Longo DL, Beckwith M et al (1994) Inhibition of human B-cell lymphoma growth by CD40 stimulation. Blood 83:2787–2794

76. Schultze JL, Michalak S, Seamon MJ et al (1997) CD40-activated human B cells: an alternative source of highly efficient antigen presenting cells to generate autologous antigen-specific T cells for adoptive immunotherapy. J Clin Invest 100:2757–2765

77. Vonderheide RH, Flaherty KT, Khalil M et al (2007) Clinical activity and immune modulation in cancer patients treated with CP-870,893, a novel CD40 agonist monoclonal antibody. J Clin Oncol 25:876–883

78. Slupsky JR, Kalbas M, Willuweit A et al (1998) Activated platelets induce tissue factor expression on human umbilical vein endothelial cells by ligation of CD40. Thromb Haemost 80:1008–1014

79. Rüter J, Antonia SJ, Burris HA et al (2010) Immune modulation with weekly dosing of an agonist CD40 antibody in a phase I study of patients with advanced solid tumors. Cancer Biol Ther 10:983–993

80. Melero I, Hirschhorn-Cymerman D, Morales-Kastresana A et al (2013) Agonist antibodies to TNFR molecules that costimulate T and NK cells. Clin Cancer Res 19:1044–1053

81. Sznol M, Hodi FS, Margolin K et al (2008) Phase I study of BMS-663513, a fully human anti-CD137 agonist monoclonal antibody, in patients with advanced cancer. J Clin Oncol 26:Abstract 3007

82. Hwu WJ (2010) Targeted therapies for melanoma: from bench to bedside. HemOnc Today (published online 25 Jun 2010). http://www.healio.com/hematology-oncology/melanoma-skin-cancer/news/print/hematology-oncology/%7B77E71A11-1FD1-4193-A2F7-7C50C6121C1F%7D/Targeted-therapy-for-metastatic-melanoma-From-bench-to-bedside. Accessed 29 Jun 2013

83. Postow MA, Callahan MK, Barker CA et al (2012) Immunologic correlates of the abscopal effect in a patient with melanoma. N Engl J Med 366:925–931

84. Ribas A, Hodi FS, Callahan M et al (2013) Hepatotoxicity with combination of vemurafenib and ipilimumab. N Engl J Med 368:1365–1366

85. Puzanov I, Callahan MK, Linette GP et al (2014) Phase 1 study of the BRAF inhibitor dabrafenib with or wihout the MEK inhibitor trametinib in combination with ipilimumab for V600E/K mutation-positive unresectable or metastatic melanoma. J Clin Oncol 32:Abstract 2511

86. Prieto PA, Yang JC, Sherry RM et al (2012) CTLA-4 blockade with ipilimumab: long-term follow-up of 177 patients with metastatic melanoma. Clin Cancer Res 18:2039–2047

Chapter 11
Targeted Therapy in Melanoma

Isabella C. Glitza, Dae Won Kim, Young Kwang Chae, and Kevin B. Kim

Abstract Melanoma has the highest mutation rate of all common cancers, and genomic research has accelerated the development of multiple new targeted therapies. The most commonly found mutations in melanoma are *BRAF*, *NRAS*, and *KIT*, and this chapter provides a detailed overview of each gene, their association with clinical features, as well as currently approved and investigational targeted approaches for each of these mutations. Safety profiles and underlying mechanisms of resistance are presented. Lastly, *GNAQ/GNA11* mutations, found in up to 80 % of uveal melanoma patients, are detailed, and new insights into the role of the PTEN/PI3K/AKT/mTOR pathway are discussed.

Keywords Melanoma • Genetic mutations • BRAF • NRAS • KIT • GNAQ • GNA11 • PI3K/AKT • Targeted therapy • Safety profile • Small-molecule inhibitors

I.C. Glitza, MD (✉)
Department of Melanoma Medical Oncology, The University of Texas MD Anderson
Cancer Center, Unit 430, 1515 Holcombe Blvd, Houston, TX 77030, USA
e-mail: icglitza@mdanderson.org

D.W. Kim, MD
Moffitt Cancer Center, 12902 Magnolia Drive, Tampa, FL 33612, USA

Y.K. Chae, MD
Division of Hematology and Oncology, Department of Medicine, Northwestern University
Feinberg School of Medicine Robert H. Lurie Comprehensive Cancer Center of Northwestern
University, 645 N. Michigan Avenue, Suite 1006,
Chicago, IL 60611, USA

K.B. Kim, MD
Department of Melanoma Medical Oncology, The University of Texas MD Anderson
Cancer Center, Unit 430, 1515 Holcombe Blvd, Houston, TX 77030, USA

California Pacific Medical Center, San Francisco, CA, USA

© Springer Science+Business Media New York 2016
C.A. Torres-Cabala, J.L. Curry (eds.), *Genetics of Melanoma*, Cancer Genetics,
DOI 10.1007/978-1-4939-3554-3_11

11.1   Introduction

The incidence of melanoma and melanoma-related deaths has both increased over the last several decades in the United States, with more than 76,000 new cases and more than 9000 deaths predicted in 2013 [1]. The vast majority of patients with malignant melanoma are diagnosed early with locally confined disease and have an excellent clinical outcome; however, patients with metastatic melanoma have a poor prognosis, with a median survival of 6–9 months [2–5]. Although surgery remains the mainstay of therapy for localized disease, the treatment for metastatic melanoma remains challenging.

Until 2011, only two drugs had received approval from the US Food and Drug Administration (FDA) for the treatment of metastatic melanoma. Dacarbazine, an alkylating agent that was approved in 1975, has response rates of only 5–12 % in large phase III clinical studies and has never shown a substantial prolongation of median progression-free survival (PFS) or overall survival (OS) [6–10]. Recombinant human interleukin-2, the second FDA-approved therapy after dacarbazine, has shown similar response rates. A pooled analysis of eight trials with a total of 270 patients treated with interleukin-2 showed a total response rate of about 16 % [11], but the most recent phase III study showed a response rate of only 6 % [11, 12]. Interleukin-2 treatment is associated with significant toxicity, including capillary leakage syndrome, and can induce long-term survival in only a small subgroup of patients, namely, those patients presenting with metastases mainly in the lungs or soft tissues, normal serum lactate dehydrogenase levels, and good overall performance status [13].

More recently, new treatment approaches, including targeted therapies and immunotherapies, have shown promising results. Ipilimumab, a monoclonal antibody targeting anti-cytotoxic T lymphocyte-associated antigen 4 (CTLA-4), was evaluated in a phase III trial in patients with metastatic melanoma who were previously treated with at least one systemic therapy. The results of the study revealed statistically significant improvement in PFS and OS over a comparison treatment (gp100 vaccine) [14] and led to the approval of this drug in 2011. Response rates to ipilimumab are low (5–16 %), but durable responses have been observed in patients who achieved complete remissions [14–16]. Despite the survival benefit of ipilimumab, however, most patients with advanced melanoma are not cured and need other effective therapies. Rapid advances in our understanding of melanoma genetics since the early 2000s have led to the successful development of targeted drugs. This chapter will discuss the development and promising clinical investigations of these small molecules targeting mutated kinases or aberrant signal transduction pathways in melanoma.

11.2   BRAF Mutation

11.2.1   Discovery of the BRAF Mutation in Melanoma

The discovery of oncogenes has accelerated translational oncology research over the past decade. One of the most significant discoveries in solid tumors was the identification of frequent mutations in the *BRAF* gene in human cancers by Davies et al. in 2002 [17]. Since their initial findings in melanoma, mutations in this specific gene have been reported in a number of additional malignancies, including papillary thyroid cancer, hairy cell leukemia, and colon cancer, and have a total incidence of 7–8 % in all human cancers [18–21]. Multiple investigators have confirmed the presence of *BRAF* mutations in approximately 50 % of all melanomas [22–25]. BRAF, a serine/threonine kinase, is one of the key elements in the mitogen-activated protein kinase (MAPK) pathway. The most common of the *BRAF* mutations (in 75–90 % of all BRAF-mutant cells) is a missense mutation at codon 600 in exon 15 that leads to the substitution of glutamic acid for valine (*V600E BRAF*) [2, 17, 25]. Other variants include *V600K* (up to 22 % of all mutations) and the rare mutations *V600R*, *V600D*, *V600M*, *L597*, and *K601E* [22, 25–29].

11.2.2   Function of BRAF

BRAF kinase, one of the three RAF kinase isoforms, is an intermediary in the MAPK pathway, which is one of the best characterized signal transduction pathways in human cancers. In general, the activation of membrane-bound receptor tyrosine kinases, either by binding to their ligands or by acquiring gene mutations, changes the RAS proteins from an inactive GDP-bound state to an active GTP-bound state, which in turn stimulates the activation of RAS downstream effectors, the RAF kinases. Subsequently, the active RAF kinases activate MAPK pathways through their only known downstream effectors, MEK1 and MEK2, and ultimately cause unregulated cell proliferation and growth (Fig. 11.1) [30–32].

In contrast with wild-type *BRAF*, mutated *BRAF* gene causes constitutive activation of the BRAF kinase independent of RAS activation or dimerization with other RAF kinases and results in MEK and ERK activation [33–36]. In particular, the *V600E BRAF* mutation results in tenfold higher basal kinase activity than that of wild-type *BRAF* [17]. Accordingly, inhibition of *V600E BRAF* kinase in cell lines leads to decreased ERK activity, resulting in rapid cell arrest, decreased transcription rates, and ultimately apoptosis, making *V600E BRAF* a desirable target for new therapeutics [33, 37].

Interestingly, *BRAF* mutations are found not only in melanoma cells but also in benign human nevi [38–40]. Further research revealed that *V600E BRAF* can cause melanocytic hyperplasia and functions as an initial step in the development of malignant melanoma, but additional genetic mutations are necessary for oncogenesis [41].

11.2.3   Characteristics and Prognosis of Patients with BRAF-Mutant Melanoma

Despite the frequent occurrence of *BRAF* mutations in melanoma, the incidence of this mutation varies significantly depending on the histopathological subtype and patient factors. The frequency of *BRAF* mutation is approximately 50 % in

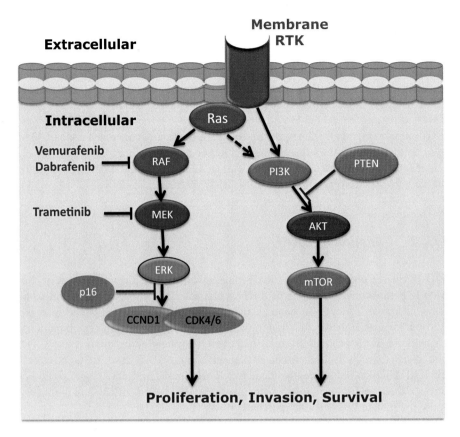

Fig. 11.1 The MAPK signal transduction pathway

primary nodular or superficial spreading melanomas originating in intermittently sun-exposed skin. A recent meta-analysis found that the frequency of *BRAF* mutation was significantly related to the location of the primary melanoma; the incidence of *BRAF* mutation was highest in the trunk (294 of 520 cases, 57 %), followed by the extremities (210 of 454, 46 %) and the face or scalp (94 of 332, 28 %) [42]. In another report of a series of 102 patients, *BRAF* mutations were present in 3 % of the melanomas of mucosal surfaces, in 21 % of acral lentiginous melanoma, in 6 % of melanomas on the skin with chronic sun-induced damage, and in 56 % of melanomas on the skin without chronic sun-induced damage [43]. *BRAF* mutations have been rarely reported in uveal melanomas [22–24, 44].

Younger age at presentation has been associated with a higher likelihood of *BRAF* mutation, with one analysis reporting that all patients <30 years old and only 25 % of patients ≥70 years old had *BRAF*-mutant metastatic melanoma [24, 45]. A recent meta-analysis did not confirm this finding when it reviewed the data of 394 patients [24, 42, 45]. Another study reported a higher proportion of *V600K* mutations in older patients [46]. In addition, patients with *BRAF*-mutant melanoma tend to have a higher number of melanocytic nevi [47].

A number of retrospective studies have suggested that the presence of a *BRAF* mutation is a potential marker of poor prognosis. A retrospective analysis at The University of Texas MD Anderson Cancer Center found a higher frequency of ulceration in *BRAF*-mutated melanomas [48]. A French review included 105 consecutive patients with stage III cutaneous melanomas. Patients with *BRAF*-mutant melanoma had a shorter median OS than patients with *BRAF* wild-type melanoma (1.4 vs. 2.8 years, $p = 0.005$) [49]. An Australian study examined 46 patients with *BRAF* mutations and found that the different genotypes within *BRAF*-mutant metastatic melanoma exhibit different biological and clinical behaviors. No survival difference was seen between the *V600K* and *V600E* mutation subtypes, but the disease-free interval was shorter for patients harboring the *V600K* mutation [24]. Patients with *BRAF*-mutant metastatic melanoma who were not treated with a BRAF inhibitor had a lower 1-year survival rate than those without this mutation. However, patients with a *BRAF* mutation who were treated with a BRAF inhibitor had significantly longer survival times [23, 25].

11.2.4 Selective BRAF Inhibitors

11.2.4.1 Clinical Efficacy

Despite its activity in in vitro and xenograft models [50–52], sorafenib, an inhibitor of CRAF, BRAF, and VEGF, failed to show clinical benefit in patients with metastatic melanoma [53–56]. In a number of clinical studies of sorafenib, patients with metastatic melanoma were enrolled regardless of their *BRAF* mutation status and treated with sorafenib as a single agent or in combination with chemotherapeutic agents, but the clinical benefit of sorafenib did not appear to correlate with BRAF status [55, 56]. The reason for these disappointing results is likely related to sorafenib's only modest inhibition of the MAPK pathway [57, 58].

Vemurafenib [PLX4032; Zelboraf (Roche, Basel, Switzerland)] is a highly potent oral BRAF inhibitor, with a biochemical half maximal inhibitory concentration (IC$_{50}$) of ~31 nM, that binds to the ATP-binding site of mutated *V600 BRAF* kinase and inhibits its activity [59]. In a phase I study, vemurafenib induced a significant decrease in p-ERK, cyclin D1, and Ki-67 expression in patients treated at the maximum tolerated dose (MTD) of 960 mg orally twice a day after only 2 weeks of treatment with a majority of patients ultimately experiencing a major clinical response [60]. However, none of the five patients with wild-type *BRAF* melanoma who received at least 240 mg of vemurafenib twice daily in the study had a clinical response. A phase II study of vemurafenib with 132 patients reported an overall response rate of 53 % (and a 6 % complete response rate) in patients with *V600 BRAF*-mutant metastatic melanoma. The median PFS was 6.8 months, and the median OS duration was 15.9 months [61].

A pivotal double-blind, randomized, phase III trial was conducted to compare the survival of patients with *V600E BRAF*-mutant advanced melanoma who received vemurafenib with that of those who received dacarbazine [7]. In this study, 675 patients were randomized to vemurafenib or dacarbazine treatment at a 1:1 ratio. The interim analysis showed that both PFS [5.3 vs. 1.6 months, hazard ratio (HR) = 0.26 [95 % confidence interval (CI), 0.20–0.33], $p < 0.001$] and OS [HR = 0.37 (95 % CI, 0.26–0.55), $p < 0.001$] were significantly longer in the vemurafenib arm. There were ten patients whose tumors were later found to also contain a *V600K BRAF* mutation; among those patients, four had a partial response, suggesting the clinical efficacy of vemurafenib in this subset of patients. An updated analysis of the study showed continued superiority of vemurafenib over dacarbazine (median PFS duration of 6.9 months vs. 1.6 months, HR = 0.38, $p < 0.001$; median OS duration of 13.6 vs. 9.7 months, HR = 0.70, $p < 0.001$) [62]. On the basis of the improved clinical outcomes in this study, vemurafenib received an approval from the FDA for the treatment of *V600 BRAF*-mutant metastatic melanoma in the United States in August 2011 (Table 11.1).

Dabrafenib [Tafinlar (GlaxoSmithKline, Brentford, UK)] is another potent selective BRAF inhibitor with IC_{50} of 0.8 nM [63]. Early phase I and II trials reported that dabrafenib was well tolerated at doses of up to 300 mg twice a day without reaching the MTD, and 150 mg twice daily was selected as the recommended dose for further studies owing to a near-maximum pharmacodynamic effect at this dose and no apparent additional clinical benefit beyond this dose [64]. Dabrafenib potently inhibited mutated *BRAF* kinase, decreased the expression of phosphorylated ERK, and induced significant tumor regression [65]. In a phase III study, 250 patients with *V600E BRAF*-mutant metastatic melanoma were randomly assigned to receive either dabrafenib (150 mg twice daily, orally) or dacarbazine, and the primary objective was to compare PFS between the two groups [66]. In an initial analysis, the median PFS was 5.1 months for dabrafenib and 2.7 months for dacarbazine [HR = 0.30 (95 % CI, 0.18–0.53), $p < 0.0001$], with response rates of 53 % and 6 % for dabrafenib and dacarbazine, respectively. These data led to the FDA's approval of dabrafenib in May 2013 for unresectable or metastatic melanoma with the *V600E BRAF* mutation. The latest update of the study, with a median follow-up of 15.2 months for dabrafenib and 12.7 months for dacarbazine, confirmed the efficacy of dabrafenib; the HR for progression was 0.37 (95 % CI, 0.23–0.57), and the median PFS was 6.9 months for dabrafenib and 2.7 months for dacarbazine [9]. Despite the fact that 59 % of the patients whose disease progressed on dacarbazine were switched to (crossover) dabrafenib, the median OS was over 18 months in the dabrafenib arm and over 15 months in the dacarbazine arm [9].

11.2.4.2 Safety Profiles

The most common adverse events associated with vemurafenib treatment in the phase II and phase III trials were arthralgia, rash, photosensitivity, fatigue, alopecia, keratoacanthoma (KA) or cutaneous squamous cell carcinoma (cSCC), nausea, and diarrhea; 38 % of patients required dose modification because of intolerable toxicity [7, 61]. The most common grade 3 adverse events were the development of cSCCs and KAs (18–25 % of patients). Grade 3 rash (8 %), arthralgia (6 %), abnormal liver

Table 11.1 Clinical efficacy data of randomized phase II and III studies of targeted therapies in melanoma

Trial and regimen	N	Treatment setting	Primary end point	Hazard ratio (95 % CI)	p value	References
BRAF mutation						
Dacarbazine	338	First line; V600E BRAF	OS (median, months)[a]			Chapman et al. [7]
			9.7	0.70 (0.57–0.87)	<0.001	
Vemurafenib	337		13.6			
Dacarbazine	338		PFS (median, months)			
			1.6	0.38 (0.32–0.46)	<0.001	
Vemurafenib	337		6.9			
Dacarbazine	63	First line; V600E BRAF	PFS (median, months)			Hauschild et al. [9]
Dabrafenib	187		2.7	0.37 (0.23–0.57)	<0.0001	
			6.9			
Chemotherapy[b]	108	≤1 prior systemic therapy; V600E/K BRAF	PFS (median, months)			Flaherty et al. [103]
Trametinib	214		1.5	0.45 (0.33–0.63)	<0.001	
			4.8			
Dabrafenib	54	V600E/K BRAF	PFS (median, months)			Flaherty et al. [106]
Dabrafenib/ trametinib[c]	54		5.8	0.39 (0.25–0.62)	<0.001	
			9.4			
Vemurafenib	132	V600E BRAF	ORR			Sosman et al. [61]
			53 % (95 % CI, 44–62)			
Dabrafenib	76	V600E BRAF	ORR			Ascierto et al. [65]
			59 % (95 % CI, 48–70)			
Trametinib	57[d] 40[e]	V600E/K BRAF	ORR			Kim et al. [102]
			25 % (95 % CI, 14–38)			
			0 %			
KIT mutation						
Imatinib	25	First line; KIT mutations and/ or amplification	ORR			Carvajal et al. [119]
			16 % (95 % CI, 2–30)			
Imatinib	43	First line; KIT mutations and/ or amplification	PFS (median, months)			Guo et al. [120]
			3.5 (range, 1.3–5.7)			
			6-month PFS rate			
			36.6 %			

(continued)

Table 11.1 (continued)

Trial and regimen	N	Treatment setting	Primary end point	Hazard ratio (95 % CI)	p value	References
Imatinib	24	First line; *KIT* mutations and/ or amplification	ORR			Hodi et al. [122]
			29 % (95 % CI, 13–51)			
			TTP (median, months)			
			3.7 (95 % CI, 2.6 to 5.6)			
Nilotinib	9	First line; *KIT* mutations and/ or amplification	PFS (median, months)			Cho et al. [121]
			2.5 (95 % CI, 0.1–5.0)			
NRAS mutation						
MEK162	30	First line; *NRAS* mutation	ORR			Ascierto et al. [105]
			20 % (95 % CI, 8–39)			
GNAQ/GNA11 mutation						
Selumetinib Temozolomide	38	Uveal melanoma[a, f]	PFS (median, weeks)			Carvajal et al. [130]
(or dacarbazine)	42		15.4	0.55 (0.34–0.87)	0.011	
			7.0			

N number of patients, *CI* confidence interval, *OS* overall survival, *PFS* progression-free survival, *ORR* overall response rate, *TTP* time to progression
[a]Crossover was allowed in the control group
[b]Dacarbazine or paclitaxel
[c]The doses were 150 mg dabrafenib twice a day and 2 mg trametinib once a day
[d]BRAF inhibitor naïve
[e]Previously treated with a BRAF inhibitor
[f]Among all patients with uveal melanoma, only those with exon 5 GNAQ/GNA11 mutation are reported in this table

enzymes (6 %), and photosensitivity (3 %) were also reported [7, 61, 67]. Adverse events led to the discontinuation of vemurafenib in 3–7 % of patients, and dose reduction was necessary in 38–45 % of the patients [8, 62].

For dabrafenib, the most common adverse reactions of any grade were hyperkeratosis, headache, pyrexia, arthralgia, papilloma, alopecia, palmar-plantar erythrodysesthesia, and rash [65, 66]. The incidence of adverse events resulting in permanent discontinuation of dabrafenib in the phase III trial was 3 %. The dose of dabrafenib was reduced in 28 % of patients. The most frequent adverse reactions leading to dose reduction of dabrafenib were pyrexia, palmar-plantar erythrodysesthesia, chills, fatigue, and headache [9, 66].

The development of cSCCs and KAs discovered during the early clinical investigation of the BRAF inhibitors was intriguing. In a search for mechanisms to explain the development of these hyperproliferative skin lesions, researchers have found that in cells without a *BRAF* mutation, especially ones containing a *RAS* mutation, BRAF inhibitors induce paradoxical activation of the MAPK pathway through a CRAF-dependent mechanism, which leads to the accelerated growth of these skin lesions and a median onset of approximately 10 weeks after start of treatment [68, 69]. Consistent with this mechanism of paradoxical activation, the addition of a MEK inhibitor to a BRAF inhibitor was shown to block the growth of skin lesions harboring an *HRAS* mutation [70].

In addition to the development of cSCCs and KAs, the diagnosis of new primary melanomas without a *BRAF* mutation, progression of *RAS*-mutant chronic myelomonocytic leukemia, and development of colonic adenomatous polyps have been reported during BRAF inhibitor treatment [71–73]. Therefore, careful surveillance for new malignancies is strongly advocated when patients are receiving a BRAF inhibitor.

11.2.4.3 Mechanisms of Resistance

Despite the fact that the majority of patients with a *BRAF* mutation respond to BRAF inhibitor treatment, most of them develop resistance to the therapy within a year, and a small subset (~10 %) of the patients have melanomas with primary resistance to BRAF inhibitor treatment [60, 74]. Intrinsic primary resistance is likely to be the result of other genetic or epigenetic aberrations leading to the activation of essential signal transduction pathways that bypass the inhibitory effect of the BRAF inhibitors on the MAPK pathway. These can include inactivation of *phosphatase and tensin homolog (PTEN)*, *cyclin-dependent kinase inhibitor 2A (CDKN2A)*, and *retinoblastoma 1 (RB1)*, among others [74–76]. Recent biomarker studies examined tumor samples collected from patients who were enrolled in phase I trials of vemurafenib or dabrafenib and showed that decreased levels of *PTEN* at baseline were predictive of a worse clinical outcome [76, 77]. In addition, higher copy numbers of *CCND1* and lower copy numbers of *CDKN2A* at baseline were significantly associated with shorter PFS [75, 76, 78].

11.2.4.4 Mechanisms of Resistance

Unlike mutation-derived resistance to other targeted therapies, such as resistance to EGFR inhibitors in non-small cell lung cancers and resistance to Bcr-abl inhibitors in chronic myelogenous leukemia, resistance to BRAF inhibitors through acquired mutations in the *BRAF* gene or a loss of *BRAF* mutation has not been found in melanoma. In general, there are two categories of resistance mechanisms to BRAF inhibitors: MEK dependent and MEK independent. In the phase I and II studies of vemurafenib or dabrafenib, marked downregulation of p-MEK and p-ERK was observed in virtually all biopsy samples after the first 2 weeks of treatment. However, at the time of disease progression, a variable degree of the MEK and ERK reactivation was found [60, 76, 77]. It is likely that the tumors with a reactivated

MAPK pathway at the time of disease progression have MEK-dependent resistance and those with a suppressed MAPK pathway have MEK-independent resistance.

MEK-dependent resistance can develop through a variety of mechanisms, including the acquisition of a new *NRAS* or *MEK* mutation [76, 77, 79], increased expression of COT-1 (a serine/threonine kinase protein) [74], upregulation of CRAF kinase [80], or dimerization of RAF kinases via alternative splicing of the *BRAF* gene [36]. These aberrations can potentially activate the MEK protein and thus the MAPK signaling pathway, despite the continued inhibition of mutated *BRAF* kinase. For patients with MEK-dependent resistance, there is a rationale to combine a MEK inhibitor with a BRAF inhibitor to prevent or delay the resistance.

In contrast, in patients with MEK-independent resistance to BRAF inhibitors, which can develop through upregulation of membrane receptor tyrosine kinases such as platelet-derived growth factor receptor (PDGFR)-β and insulin-like growth factor 1 receptor (IGF-1R) [79, 81] or a loss of PTEN function [76, 77], the addition of a MEK inhibitor is not likely to significantly prolong the duration of disease control due to the activation of alternative signaling pathways. For melanomas with these genetic or epigenetic abnormalities, there is great interest in investigating the combination of BRAF inhibitors with inhibitors of the receptor tyrosine kinase or the phosphatidylinositol 3-kinase (PI3K)/AKT (also known as protein kinase B)/mammalian target of rapamycin (mTOR) pathway.

In addition to the resistance mechanisms occurring within the tumor cells, resistance to BRAF inhibitors can develop via the interactions with stromal cells. Straussman and colleagues [82] demonstrated that hepatocyte growth factor secreted by stromal cells activates its receptor, MET kinase, in melanoma cells, which results in the activation of both the MAPK and PI3K/AKT signal transduction pathways. They showed that the inhibition of both mutated BRAF kinase and hepatocyte growth factor or MET kinase reverses the resistance to BRAF inhibitors [82].

11.2.5   Selective MEK Inhibitors

Because of the central role played by MEK protein in the MAPK signaling pathway, especially in melanoma cells harboring a *BRAF* or *NRAS* mutation, targeting MEK has become an appealing approach for targeted therapy in melanoma. A number of MEK inhibitors have promising antitumor activity in *BRAF*- or *NRAS*-mutant cell lines [83–85]. On the basis of their selective activities against multiple tumor types with constitutively activated ERK protein, CI-1040 (Pfizer, Inc., New York, NY) and PD-0325901 (Pfizer, Inc.), both selective non-ATP-competitive inhibitors of MEK1 and MEK2, were tested in clinical studies in patients with advanced solid tumors [86–91]. However, because of a lack of clinical activity for CI-1040 and a high frequency of neurologic, musculoskeletal, and ocular toxicities for PD-0325901, further clinical development of these agents was discontinued.

Selumetinib [ARRY-142886 (AstraZeneca, PLC., London, UK)] is a highly selective allosteric inhibitor of both MEK1 and MEK2. In preclinical studies, selumetinib induced more significant inhibition of ERK activity and growth in various tumor cells harboring *BRAF* or *RAS* mutations than in those without *BRAF* or *RAS* mutations and also inhibited tumor growth in xenograft models harboring a *V600E BRAF* mutation [92, 93]. In a phase I study of selumetinib (free-base formulation), 9 of 20 patients with metastatic melanoma had long-term disease stabilization [94]. Common adverse events included fatigue, rash, diarrhea, peripheral edema, and nausea, and 100 mg twice a day was determined to be the MTD. Despite its promising efficacy in the phase I study, however, a randomized phase II trial revealed that there was no significant difference in clinical efficacy between selumetinib (free base) and temozolomide among 200 chemotherapy-naïve patients with advanced melanoma [95]. Only 6 % of the patients who received selumetinib had a clinical response, and even among those with *BRAF*-mutant melanoma, the response rate was 11 %.

A hydrogen-sulfate formulation of selumetinib, which has more favorable pharmacokinetic properties than the free-base formulation, has also been investigated in a clinical setting, and the MTD was 75 mg twice a day [96]. In a phase I study in which patients received various regimens containing the hydrogen-sulfate formulation of selumetinib, patients with a *BRAF* mutation had higher response rates and a longer time to progression than patients with wild-type *BRAF*, suggesting selective activity against *BRAF*-mutant melanoma [97]. Recently, a randomized phase II study was conducted to evaluate the clinical benefit of selumetinib (hydrogen-sulfate) in patients with metastatic melanoma harboring a *BRAF* mutation [98]. In this study, 91 patients were randomized to either a combination of dacarbazine and selumetinib or dacarbazine with placebo. Patients who received the combination of the dacarbazine and selumetinib had a longer PFS duration [5.6 vs. 3.0 months for dacarbazine alone, HR=0.63 (80 % CI, 0.47–0.84), $p=0.021$] and a higher confirmed response rate (29 vs. 13 % for dacarbazine alone).

Trametinib [Mekinist (GlaxoSmithKline, Brentford, UK)] is another orally available potent allosteric inhibitor of MEK1 and MEK2. It inhibits the catalytic activity of MEK1/MEK2 and inhibits phosphorylation at serine 217, which results in a predominantly monophosphorylated protein at serine 221 that leads to lower kinase activity [99]. Like other MEK inhibitors, trametinib showed significant growth inhibition in multiple tumor xenografts and particularly in those harboring activating mutations in *BRAF* or *RAS* tumor regression in xenograft models of *BRAF*-mutant melanoma than in wild-type *BRAF* tumors [99]. In a phase I study, trametinib was well tolerated, and the MTD was established as 3 mg once daily [100, 101]. However, a dose of 2 mg once daily was selected for further clinical investigation on the basis of optimal pharmacokinetic, safety, and activity profiles at this dose.

A phase II study of trametinib included 57 patients with *BRAF*-mutant melanoma not previously treated with a BRAF inhibitor; the response rate was 25, and 51 % of the patients had disease stabilization [102]. The promising results in the phase II study promptly led to a randomized phase III study to evaluate the PFS advantage of trametinib over chemotherapy approaches in patients with metastatic melanoma harboring a *BRAF* mutation. In this phase III study, a total of 322 patients

248   I.C. Glitza et al.

with *V600E* or *V600K* *BRAF*-mutant melanoma were randomized to either trametinib (2 mg once daily) or chemotherapy (dacarbazine or paclitaxel) at a 2:1 ratio, and patients in the control chemotherapy arm were allowed to cross over to receive trametinib at the time of disease progression [103]. The HR for PFS, which was the primary end point of the trial, was 0.45 (95 % CI, 0.33–0.63, $p<0.001$) in the trametinib arm, and the median PFS durations were 4.8 months and 1.5 months for the trametinib and chemotherapy arms, respectively.

Despite the fact that 47 % of the patients in the chemotherapy arm were crossed over to receive trametinib, reduction in the risk of death was observed in the patients receiving trametinib [HR = 0.54 (95 % CI, 0.32–0.92), $p=0.01$]. The median OS duration was not reached at the time of the data analysis for both arms. The positive study results of this pivotal trial led to the approval of trametinib by the FDA for the treatment of *V600E/K* *BRAF*-mutant metastatic melanoma in the United States in May 2013. However, it is important to note that trametinib does not have clinical activity in patients whose melanoma is resistant to BRAF inhibitor treatment. In the phase II study of trametinib, a cohort of 40 patients who had previously received a selective BRAF inhibitor was evaluated for clinical efficacy, and none of the patients had confirmed responses [102], indicating that trametinib as single agent must not be used as a salvage therapy for patients with melanoma that is resistant to BRAF inhibitors.

Safety data have indicated that trametinib is well tolerated. At the approved dose of 2 mg once daily, the most common adverse events are skin rash, diarrhea, peripheral edema, fatigue, and nausea, and most cases are mild in severity, with grade 3 or 4 instances of these events occurring in less than 10 % of the patients [102, 103]. The certain class effects of MEK inhibitors, such as decreased left ventricular ejection fraction and ocular toxicity (central serous retinopathy or retinal vein occlusion), occur uncommonly, and in almost all cases, these side effects are reversible upon drug discontinuation. Although only 15 % of the 211 patients who were randomized to the trametinib arm in the phase III study experienced hypertension, most of the instances of this side effect were grade 3 [103]; therefore, blood pressure must be closely monitored while patients are on trametinib treatment.

Another selective non-ATP-competitive inhibitor, MEK162 (Novartis, Basel, Switzerland), also has shown promising clinical activity in early-phase studies. In a phase I study of MEK162, the MTD was established at 60 mg twice a day [104]. In a phase II study of MEK162, 8 (20 %) of 41 patients with *V600 BRAF*-mutant melanoma had a partial response (both confirmed and unconfirmed), with a median PFS duration of 3.6 months [105], suggesting that this drug could be beneficial in patients with *BRAF*-mutant advanced melanoma and that further clinical evaluation is warranted.

11.2.6   Combined BRAF and MEK Inhibition

Based on the data that a significant proportion of the mechanisms for BRAF inhibitor resistance is associated with reactivation of the MAPK pathway, an approach to combine a BRAF inhibitor with a MEK inhibitor has garnered great interest among melanoma researchers. Proof of this concept was tested in a phase I/II study of the combination of dabrafenib and trametinib in patients with *V600 BRAF*-mutant metastatic melanoma. During the dose escalation portion of this study, the full doses of both drugs in combination (150 mg of dabrafenib twice a day and 2 mg of trametinib once a day) were well tolerated [106]. In the dose expansion portion of the study, 162 patients were randomized to dabrafenib treatment alone or two different doses of the combination regimen. The response rates were 76 % and 54 % in the full-dose combination therapy arm and the dabrafenib treatment arm, respectively ($p = 0.03$), and the median PFS duration in the combination group was also significantly better [9.4 months vs. 5.8 months, with an HR of 0.39 (95 % CI, 0.25–0.62), $p < 0.001$]. In regard to the toxicity profile, the incidence of proliferative skin lesions, including cSCC, KA, and hyperkeratosis, was lower in the combination therapy arm, as was predicted by preclinical studies. In a different phase I study, the safety and effectiveness of the combination of vemurafenib and GDC-0973, a selective MEK inhibitor, were evaluated [107]. In that study, only 1 of 44 evaluated patients developed cSCC, which was suggestive of inhibition of MEK inhibitor-induced paradoxical activation of the MAPK pathway. Preliminary efficacy data in 25 evaluable BRAF inhibitor-naïve patients showed that all 25 had tumor reduction with the combined therapy [107]. These studies suggest that a combination approach may be superior to single-agent treatment with a BRAF inhibitor. Several phase III trials of the dual inhibition of BRAF and MEK are currently under way to evaluate the concomitant inhibition of BRAF and MEK.

11.3 KIT Mutation

KIT is a type III transmembrane receptor tyrosine kinase, and binding of its ligand, stem cell factor, induces cell survival and cell proliferation by activation of several signaling pathways, such as MAPK, PI3K, phospholipase C-γ, and JAK/STAT [108]. Emerging data suggest *KIT* mutations as an oncogenic driver in melanoma. The two most common *KIT* mutations in melanoma are *L576P* (34 %) and *K642E* (15 %) in exon 11 and 13, respectively, and 70 % of *KIT* mutations occur in exon 11, which encodes the juxtamembrane domain that inhibits the receptor, while *KIT* is not bound to its ligand [109]. Therefore, *KIT* mutations in exon 11 are likely to prevent the juxtamembrane domain's inhibitory function and induce the constitutive activation of the associated signaling pathway. The analysis of 102 primary melanomas showed mutations and/or copy number increases of *KIT* in 39 % of mucosal melanomas, 36 % of acral melanomas, and 28 % of melanomas on chronically sun-damaged skin, which are less likely to harbor *BRAF* or *NRAS* mutations [43].

Several in vitro studies have shown sensitivity of *KIT*-mutant cells to *KIT* inhibitors in melanoma [110, 111]. Woodman and colleagues reported marked tumor reduction (>50 %) in two patients with metastatic melanoma harboring an *L567P KIT* mutation after treatment with dasatinib [110]. A number of other case reports also demonstrated remarkable tumor responses to imatinib in patients with metastatic melanoma with a 7-codon duplication in exon 11, *L567P KIT* in exon 11, or *K642E*

KIT in exon 13 [112–114]. Initially, three trials of imatinib failed to show clinical efficacy in patients with metastatic melanoma who were enrolled without testing for *KIT* mutations [115–117]. In these three studies, among a total of 65 advanced melanoma patients who received imatinib, only 1 patient had a durable clinical response. Likewise, a phase II study of dasatinib reported only 2 partial responses among 36 evaluable advanced melanoma patients [118]. In these early studies, *KIT* mutations or amplification were not required for eligibility, and most patients were likely to have wild-type *KIT*, which was thought to be the main reason for the studies' negative results.

On the basis of more recent promising preclinical data and early case reports of *KIT* inhibitors in *KIT*-mutant melanomas, a number of clinical trials were designed and conducted in only selected patients with *KIT* aberrations. In one open-label phase II study, 28 melanoma patients with *KIT* mutations and/or amplification were treated with 400 mg imatinib twice daily [119]. Two complete responses, two durable partial responses, and two transient responses among the 25 evaluable patients were observed in the study. Interestingly, all responders had the *L576P* mutation in exon 11 or the *K642E* mutation in exon 13. In a single-arm, open-label phase II study in Asian patients, 43 patients with metastatic melanoma harboring *KIT* mutations or amplification were treated with 400 mg imatinib daily [120]. Ten (23 %) partial responses were observed: nine of the partial responders had *KIT* mutations in exon 11 or 13 and the other patients had *KIT* amplification without a mutation. In a phase II study evaluating nilotinib in Asian patients with metastatic melanoma harboring a *KIT* aberration, two of nine patients had a partial response. Both responders had the *L576P* or *V559A* mutation in exon 11 [121]. In a recent multicenter phase II trial, metastatic melanoma patients with *KIT* mutations and/or amplification received 400 mg imatinib once a day or twice a day if there was no initial response to the once-daily dosing schedule [122]. In the study, 7 of 24 evaluable patients achieved a partial response, and all responders had a *KIT* mutation in exon 11, exon 13, or exon 17. No objective response was observed in patients with *KIT* amplification without *KIT* mutations. These studies suggest that *KIT* may be an effective therapeutic target in a subset of advanced melanoma patients with mutations in exon 11 or 13.

11.4 NRAS Mutation

NRAS is an upstream GTPase of the MAPK and PI3K/AKT pathway and is associated with cell proliferation, survival, and migration. Point mutations in the *NRAS* gene, which have been reported in 20 % of melanomas, constitutively activate the MAPK pathway and lead to unregulated cell proliferation and tumor formation [25]. *NRAS* mutations are generally mutually exclusive with *BRAF* mutations and *PTEN* loss [25], which suggests that *NRAS* mutations may activate multiple pathways, including the MAPK and the PI3K/AKT pathways [123]. Clinically, *NRAS* mutations in melanoma are associated with a higher rate of mitosis, greater Breslow depth, shorter overall survival, more advanced stage, and higher risk of central nervous system involvement than wild-type *NRAS* [25, 48, 124]. Because of the critical role of *NRAS* mutations in melanoma progression, therapeutic targeting of *NRAS* mutations in advanced melanoma is of great interest. However, because directly targeting mutated *NRAS* is challenging owing to the difficult nature of pharmacologically targeting impaired GTPase activity [125], therapeutic targets downstream of *NRAS* have been studied.

In a phase I study targeting the MAPK pathway with trametinib, seven patients with *NRAS*-mutated melanoma received the treatment, but none had a clinical response [100]. In a randomized open-label phase II study of selumetinib versus temozolomide in patients with advanced melanoma, ten patients who received selumetinib had *NRAS*-mutant melanoma, but no objective clinical response was observed among the ten patients [95]. One of the possible explanations for the disappointing initial results is the activation of multiple pathways besides the MAPK pathway by *NRAS* mutations. However, a recent phase II study of MEK162 demonstrated that 6 (20 %) of 30 patients with *NRAS*-mutated melanoma had a partial response, among which 3 had a confirmed response [105]. The median PFS for the *NRAS* mutation cohort was 3.65 months. On the basis of this result, a phase III study comparing MEK162 and chemotherapy is under way for patients with *NRAS*-mutant advanced melanoma. In addition, the combined inhibition of two different signaling pathways activated by *NRAS* mutations is being investigated. Phase I studies of combinations of a MEK inhibitor and a PI3K inhibitor as well as a MEK inhibitor and a cyclin-dependent kinase 4 (CDK4) inhibitor are currently under way. Those ongoing studies may offer a future direction for therapeutic strategy in the treatment of *NRAS* mutations in melanoma (Table 11.2).

Table 11.2 Ongoing phase II and III studies of targeted drugs in melanoma

Trial and regimen	Phase	Treatment setting	Mutation criteria	Primary end point	N
BRAF mutation					
NCT01584648 Dabrafenib + trametinib versus dacarbazine	III	Front line	*V600E/K BRAF*	PFS	340
NCT01597908 Dabrafenib + trametinib versus vemurafenib	III	Front line	*V600E/K BRAF*	OS	694
NCT01689519 Vemurafenib + GDC-0973 versus vemurafenib	III	Front line	*V600*	PFS	500
NCT01909453 LGX818 + MEK162 versus LGX818 versus vemurafenib	III	Front line	*V600E/K BRAF*	PFS	900

(continued)

Table 11.2 (continued)

Trial and regimen	Phase	Treatment setting	Mutation criteria	Primary end point	N
NCT01586195 Vemurafenib	II	Any	*BRAF* mutation other than *V600E*	ORR	50
NCT01619774 Dabrafenib + trametinib	II	For BRAF inhibitor-resistant melanoma	*V600E/K BRAF*	ORR	30
NCT01767454 Dabrafenib + ipilimumab ± trametinib	I	≤1 prior systemic therapy	*V600E/K BRAF*	Safety	72
NCT01656642 Vemurafenib + MPDL3280A (anti-PD-L1 antibody)	I	Front line	*V600 BRAF*	Safety	44
NCT01754376 Vemurafenib + interleukin-2	II	No prior interleukin-2 therapy	*V600E BRAF*	PFS	49
NCT01659151 Adoptive lymphodepletion cell therapy with TIL infusion, interleukin-2, vemurafenib	II	Any	*V600E/D/K BRAF*	ORR	60
NCT01781026 Vemurafenib	II	Neoadjuvant; active brain metastasis	*V600E/K BRAF*	ORR	34
NCT01667419 Vemurafenib versus placebo	III	Adjuvant	*V600E BRAF*	DFS	725
NCT01682083 Dabrafenib + trametinib versus placebo	III	Adjuvant	*V600E/K BRAF*	RFS	852
KIT mutation					
NCT01280565 Masitinib versus dacarbazine	III	No prior KIT inhibitors	*KIT* mutation	PFS	200
NCT01028222 Nilotinib	II	No prior tyrosine kinase inhibitors	*KIT* mutation of exon 9, 11, or 13 or mutations Y822D and D820Y, Y823D of exon 17	ORR	55
NCT00788775 Nilotinib	II	Must have had prior tyrosine kinase inhibitors, including, but not limited to, KIT inhibitors	*KIT* mutation or amplification	PFS	35
NCT00700882 Dasatinib	II	No prior KIT/PDGFR inhibitors	*KIT* mutation	ORR	87

(continued)

Table 11.2 (continued)

Trial and regimen	Phase	Treatment setting	Mutation criteria	Primary end point	N
NRAS mutation					
NCT01763164 MEK162 versus dacarbazine	III	Front line; previous immunotherapy allowed	*Q61 NRAS* mutation	PFS	393
NCT00866177 Selumetinib	II	Any	*V600E/K* BRAF or *NRAS* mutation at codons 12, 13, or 61	ORR	40
NCT01781572 MEK162+LEE011	IB/II	Any	*NRAS*	DLT/ ORR	58
NCT01693068 Pimasertib versus dacarbazine	II	Front line	*NRAS*	PFS	184
GNAQ/GNA11 mutation					
NCT01143402 Selumetinib versus temozolomide	II	Any; no prior MEK inhibitors	*GNAQ/ GNA11* wild type or mutant	PFS	159

N number of patients, *PFS* progression-free survival, *OS* overall survival, *ORR* overall response rate, *TIL* tumor-infiltrating lymphocytes, *DFS* disease-free survival, *RFS* relapse-free survival

11.5 GNAQ/GNA11 Mutation

Approximately 80 % of primary uveal melanomas, which rarely harbor *BRAF* or *NRAS* mutations, have oncogenic *Q209* (exon 5) mutations in *GNAQ* or *GNA11* [126]. GNAQ and GNA11 are both alpha subunits of heterotrimeric G proteins, which couple 7-pass transmembrane domain receptors to intracellular signaling pathways [127]. Several in vivo and in vitro studies suggest that *GNAQ/GNA11* mutations are associated with the activation of the MAPK pathway and critical for the development and progression of uveal melanoma [126, 128, 129]. Owing to the oncogenic function of *GNAQ* or *GNA11* mutations in uveal melanoma, therapeutic targeting of *GNAQ/GNA11* mutations has been of great interest. Because direct pharmacologic targeting of *GNAQ/GNA11* is not available, inhibition of key downstream effectors, such as the MAPK pathway, has been studied. In a phase I study of trametinib, no objective clinical responses were observed among 16 metastatic uveal melanoma patients, including 2 with *GNAQ* and 2 with *GNA11* mutations [100]. In a randomized phase II study of selumetinib versus temozolomide, 20 patients had advanced uveal melanoma, but none of those who received selumetinib experienced a clinical response [95].

Although these two small studies with selective MEK inhibitors failed to show clinical responses, a prospective randomized phase II trial in which patients with metastatic uveal melanoma with *GNAQ* or *GNA11* mutations were randomly assigned to either selumetinib or temozolomide (or dacarbazine) showed a possible clinical benefit of MEK inhibitors for this class of melanomas [130]. At interim analysis, among patients with exon 5 *GNAQ* or *GNA11* mutations, the median PFS duration was 15.4 weeks (95 % CI, 8.1–16.9), and the median OS duration was 10.2 months (95 % CI, 7.0–12.6) in the selumetinib group ($n = 38$), whereas the temozolomide group ($n = 42$) had a median PFS and OS duration of 7.0 weeks (95 % CI, 4.3–11.9) and 9.5 months (95 % CI, 6.1–13.9), respectively. The HR for progression was 0.55 (95 % CI, 0.34–0.87, $p = 0.011$) and for OS was 1.05 (95 % CI, 0.59–1.88, $p = 0.88$) for the selumetinib group. The final results of the study will offer better insight on the role of MEK inhibitors in the management of patients with *GNAQ/GNA11* mutations. Despite the promising results of the study, it is likely that a MEK inhibitor-based drug combination, rather than single-agent MEK inhibitors, will be necessary to have clinically meaningful success in this disease.

11.6 PTEN/PI3K/AKT/mTOR Pathway

The PTEN/PI3K/AKT/mTOR pathway regulates essential cellular functions such as cell metabolism, cell survival, growth, cell cycle progression, and migration [131]. Furthermore, its role in DNA repair, stem cell proliferation, and epithelial-mesenchymal transition has recently been under investigation [132]. Typically, PI3K is activated by various growth factor receptor proteins and cell-cell contacts [133]. The activated PI3K phosphorylates phosphatidylinositol 4,5-bisphosphate [PI(4,5)P2] and converts it into phosphatidylinositol 3,4,5-trisphosphate [PI(3,4,5) P3], which in turn binds to its downstream effector, AKT kinase, and recruits the complex to the plasma membrane. This process is negatively regulated by the tumor suppressor PTEN. Once translocated to the plasma membrane, AKT is activated through phosphorylation, and activated AKT regulates a wide range of proteins, including forkhead transcription factors, NF-κB, BAD, mTOR, and glycogen synthase kinase 3 beta (GSK-3β) [134–139]. One of the major downstream effectors of AKT is mTOR, which encompasses two distinct protein complexes: mTOR complex 1 (mTORC1) and mTOR complex 2 (mTORC2). mTORC1 is a critical regulator of ribosomal biogenesis and protein synthesis through phosphorylation of its downstream effectors S6K and 4EBP1 [140]. It is not entirely clear how the activated AKT regulates mTORC1; however, it has been shown that AKT activates mTORC1 indirectly by inhibiting the function of tuberous sclerosis complex 2 (TSC2), which is a negative regulator of mTORC1 signaling [141]. mTORC2 is activated by the stimulation of growth factor receptor proteins and can phosphorylate protein kinase Cα, AKT, and paxillin and ultimately regulates cell survival, migration, and regulation of actin [142–144].

The PTEN/PI3K/AKT/mTOR signal transduction pathway is frequently altered and activated in human cancer and is also constitutively active in a large percentage of melanomas [145]. These data are supported by the finding that AKT kinase is activated in approximately two-thirds of melanomas [146]. Deregulated AKT3, one of the three isoforms of AKT, promotes the development of malignant melanoma [147]. In addition, the expression of PTEN, which inhibits cell growth by increasing the susceptibility of melanoma cells to apoptosis [148], is lost in 10–30 % of melanomas [149] and is associated with the activation of the PI3K/AKT/mTOR pathway in melanoma specimens [150, 151]. Furthermore, low PTEN expression correlates with the shorter duration of disease control by BRAF inhibitors [76, 77], which suggests that the PTEN/PI3K/AKT signaling axis is an important factor in the resistance to BRAF inhibitors. Despite the essential role this PI3K/AKT/mTOR pathway plays in melanomagenesis and melanoma progression, activating mutations in the kinases within this pathway is relatively uncommon, with a prevalence of 1–3 % in melanoma [152–154]. However, inhibition of AKT3 activity or overexpression of active PTEN protein stimulates apoptosis in melanoma cells [147]. This suggests that the PTEN/PI3K/AKT/mTOR signaling axis is an attractive target for melanoma therapy.

It has been suggested that delivering functional PTEN into melanoma cells could theoretically be an effective treatment for melanoma. However, achieving successful systemic delivery of the PTEN gene in a human is challenging. Therefore, the current strategy for targeting the PTEN/PI3K/AKT/mTOR signaling pathway is to directly inhibit the PI3K, AKT, or mTOR kinases.

Isoselenocyanates are synthetic compounds that combine selenium [155] and isothiocyanates [156], both of which have been shown to downregulate AKT activity. Two of the isoselenocyanates, ISC-4 and ISC-6, decreased melanoma tumorigenesis and increased apoptosis threefold via AKT inhibition in preclinical models [157]. BI-69A11 (Howfond Inc., Westford, MA), another AKT inhibitor, has also shown antitumor activity in melanoma in vitro and in vivo through suppression of both the AKT and NF-κB pathways [158]. A number of selective AKT inhibitors, such as perifosine [159], MK-2206 (Merck and Co, Whitehouse Station, NJ) [160], and GSK-2141795 (GlaxoSmithKline) [161], have been evaluated in patients with metastatic solid tumors in a phase I study setting. However, no AKT inhibitors have shown substantial clinical activity in patients with metastatic melanoma to date. These limited clinical data suggest that AKT inhibitors as a single therapeutic agent are not likely sufficient to regress tumors in most patients with metastatic melanoma.

The current focus in AKT pathway research is on restoring sensitivity to other targeted agents. It is postulated that the AKT pathway may have effects on the resistance of melanoma cells to inhibitors of the MAPK pathway [162]. In vitro studies demonstrated that BRAF or MEK inhibitors induce apoptosis in *BRAF*-mutant cell lines with normal PTEN, whereas they induce only cell cycle arrest with minimal apoptosis in *BRAF*-mutant PTEN-null cell lines [163].

Accordingly, AKT and PI3K inhibition have been implicated in overcoming resistance to BRAF or MEK inhibitors in melanoma cell lines [163, 164]. Currently, several trials on combinations of BRAF inhibitors and AKT or PI3K inhibitors are under way.

Small-molecule drugs that inhibit the activation of mTOR have been evaluated in patients with metastatic melanoma over the years. However, two of the mTOR inhibitors, temsirolimus and everolimus, had only minimal clinical activity in patients with advanced melanoma [165, 166]. In addition, temsirolimus in combination with sorafenib resulted in modest antitumor efficacy in two phase II clinical trials [58, 167]. Similarly, a combination of everolimus and bevacizumab in a phase II study had only modest activity in patients with metastatic melanoma [168].

Despite the discouraging clinical results of these studies, mTOR inhibition may still have significant implications in melanoma therapy. For example, durable activation of the mTOR signaling pathway was observed in *BRAF*-mutant human melanoma cell lines with de novo resistance to vemurafenib [169]. In this in vitro model, targeting both mTOR and AKT led to cell death when combined with a BRAF inhibitor, implying a complex feedback mechanism in the AKT/mTOR pathway [169]. This complex network of signaling pathways must be carefully investigated in future clinical trials.

11.7 Cell Cycle Pathway Inhibition

Patients with familial malignant melanoma are known to have a germ line mutation in *CDKN2A* (*p16INK4A*) [170, 171]. This gene encodes the p16 protein, which, when mutated, is incapable of inhibiting CDK4 and inducing regulatory arrest of the cell cycle. This permits unchecked progression through the cell cycle.

CDK4 is a member of the cyclin-dependent protein kinase family and is involved in the control of cell proliferation during the G1 phase of the cell cycle [172]. CDK4 mediates phosphorylation of the Rb protein, which drives cells into G1/S phase transition by releasing E2F transcription factor [173]. In addition, the complex formed by CDK4 and cyclin D1 has been implicated in the control of cell proliferation [174]. Somatic mutations in both *CDKN2A* and *CDK4* have also been observed in sporadic melanomas [175], and increased cyclin D1 protein expression was observed in one-third of melanoma cases [176]. Accordingly, the CDKN2A/CDK4/Rb pathway functions as a vital gatekeeper in cell cycle progression and plays a role in melanoma tumorigenesis. Therefore, therapeutic targeting of this cell cycle pathway may be possible with the development of effective CDK4 inhibitors.

P276-00 (Piramal Enterprises Limited, Mumbai, India) is a novel, potent small-molecule inhibitor of CDK4-D1, CDK1-B, and CDK9-T [176]. It causes a significant and selective antiproliferative effect by inducing G0-G1 arrest in vitro and in vivo [176, 177]. On the basis of promising preclinical proofs of concept, a variety of CDK inhibitors are undergoing clinical evaluation either as single agents or in combination with other approved agents in patients with advanced solid tumors. In patients with advanced malignant melanoma, a phase II study of P276-00 in tumors with cyclin D1-positive protein expression profiles has just been completed (NCT00835419), and results of the study will be available soon. In a phase I study, PD0332991 (Pfizer, Inc.), an oral CDK4/CDK6 inhibitor, was found to be well tolerated in solid tumors, including melanoma [178]. In addition, phase I studies of a number of oral CDK4 inhibitors, including LEE011 (GlaxoSmithKline) and LY2835219 (Eli Lilly, Indianapolis, IN), in combination with either a BRAF inhibitor or a MEK inhibitor, are currently ongoing in patients with metastatic melanoma.

11.8   Conclusions

Advances in our knowledge regarding the molecular biology of melanomas and the development of innovative molecular analytic techniques have resulted in recent successes in melanoma-targeted therapy. Both selective BRAF inhibitors and MEK inhibitors were approved by the FDA for the treatment of *BRAF*-mutant advanced melanoma on the basis of survival advantages over conventional chemotherapy drugs, giving hope to many patients with advanced melanoma. In addition, KIT inhibitors for *KIT*-mutant melanomas and MEK inhibitors for *NRAS*- and *GNA*-mutant melanomas appear promising in early-phase clinical trials. However, the cure or long-term control of advanced melanoma with single-agent small-molecule therapies is unlikely due to rapid development of drug resistance through complex compensatory molecular mechanisms. A recent systematic approach of combining drugs inhibiting different kinases on the basis of sound scientific rationale and robust preclinical data has shown great promise, especially in the case of combined BRAF and MEK inhibitors. Therefore, it is essential to assess the relevant genetic or epigenetic aberrations in each patient's melanoma to determine the optimal targeted therapy options. Further understanding of the complex network of the signal transduction pathways in melanoma will certainly enable us to treat patients with more effective targeted therapies on an individual basis and hopefully with less toxicity.

References

1. Siegel R, Naishadham D, Jemal A (2013) Cancer statistics, 2013. CA Cancer J Clin 63: 11–30
2. Jang S, Atkins MB (2013) Which drug, and when, for patients with BRAF-mutant melanoma? Lancet Oncol 14:e60–e69
3. Dean E, Lorigan P (2012) Advances in the management of melanoma: targeted therapy, immunotherapy and future directions. Expert Rev Anticancer Ther 12:1437–1448
4. Mackiewicz-Wysocka M, Zolnierek J, Wysocki PJ (2013) New therapeutic options in systemic treatment of advanced cutaneous melanoma. Expert Opin Investig Drugs 22:181–190
5. Balch CM, Soong SJ, Atkins MB et al (2004) An evidence-based staging system for cutaneous melanoma. CA Cancer J Clin 54:131–149, quiz 182-4
6. Bedikian AY, Millward M, Pehamberger H et al (2006) Bcl-2 antisense (oblimersen sodium) plus dacarbazine in patients with advanced melanoma: the oblimersen melanoma study group. J Clin Oncol 24:4738–4745
7. Chapman PB, Hauschild A, Robert C et al (2011) Improved survival with vemurafenib in melanoma with BRAF V600E mutation. N Engl J Med 364:2507–2516

8. Chapman PB, Einhorn LH, Meyers ML et al (1999) Phase III multicenter randomized trial of the Dartmouth regimen versus dacarbazine in patients with metastatic melanoma. J Clin Oncol 17:2745–2751

9. Hauschild A, Grob JJ, Demidov LV et al (2013) An update on BREAK-3, a phase III, randomized trial: dabrafenib versus dacarbazine in patients with BRAF V600E-positive mutation metastatic melanoma J Clin Oncol 31(Suppl):Abstr 9013

10. Hill GJ 2nd, Krementz ET, Hill HZ (1984) Dimethyl triazeno imidazole carboxamide and combination therapy for melanoma. IV. Late results after complete response to chemotherapy (Central Oncology Group protocols 7130, 7131, and 7131A). Cancer 53:1299–1305

11. Atkins MB, Lotze MT, Dutcher JP et al (1999) High-dose recombinant interleukin 2 therapy for patients with metastatic melanoma: analysis of 270 patients treated between 1985 and 1993. J Clin Oncol 17:2105–2116

12. Schwartzentruber DJ, Lawson DH, Richards JM et al (2011) gp100 peptide vaccine and interleukin-2 in patients with advanced melanoma. N Engl J Med 364:2119–2127

13. Phan GQ, Attia P, Steinberg SM et al (2001) Factors associated with response to high-dose interleukin-2 in patients with metastatic melanoma. J Clin Oncol 19:3477–3482

14. Hodi FS, O'Day SJ, McDermott DF et al (2010) Improved survival with ipilimumab in patients with metastatic melanoma. N Engl J Med 363:711–723

15. Hersh EM, O'Day SJ, Powderly J et al (2011) A phase II multicenter study of ipilimumab with or without dacarbazine in chemotherapy-naive patients with advanced melanoma. Invest New Drugs 29:489–498

16. Weber J, Thompson JA, Hamid O et al (2009) A randomized, double-blind, placebo-controlled, phase II study comparing the tolerability and efficacy of ipilimumab administered with or without prophylactic budesonide in patients with unresectable stage III or IV melanoma. Clin Cancer Res 15:5591–5598

17. Davies H, Bignell GR, Cox C et al (2002) Mutations of the BRAF gene in human cancer. Nature 417:949–954

18. Cappola AR, Mandel SJ (2013) Molecular testing in thyroid cancer: BRAF mutation status and mortality. JAMA 309:1529–1530

19. Dietrich S, Glimm H, Andrulis M et al (2012) BRAF inhibition in refractory hairy-cell leukemia. N Engl J Med 366:2038–2040

20. Oikonomou E, Pintzas A (2006) Cancer genetics of sporadic colorectal cancer: BRAF and PI3KCA mutations, their impact on signaling and novel targeted therapies. Anticancer Res 26:1077–1084

21. Garnett MJ, Marais R (2004) Guilty as charged: B-RAF is a human oncogene. Cancer Cell 6:313–319

22. Curtin JA, Fridlyand J, Kageshita T et al (2005) Distinct sets of genetic alterations in melanoma. N Engl J Med 353:2135–2147

23. Long GV, Menzies AM, Nagrial AM et al (2011) Prognostic and clinicopathologic associations of oncogenic BRAF in metastatic melanoma. J Clin Oncol 29:1239–1246

24. Menzies AM, Haydu LE, Visintin L et al (2012) Distinguishing clinicopathologic features of patients with V600E and V600K BRAF-mutant metastatic melanoma. Clin Cancer Res 18:3242–3249

25. Jakob JA, Bassett RL Jr, Ng CS et al (2012) NRAS mutation status is an independent prognostic factor in metastatic melanoma. Cancer 118:4014–4023

26. Greaves WO, Verma S, Patel KP et al (2013) Frequency and spectrum of BRAF mutations in a retrospective, single-institution study of 1112 cases of melanoma. J Mol Diagn 15:220–226

27. Lovly CM, Dahlman KB, Fohn LE et al (2012) Routine multiplex mutational profiling of melanomas enables enrollment in genotype-driven therapeutic trials. PLoS One 7:e35309

28. Wagle N, Emery C, Berger MF et al (2011) Dissecting therapeutic resistance to RAF inhibition in melanoma by tumor genomic profiling. J Clin Oncol 29:3085–3096

29. Klein O, Clements A, Menzies AM et al (2013) BRAF inhibitor activity in V600R metastatic melanoma. Eur J Cancer 49:1073–1079

30. Robinson MJ, Cobb MH (1997) Mitogen-activated protein kinase pathways. Curr Opin Cell Biol 9:180–186
31. McCubrey JA, Steelman LS, Chappell WH et al (2007) Roles of the Raf/MEK/ERK pathway in cell growth, malignant transformation and drug resistance. Biochim Biophys Acta 1773:1263–1284
32. Steelman LS, Abrams SL, Shelton JG et al (2010) Dominant roles of the Raf/MEK/ERK pathway in cell cycle progression, prevention of apoptosis and sensitivity to chemotherapeutic drugs. Cell Cycle 9:1629–1638
33. Joseph EW, Pratilas CA, Poulikakos PI et al (2010) The RAF inhibitor PLX4032 inhibits ERK signaling and tumor cell proliferation in a V600E BRAF-selective manner. Proc Natl Acad Sci USA 107:14903–14908
34. Weber CK, Slupsky JR, Kalmes HA et al (2001) Active Ras induces heterodimerization of cRaf and BRaf. Cancer Res 61:3595–3598
35. Rajakulendran T, Sahmi M, Lefrancois M et al (2009) A dimerization-dependent mechanism drives RAF catalytic activation. Nature 461:542–545
36. Poulikakos PI, Persaud Y, Janakiraman M et al (2011) RAF inhibitor resistance is mediated by dimerization of aberrantly spliced BRAF(V600E). Nature 480:387–390
37. Hoeflich KP, Gray DC, Eby MT et al (2006) Oncogenic BRAF is required for tumor growth and maintenance in melanoma models. Cancer Res 66:999–1006
38. Michaloglou C, Vredeveld LC, Soengas MS et al (2005) BRAFE600-associated senescence-like cell cycle arrest of human naevi. Nature 436:720–724
39. Pollock PM, Harper UL, Hansen KS et al (2003) High frequency of BRAF mutations in nevi. Nat Genet 33:19–20
40. Yazdi AS, Palmedo G, Flaig MJ et al (2003) Mutations of the BRAF gene in benign and malignant melanocytic lesions. J Invest Dermatol 121:1160–1162
41. Dankort D, Curley DP, Cartlidge RA et al (2009) Braf(V600E) cooperates with Pten loss to induce metastatic melanoma. Nat Genet 41:544–552
42. Lee JH, Choi JW, Kim YS (2011) Frequencies of BRAF and NRAS mutations are different in histological types and sites of origin of cutaneous melanoma: a meta-analysis. Br J Dermatol 164:776–784
43. Curtin JA, Busam K, Pinkel D et al (2006) Somatic activation of KIT in distinct subtypes of melanoma. J Clin Oncol 24:4340–4346
44. Maat W, Kilic E, Luyten GP et al (2008) Pyrophosphorolysis detects B-RAF mutations in primary uveal melanoma. Invest Ophthalmol Vis Sci 49:23–27
45. Bauer J, Buttner P, Murali R et al (2011) BRAF mutations in cutaneous melanoma are independently associated with age, anatomic site of the primary tumor, and the degree of solar elastosis at the primary tumor site. Pigment Cell Melanoma Res 24:345–351
46. Bucheit AD, Syklawer E, Jakob JA et al (2013) Clinical characteristics and outcomes with specific BRAF and NRAS mutations in patients with metastatic melanoma. Cancer 119(21):3821–3829
47. Thomas NE (2006) BRAF somatic mutations in malignant melanoma and melanocytic naevi. Melanoma Res 16:97–103
48. Ellerhorst JA, Greene VR, Ekmekcioglu S et al (2011) Clinical correlates of NRAS and BRAF mutations in primary human melanoma. Clin Cancer Res 17:229–235
49. Moreau S, Saiag P, Aegerter P et al (2012) Prognostic value of BRAF(V(6)(0)(0)) mutations in melanoma patients after resection of metastatic lymph nodes. Ann Surg Oncol 19:4314–4321
50. Sharma A, Trivedi NR, Zimmerman MA et al (2005) Mutant V599EB-Raf regulates growth and vascular development of malignant melanoma tumors. Cancer Res 65:2412–2421
51. Mangana J, Levesque MP, Karpova MB et al (2012) Sorafenib in melanoma. Expert Opin Investig Drugs 21:557–568
52. Wilhelm SM, Carter C, Tang L et al (2004) BAY 43-9006 exhibits broad spectrum oral antitumor activity and targets the RAF/MEK/ERK pathway and receptor tyrosine kinases involved in tumor progression and angiogenesis. Cancer Res 64:7099–7109

53. Eisen T, Marais R, Affolter A et al (2011) Sorafenib and dacarbazine as first-line therapy for advanced melanoma: phase I and open-label phase II studies. Br J Cancer 105:353–359
54. Eisen T, Ahmad T, Flaherty KT et al (2006) Sorafenib in advanced melanoma: a Phase II randomised discontinuation trial analysis. Br J Cancer 95:581–586
55. Hauschild A, Agarwala SS, Trefzer U et al (2009) Results of a phase III, randomized, placebo-controlled study of sorafenib in combination with carboplatin and paclitaxel as second-line treatment in patients with unresectable stage III or stage IV melanoma. J Clin Oncol 27:2823–2830
56. Flaherty KT, Lee SJ, Zhao F et al (2013) Phase III trial of carboplatin and paclitaxel with or without sorafenib in metastatic melanoma. J Clin Oncol 31:373–379
57. Ott PA, Hamilton A, Min C et al (2010) A phase II trial of sorafenib in metastatic melanoma with tissue correlates. PLoS One 5:e15588
58. Davies MA, Fox PS, Papadopoulos NE et al (2012) Phase I study of the combination of sorafenib and temsirolimus in patients with metastatic melanoma. Clin Cancer Res 18: 1120–1128
59. Bollag G, Hirth P, Tsai J et al (2010) Clinical efficacy of a RAF inhibitor needs broad target blockade in BRAF-mutant melanoma. Nature 467:596–599
60. Flaherty KT, Puzanov I, Kim KB et al (2010) Inhibition of mutated, activated BRAF in metastatic melanoma. N Engl J Med 363:809–819
61. Sosman JA, Kim KB, Schuchter L et al (2012) Survival in BRAF V600-mutant advanced melanoma treated with vemurafenib. N Engl J Med 366:707–714
62. Chapman PB, Hauschild A, Robert C et al (2012) Updated overall survival (OS) results for BRIM-3, a phase III randomized, open-label, multicenter trial comparing BRAF inhibitor vemurafenib (vem) with dacarbazine (DTIC) in previously untreated patients with BRAFV600E-mutated melanoma. J Clin Oncol 30(Suppl):Abstr 8502
63. Gibney GT, Zager JS (2013) Clinical development of dabrafenib in BRAF mutant melanoma and other malignancies. Expert Opin Drug Metab Toxicol 9:893–899
64. Falchook GS, Long GV, Kurzrock R et al (2012) Dabrafenib in patients with melanoma, untreated brain metastases, and other solid tumours: a phase 1 dose-escalation trial. Lancet 379:1893–1901
65. Ascierto PA, Minor D, Ribas A et al (2013) Phase II trial (BREAK-2) of the BRAF inhibitor dabrafenib (GSK2118436) in patients with metastatic melanoma. J Clin Oncol 31(26): 3205–3211
66. Hauschild A, Grob JJ, Demidov LV et al (2012) Dabrafenib in BRAF-mutated metastatic melanoma: a multicentre, open-label, phase 3 randomised controlled trial. Lancet 380: 358–365
67. Su F, Bradley WD, Wang Q et al (2012) Resistance to selective BRAF inhibition can be mediated by modest upstream pathway activation. Cancer Res 72:969–978
68. Hatzivassiliou G, Song K, Yen I et al (2010) RAF inhibitors prime wild-type RAF to activate the MAPK pathway and enhance growth. Nature 464:431–435
69. Yang H, Higgins B, Kolinsky K et al (2010) RG7204 (PLX4032), a selective BRAFV600E inhibitor, displays potent antitumor activity in preclinical melanoma models. Cancer Res 70:5518–5527
70. Su F, Viros A, Milagre C et al (2012) RAS mutations in cutaneous squamous-cell carcinomas in patients treated with BRAF inhibitors. N Engl J Med 366:207–215
71. Long GV, Wilmott JS, Haydu LE et al (2013) Effects of BRAF inhibitors on human melanoma tissue before treatment, early during treatment, and on progression. Pigment Cell Melanoma Res 26:499–508
72. Zimmer L, Hillen U, Livingstone E et al (2012) Atypical melanocytic proliferations and new primary melanomas in patients with advanced melanoma undergoing selective BRAF inhibition. J Clin Oncol 30:2375–2383
73. Callahan MK, Rampal R, Harding JJ et al (2012) Progression of RAS-mutant leukemia during RAF inhibitor treatment. N Engl J Med 367:2316–2321

74. Johannessen CM, Boehm JS, Kim SY et al (2010) COT drives resistance to RAF inhibition through MAP kinase pathway reactivation. Nature 468:968–972

75. Xing F, Persaud Y, Pratilas CA et al (2012) Concurrent loss of the PTEN and RB1 tumor suppressors attenuates RAF dependence in melanomas harboring (V600E)BRAF. Oncogene 31:446–457

76. Nathanson KL, Martin AM, Wubbenhorst B et al (2013) Tumor genetic analyses of patients with metastatic melanoma treated with the BRAF inhibitor dabrafenib (GSK2118436). Clin Cancer Res 19(17):4868–4878

77. Trunzer K, Pavlick AC, Schuchter L et al (2013) Pharmacodynamic effects and mechanisms of resistance to vemurafenib in patients with metastatic melanoma. J Clin Oncol 31(14): 1767–1774

78. Paraiso KH, Xiang Y, Rebecca VW et al (2011) PTEN loss confers BRAF inhibitor resistance to melanoma cells through the suppression of BIM expression. Cancer Res 71: 2750–2760

79. Villanueva J, Vultur A, Lee JT et al (2010) Acquired resistance to BRAF inhibitors mediated by a RAF kinase switch in melanoma can be overcome by cotargeting MEK and IGF-1R/PI3K. Cancer Cell 18:683–695

80. Montagut C, Sharma SV, Shioda T et al (2008) Elevated CRAF as a potential mechanism of acquired resistance to BRAF inhibition in melanoma. Cancer Res 68:4853–4861

81. Nazarian R, Shi H, Wang Q et al (2010) Melanomas acquire resistance to B-RAF(V600E) inhibition by RTK or N-RAS upregulation. Nature 468:973–977

82. Straussman R, Morikawa T, Shee K et al (2012) Tumour micro-environment elicits innate resistance to RAF inhibitors through HGF secretion. Nature 487:500–504

83. von Euw E, Atefi M, Attar N et al (2012) Antitumor effects of the investigational selective MEK inhibitor TAK733 against cutaneous and uveal melanoma cell lines. Mol Cancer 11:22

84. Greger JG, Eastman SD, Zhang V et al (2012) Combinations of BRAF, MEK, and PI3K/mTOR inhibitors overcome acquired resistance to the BRAF inhibitor GSK2118436 dabrafenib, mediated by NRAS or MEK mutations. Mol Cancer Ther 11:909–920

85. Conrad WH, Swift RD, Biechele TL et al (2012) Regulating the response to targeted MEK inhibition in melanoma: enhancing apoptosis in NRAS- and BRAF-mutant melanoma cells with Wnt/beta-catenin activation. Cell Cycle 11:3724–3730

86. Lorusso PM, Adjei AA, Varterasian M et al (2005) Phase I and pharmacodynamic study of the oral MEK inhibitor CI-1040 in patients with advanced malignancies. J Clin Oncol 23:5281–5293

87. LoRusso PM, Krishnamurthi SS, Rinehart JJ et al (2010) Phase I pharmacokinetic and pharmacodynamic study of the oral MAPK/ERK kinase inhibitor PD-0325901 in patients with advanced cancers. Clin Cancer Res 16:1924–1937

88. Rinehart J, Adjei AA, Lorusso PM et al (2004) Multicenter phase II study of the oral MEK inhibitor, CI-1040, in patients with advanced non-small-cell lung, breast, colon, and pancreatic cancer. J Clin Oncol 22:4456–4462

89. Brown AP, Carlson TC, Loi CM et al (2007) Pharmacodynamic and toxicokinetic evaluation of the novel MEK inhibitor, PD0325901, in the rat following oral and intravenous administration. Cancer Chemother Pharmacol 59:671–679

90. Haura EB, Ricart AD, Larson TG et al (2010) A phase II study of PD-0325901, an oral MEK inhibitor, in previously treated patients with advanced non-small cell lung cancer. Clin Cancer Res 16:2450–2457

91. Boasberg PD, Redfern CH, Daniels GA et al (2011) Pilot study of PD-0325901 in previously treated patients with advanced melanoma, breast cancer, and colon cancer. Cancer Chemother Pharmacol 68:547–552

92. Yeh TC, Marsh V, Bernat BA et al (2007) Biological characterization of ARRY-142886 (AZD6244), a potent, highly selective mitogen-activated protein kinase kinase 1/2 inhibitor. Clin Cancer Res 13:1576–1583

93. Haass NK, Sproesser K, Nguyen TK et al (2008) The mitogen-activated protein/extracellular signal-regulated kinase kinase inhibitor AZD6244 (ARRY-142886) induces growth arrest in

melanoma cells and tumor regression when combined with docetaxel. Clin Cancer Res 14:230–239

94. Adjei AA, Cohen RB, Franklin W et al (2008) Phase I pharmacokinetic and pharmacodynamic study of the oral, small-molecule mitogen-activated protein kinase kinase 1/2 inhibitor AZD6244 (ARRY-142886) in patients with advanced cancers. J Clin Oncol 26:2139–2146

95. Kirkwood JM, Bastholt L, Robert C et al (2012) Phase II, open-label, randomized trial of the MEK1/2 inhibitor selumetinib as monotherapy versus temozolomide in patients with advanced melanoma. Clin Cancer Res 18:555–567

96. Banerji U, Camidge DR, Verheul HM et al (2010) The first-in-human study of the hydrogen sulfate (Hyd-sulfate) capsule of the MEK1/2 inhibitor AZD6244 (ARRY-142886): a phase I open-label multicenter trial in patients with advanced cancer. Clin Cancer Res 16: 1613–1623

97. Patel SP, Lazar AJ, Papadopoulos NE et al (2013) Clinical responses to selumetinib (AZD6244; ARRY-142886)-based combination therapy stratified by gene mutations in patients with metastatic melanoma. Cancer 119:799–805

98. Robert C, Dummer R, Gutzmer R et al (2013) Selumetinib plus dacarbazine versus placebo plus dacarbazine as first-line treatment for BRAF-mutant metastatic melanoma: a phase 2 double-blind randomised study. Lancet Oncol 14:733–740

99. Gilmartin AG, Bleam MR, Groy A et al (2011) GSK1120212 (JTP-74057) is an inhibitor of MEK activity and activation with favorable pharmacokinetic properties for sustained in vivo pathway inhibition. Clin Cancer Res 17:989–1000

100. Falchook GS, Lewis KD, Infante JR et al (2012) Activity of the oral MEK inhibitor trametinib in patients with advanced melanoma: a phase 1 dose-escalation trial. Lancet Oncol 13:782–789

101. Infante JR, Fecher LA, Falchook GS et al (2012) Safety, pharmacokinetic, pharmacodynamic, and efficacy data for the oral MEK inhibitor trametinib: a phase 1 dose-escalation trial. Lancet Oncol 13:773–781

102. Kim KB, Kefford R, Pavlick AC et al (2013) Phase II study of the MEK1/MEK2 inhibitor Trametinib in patients with metastatic BRAF-mutant cutaneous melanoma previously treated with or without a BRAF inhibitor. J Clin Oncol 31:482–489

103. Flaherty KT, Robert C, Hersey P et al (2012) Improved survival with MEK inhibition in BRAF-mutated melanoma. N Engl J Med 367:107–114

104. Bendell JPK, Jones S et al (2011) A phase 1 dose-escalation study of MEK inhibitor MEK162 (ARRY-438162) in patients with advanced solid tumors. In: Presented at the AACR-NCI-EORTC international conference on molecular targets and cancer therapeutics, San Francisco, 12–15 Nov 2011

105. Ascierto PA, Schadendorf D, Berking C et al (2013) MEK162 for patients with advanced melanoma harbouring NRAS or Val600 BRAF mutations: a non-randomised, open-label phase 2 study. Lancet Oncol 14:249–256

106. Flaherty KT, Infante JR, Daud A et al (2012) Combined BRAF and MEK inhibition in melanoma with BRAF V600 mutations. N Engl J Med 367:1694–1703

107. Gonzalez R, Ribas A, Daud A et al (2012) Phase IB study of vemurafenib in combination with the MEK inhibitor, GDC-0973, in patients (pts) with unresectable or metastatic BRAFV600 mutated melanoma (BRIM7). ESMO 2744

108. Ronnstrand L (2004) Signal transduction via the stem cell factor receptor/c-Kit. Cell Mol Life Sci 61:2535–2548

109. Woodman SE, Davies MA (2010) Targeting KIT in melanoma: a paradigm of molecular medicine and targeted therapeutics. Biochem Pharmacol 80:568–574

110. Woodman SE, Trent JC, Stemke-Hale K et al (2009) Activity of dasatinib against L576P KIT mutant melanoma: molecular, cellular, and clinical correlates. Mol Cancer Ther 8: 2079–2085

111. Jiang X, Zhou J, Yuen NK et al (2008) Imatinib targeting of KIT-mutant oncoprotein in melanoma. Clin Cancer Res 14:7726–7732

112. Hodi FS, Friedlander P, Corless CL et al (2008) Major response to imatinib mesylate in KIT-mutated melanoma. J Clin Oncol 26:2046–2051
113. Lutzky J, Bauer J, Bastian BC (2008) Dose-dependent, complete response to imatinib of a metastatic mucosal melanoma with a K642E KIT mutation. Pigment Cell Melanoma Res 21:492–493
114. Satzger I, Kuttler U, Volker B et al (2010) Anal mucosal melanoma with KIT-activating mutation and response to imatinib therapy—case report and review of the literature. Dermatology 220:77–81
115. Ugurel S, Hildenbrand R, Zimpfer A et al (2005) Lack of clinical efficacy of imatinib in metastatic melanoma. Br J Cancer 92:1398–1405
116. Wyman K, Atkins MB, Prieto V et al (2006) Multicenter Phase II trial of high-dose imatinib mesylate in metastatic melanoma: significant toxicity with no clinical efficacy. Cancer 106:2005–2011
117. Kim KB, Eton O, Davis DW et al (2008) Phase II trial of imatinib mesylate in patients with metastatic melanoma. Br J Cancer 99:734–740
118. Kluger HM, Dudek AZ, McCann C et al (2011) A phase 2 trial of dasatinib in advanced melanoma. Cancer 117:2202–2208
119. Carvajal RD, Antonescu CR, Wolchok JD et al (2011) KIT as a therapeutic target in metastatic melanoma. JAMA 305:2327–2334
120. Guo J, Si L, Kong Y et al (2011) Phase II, open-label, single-arm trial of imatinib mesylate in patients with metastatic melanoma harboring c-Kit mutation or amplification. J Clin Oncol 29:2904–2909
121. Cho JH, Kim KM, Kwon M et al (2012) Nilotinib in patients with metastatic melanoma harboring KIT gene aberration. Invest New Drugs 30:2008–2014
122. Hodi FS, Corless CL, Giobbie-Hurder A et al (2013) Imatinib for melanomas harboring mutationally activated or amplified KIT arising on mucosal, acral, and chronically sun-damaged skin. J Clin Oncol 31:3182–3190
123. Jaiswal BS, Janakiraman V, Kljavin NM et al (2009) Combined targeting of BRAF and CRAF or BRAF and PI3K effector pathways is required for efficacy in NRAS mutant tumors. PLoS One 4:e5717
124. Devitt B, Liu W, Salemi R et al (2011) Clinical outcome and pathological features associated with NRAS mutation in cutaneous melanoma. Pigment Cell Melanoma Res 24:666–672
125. Diaz-Flores E, Shannon K (2007) Targeting oncogenic Ras. Genes Dev 21:1989–1992
126. Van Raamsdonk CD, Griewank KG, Crosby MB et al (2010) Mutations in GNA11 in uveal melanoma. N Engl J Med 363:2191–2199
127. Neves SR, Ram PT, Iyengar R (2002) G protein pathways. Science 296:1636–1639
128. Van Raamsdonk CD, Bezrookove V, Green G et al (2009) Frequent somatic mutations of GNAQ in uveal melanoma and blue naevi. Nature 457:599–602
129. Ambrosini G, Pratilas CA, Qin LX et al (2012) Identification of unique MEK-dependent genes in GNAQ mutant uveal melanoma involved in cell growth, tumor cell invasion, and MEK resistance. Clin Cancer Res 18:3552–3561
130. Carvajal RD, Sosman JA, Quevedo F et al (2013) Phase II study of selumetinib (sel) versus temozolomide (TMZ) in gnaq/Gna11 (Gq/11) mutant (mut) uveal melanoma (UM). J Clin Oncol 31(Suppl):Abstr CRA9003
131. Fresno Vara JA, Casado E, de Castro J et al (2004) PI3K/Akt signalling pathway and cancer. Cancer Treat Rev 30:193–204
132. Engelman JA, Luo J, Cantley LC (2006) The evolution of phosphatidylinositol 3-kinases as regulators of growth and metabolism. Nat Rev Genet 7:606–619
133. Downward J (2004) PI 3-kinase, Akt and cell survival. Semin Cell Dev Biol 15:177–182
134. Brunet A, Bonni A, Zigmond MJ et al (1999) Akt promotes cell survival by phosphorylating and inhibiting a forkhead transcription factor. Cell 96:857–868
135. Datta SR, Dudek H, Tao X et al (1997) Akt phosphorylation of BAD couples survival signals to the cell-intrinsic death machinery. Cell 91:231–241

136. Romashkova JA, Makarov SS (1999) NF-kappaB is a target of AKT in anti-apoptotic PDGF signalling. Nature 401:86–90
137. Dhawan P, Singh AB, Ellis DL et al (2002) Constitutive activation of Akt/protein kinase B in melanoma leads to up-regulation of nuclear factor-kappaB and tumor progression. Cancer Res 62:7335–7342
138. Sekulic A, Hudson CC, Homme JL et al (2000) A direct linkage between the phosphoinositide 3-kinase-AKT signaling pathway and the mammalian target of rapamycin in mitogen-stimulated and transformed cells. Cancer Res 60:3504–3513
139. Cross DA, Alessi DR, Cohen P et al (1995) Inhibition of glycogen synthase kinase-3 by insulin mediated by protein kinase B. Nature 378:785–789
140. Hay N, Sonenberg N (2004) Upstream and downstream of mTOR. Genes Dev 18:1926–1945
141. Inoki K, Li Y, Zhu T et al (2002) TSC2 is phosphorylated and inhibited by Akt and suppresses mTOR signalling. Nat Cell Biol 4:648–657
142. Sarbassov DD, Ali SM, Sengupta S et al (2006) Prolonged rapamycin treatment inhibits mTORC2 assembly and Akt/PKB. Mol Cell 22:159–168
143. Sarbassov DD, Ali SM, Kim DH et al (2004) Rictor, a novel binding partner of mTOR, defines a rapamycin-insensitive and raptor-independent pathway that regulates the cytoskeleton. Curr Biol 14:1296–1302
144. Hresko RC, Mueckler M (2005) mTOR.RICTOR is the Ser473 kinase for Akt/protein kinase B in 3T3-L1 adipocytes. J Biol Chem 280:40406–40416
145. Russo AE, Torrisi E, Bevelacqua Y et al (2009) Melanoma: molecular pathogenesis and emerging target therapies (Review). Int J Oncol 34:1481–1489
146. Robertson GP (2005) Functional and therapeutic significance of Akt deregulation in malignant melanoma. Cancer Metastasis Rev 24:273–285
147. Stahl JM, Sharma A, Cheung M et al (2004) Deregulated Akt3 activity promotes development of malignant melanoma. Cancer Res 64:7002–7010
148. Lu Y, Lin YZ, LaPushin R et al (1999) The PTEN/MMAC1/TEP tumor suppressor gene decreases cell growth and induces apoptosis and anoikis in breast cancer cells. Oncogene 18:7034–7045
149. Tsao H, Zhang X, Benoit E et al (1998) Identification of PTEN/MMAC1 alterations in uncultured melanomas and melanoma cell lines. Oncogene 16:3397–3402
150. Stahl JM, Cheung M, Sharma A et al (2003) Loss of PTEN promotes tumor development in malignant melanoma. Cancer Res 63:2881–2890
151. Davies MA, Stemke-Hale K, Lin E et al (2009) Integrated molecular and clinical analysis of AKT activation in metastatic melanoma. Clin Cancer Res 15:7538–7546
152. Curtin JA, Stark MS, Pinkel D et al (2006) PI3-kinase subunits are infrequent somatic targets in melanoma. J Invest Dermatol 126:1660–1663
153. Davies MA, Stemke-Hale K, Tellez C et al (2008) A novel AKT3 mutation in melanoma tumours and cell lines. Br J Cancer 99:1265–1268
154. Omholt K, Krockel D, Ringborg U et al (2006) Mutations of PIK3CA are rare in cutaneous melanoma. Melanoma Res 16:197–200
155. Bandura L, Drukala J, Wolnicka-Glubisz A et al (2005) Differential effects of selenite and selenate on human melanocytes, keratinocytes, and melanoma cells. Biochem Cell Biol 83:196–211
156. Keum YS, Jeong WS, Kong AN (2004) Chemoprevention by isothiocyanates and their underlying molecular signaling mechanisms. Mutat Res 555:191–202
157. Sharma A, Sharma AK, Madhunapantula SV et al (2009) Targeting Akt3 signaling in malignant melanoma using isoselenocyanates. Clin Cancer Res 15:1674–1685
158. Feng Y, Barile E, De SK et al (2011) Effective inhibition of melanoma by BI-69A11 is mediated by dual targeting of the AKT and NF-kappaB pathways. Pigment Cell Melanoma Res 24:703–713

159. Van Ummersen L, Binger K, Volkman J et al (2004) A phase I trial of perifosine (NSC 639966) on a loading dose/maintenance dose schedule in patients with advanced cancer. Clin Cancer Res 10:7450–7456
160. Yap TA, Yan L, Patnaik A et al (2011) First-in-man clinical trial of the oral pan-AKT inhibitor MK-2206 in patients with advanced solid tumors. J Clin Oncol 29:4688–4695
161. Burris H, Siu L, Infante J et al (2011) Safety, pharmacokinetics (PK), pharmacodynamics (PD), and clinical activity of the oral AKT inhibitor GSK2141795 (GSK795) in a phase I first-in-human study. J Clin Oncol 29 (Suppl); Abstr 3003
162. Atefi M, von Euw E, Attar N et al (2011) Reversing melanoma cross-resistance to BRAF and MEK inhibitors by co-targeting the AKT/mTOR pathway. PLoS One 6:e28973
163. Gopal YN, Deng W, Woodman SE et al (2010) Basal and treatment-induced activation of AKT mediates resistance to cell death by AZD6244 (ARRY-142886) in Braf-mutant human cutaneous melanoma cells. Cancer Res 70:8736–8747
164. Mitsiades N, Chew SA, He B et al (2011) Genotype-dependent sensitivity of uveal melanoma cell lines to inhibition of B-Raf, MEK, and Akt kinases: rationale for personalized therapy. Invest Ophthalmol Vis Sci 52:7248–7255
165. Margolin K, Longmate J, Baratta T et al (2005) CCI-779 in metastatic melanoma: a phase II trial of the California Cancer Consortium. Cancer 104:1045–1048
166. Rao R, Windschitl H, Allred J et al (2006) Phase II trial of the mTOR inhibitor everolimus (RAD-001) in metastatic melanoma. J Clin Oncol 24, 2006 ASCO Annual Meeting Proceedings (Post-Meeting Edition). Vol 24, No 18S (June 20 Supplement), 2006:8043
167. Margolin KA, Moon J, Flaherty LE et al (2012) Randomized phase II trial of sorafenib with temsirolimus or tipifarnib in untreated metastatic melanoma (S0438). Clin Cancer Res 18:1129–1137
168. Hainsworth JD, Infante JR, Spigel DR et al (2010) Bevacizumab and everolimus in the treatment of patients with metastatic melanoma: a phase 2 trial of the Sarah Cannon oncology research consortium. Cancer 116:4122–4129
169. Deng W, Gopal YN, Scott A et al (2012) Role and therapeutic potential of PI3K-mTOR signaling in de novo resistance to BRAF inhibition. Pigment Cell Melanoma Res 25:248–258
170. Hussussian CJ, Struewing JP, Goldstein AM et al (1994) Germline p16 mutations in familial melanoma. Nat Genet 8:15–21
171. Goldstein AM, Chan M, Harland M et al (2007) Features associated with germline CDKN2A mutations: a GenoMEL study of melanoma-prone families from three continents. J Med Genet 44:99–106
172. Harbour JW, Dean DC (2000) The Rb/E2F pathway: expanding roles and emerging paradigms. Genes Dev 14:2393–2409
173. Sherr CJ (2001) The INK4a/ARF network in tumour suppression. Nat Rev Mol Cell Biol 2:731–737
174. Harbour JW, Luo RX, Dei Santi A et al (1999) Cdk phosphorylation triggers sequential intramolecular interactions that progressively block Rb functions as cells move through G1. Cell 98:859–869
175. Gast A, Scherer D, Chen B et al (2010) Somatic alterations in the melanoma genome: a high-resolution array-based comparative genomic hybridization study. Genes Chromosomes Cancer 49:733–745
176. Joshi KS, Rathos MJ, Joshi RD et al (2007) In vitro antitumor properties of a novel cyclin-dependent kinase inhibitor, p 276–00. Mol Cancer Ther 6:918–925
177. Joshi KS, Rathos MJ, Mahajan P et al (2007) P 276–00, a novel cyclin-dependent inhibitor induces G1–G2 arrest, shows antitumor activity on cisplatin-resistant cells and significant in vivo efficacy in tumor models. Mol Cancer Ther 6:926–934
178. Schwartz GK, LoRusso PM, Dickson MA et al (2011) Phase I study of PD 0332991, a cyclin-dependent kinase inhibitor, administered in 3-week cycles (Schedule 2/1). Br J Cancer 104:1862–1868

Chapter 12
Dermatologic Toxicities
to Melanoma Targeted Therapies

**Jonathan L. Curry, Ana M. Ciurea, Priyadharsini Nagarajan, and
Carlos A. Torres-Cabala**

Abstract The development of targeted therapeutic agents has revolutionized the
medical treatment of melanoma. Compared to chemotherapy, patients treated with
targeted therapy benefit from reduction in tumor burden and improved overall
survival.

   While the treatment benefits of targeted therapy hold promise, the development
of dermatologic toxicity is an unforeseeable consequence. Recognition of these
cutaneous adverse side effects will be important as we see expansion in the types of
targeted therapeutic agents available for melanoma. We will examine common dermatologic toxicities associated with melanoma-targeted therapy using BRAF inhibitors (e.g., vemurafenib) and MEK inhibitors (e.g., trametinib) and immune
checkpoint antibodies with anti-CTLA-4 (e.g., ipilimumab) and anti-PD-1 (e.g.,
nivolumab).

Keywords Dermatologic toxicity • Adverse reactions • Squamous cell carcinoma
• Keratoacanthoma • Dermatitis • BRAF inhibitors • Targeted therapy • MEK
inhibitors • Anti-PD-1 • Anti-CTLA-4 • Immune checkpoint blockade

J.L. Curry, MD (✉) • C.A. Torres-Cabala
Department of Pathology, The University of Texas MD Anderson Cancer Center,
Houston, TX, USA

Department of Dermatology, The University of Texas MD Anderson Cancer Center, Houston,
TX, USA
e-mail: jlcurry@mdanderson.org

A.M. Ciurea
Department of Dermatology, The University of Texas MD Anderson Cancer Center, Houston,
TX, USA

P. Nagarajan
Department of Pathology, The University of Texas MD Anderson Cancer Center,
Houston, TX, USA

© Springer Science+Business Media New York 2016   267
C.A. Torres-Cabala, J.L. Curry (eds.), *Genetics of Melanoma*, Cancer Genetics,
DOI 10.1007/978-1-4939-3554-3_12

Advanced-stage melanoma is notorious for its therapeutic challenges with standard chemotherapy and interferon (IFN) alpha-2b [1–3]. The development of small-molecule inhibitors that selectively target susceptible proteins involved in the genetic signaling network of melanoma (e.g., BRAF) or monoclonal antibodies that reclaim the host immune function (e.g., anti-PD-1 antibody) from tumor cells has transformed the medical treatment of melanoma [4, 5]. Patients treated with BRAF inhibitor (BRAFi) (e.g., vemurafenib) had better clinical response and overall survival rates than patients treated with chemotherapy, although much of the clinical benefits were transient and met with the development of resistance [6, 7]. Patients treated with anti-CTLA-4 (e.g., ipilimumab) or anti-PD-1 (e.g., nivolumab) monoclonal antibody demonstrated tumor regression and improved survival [5, 8–11].

The emergence of dermatologic toxicities to novel therapeutic agents is an important component in the management of patients on targeted therapy. Given the highly interconnected cross talk of the genetic signaling network in melanoma, different classes of therapeutic agents may target molecules that impact common cellular pathways—translating into shared cutaneous toxicity profiles [12]. We will review the dermatologic toxicities in patients treated with BRAFi, MEKi, and immune checkpoint monoclonal antibodies summarized in Table 12.1.

Table 12.1 Histopathologic category of dermatologic toxicity and associated targeted therapeutic agent

Dermatologic toxicity	Class of targeted therapy	Drug
Inflammatory		
Acute folliculitis	BRAFi, MEKi	Vemurafenib, dabrafenib, selumetinib, trametinib, pimasertib
DHR	BRAFi, MEKi, Anti-CTLA-4, Anti-PD-1	Vemurafenib, dabrafenib, selumetinib, trametinib, pimasertib ipilimumab nivolumab, pembrolizumab
Neutrophilic dermatosis	BRAFi	Vemurafenib, dabrafenib
Panniculitis	BRAFi	Vemurafenib, dabrafenib
Vesiculobullous	Anti-PD-1	Nivolumab, pembrolizumab
Neoplastic		
Keratinocytic		
Benign: KP, FC, AK, VV, KA	BRAFi	Vemurafenib, dabrafenib
Melanocytic		
Benign: BN, DN, Nevi with atypia	BRAFi	Vemurafenib, dabrafenib
Malignant: MIS, inv. melanoma	BRAFi	Vemurafenib, dabrafenib

DHR dermal hypersensitivity reaction, *KP* keratosis pilaris, *FC* follicular cyst, *AK* actinic keratosis, *VV* verruca, *KA* keratoacanthoma, *BN* blue nevus, *DN* dysplastic nevus, *MIS* melanoma in situ, *inv.* invasive

12.1   Dermatologic Toxicities to BRAF Inhibitor

Patients treated with BRAFi (e.g., vemurafenib) therapy may develop a variety of dermatologic toxicities (DT) in the form of cutaneous epithelial and melanocytic proliferations (e.g., SCC and melanoma) or inflammatory disorders [4]. Cutaneous epithelial proliferations (CEP) include lesions such as keratosis pilaris (KP), actinic keratosis (AK), acantholytic dyskeratosis (AD), verruca, keratoacanthomas (KA), and squamous cell carcinomas (SCC). Melanocytic lesions including second primary melanomas, dysplastic nevi, nevi with cytologic atypia, and banal nevi also have been reported in association with BRAFi therapy [13–15].

In our experience, the median onset of lesions that developed in patients during BRAFi therapy was 3 months. Majority of patients (79 %) were likely to have between 1 and 5 lesions biopsied at one visit. Lesions that most frequently prompt a skin biopsy due to abnormal clinical appearance were keratinocytic lesions (~85 % of lesions biopsied). Warty papules with histologic features of verruca accounted for ~40 % of the lesions biopsied followed by invasive SCC in 24 % of lesions (Fig. 12.1) [16]. KA accounted for a minority (3 %) of the lesions biopsied.

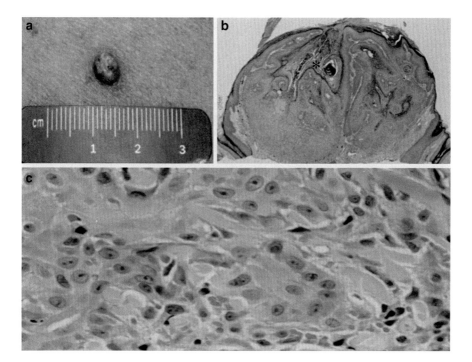

Fig. 12.1 Cutaneous epithelial proliferation seen with BRAFi therapy. (**a**) Erythematous papule with scale. (**b**) Invasive well-differentiated squamous cell carcinoma with cup-shaped, keratoacanthoma-like pattern of growth. The surface of the lesion demonstrates hyperkeratosis and papillomatosis (*asterisk*) (hematoxylin and eosin ×20). (**c**) Invasive tumor cells in the dermis infiltrate between collagen bundles (hematoxylin and eosin ×400)

Histologically, BRAFi-associated keratinocytic proliferations demonstrated similar morphologic features that included papillomatosis, hyperkeratosis, and hypergranulosis with an endophytic/exophytic cupped architecture. Lesions with predominantly endophytic growth pattern had features of KA; however, in our practice, evaluation of the base of the lesion is critical in distinction of KA versus invasive SCC with KA-like architecture. Lesions with an infiltrative border with architectural pattern of KA meet our criteria for an invasive SCC with KA-like features. In contrast lesions that demonstrate more of a pushing border meet the criteria for a KA. Lesions were commonly associated with abnormality of the follicular unit characterized by acanthosis of the follicular epithelium, distortion or rupture of the follicle. The median tumor thickness of invasive carcinoma was 2.6 mm indicating that BRAFi-associated SCC are relatively thick lesions and a deep shave or skin punch to evaluate the base of the lesion will further aid in differentiating KA-associated BRAFi lesions from invasive SCC [16]. Treatment with combinatorial therapy of isotretinoin and 5-fluorouracil may be beneficial in medical treatment of these types of DT [17].

Inflammatory dermatologic toxicities accounted for ~15 % of the lesions and included dermal hypersensitivity reaction (DHR), folliculitis, granulomas, and panniculitis [16]. Various forms of panniculitis and neutrophilic dermatosis or Sweet-like eruption are now recognized toxicities to BRAFi [18–22]. Panniculitis associated with BRAFi can present with granulomatous necrotizing inflammation, mimicking infectious processes [19]. As in the cases of neutrophilic dermatoses, special studies performed on biopsy sections and/or tissue cultures are needed to rule out infectious etiologies in these cases (Fig. 12.2).

The development of new or altered melanocytic lesions in patients on BRAFi therapy is an emerging toxicity profile [13–15]. Melanocytic lesions accounted for

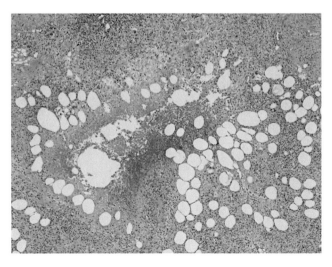

Fig. 12.2 BRAFi therapy-induced panniculitis. (**a**) Subcutaneous nodules on a patient with metastatic melanoma. (**b**) On histological examination, a necrotizing granulomatous process involving subcutis is seen. Special stains and tissue cultures were negative for bacterial and fungal microorganisms (hematoxylin and eosin ×40)

Fig. 12.3 Melanocytic proliferation seen with BRAFi therapy. Invasive melanoma (M) associated with nevus (N) and background verrucous epithelial changes of papillomatosis, hyperkeratosis, hypergranulosis, and acanthosis. Confluent proliferation of melanocytes (*arrows*) with pagetoid spread in the epidermis (hematoxylin and eosin, ×100)

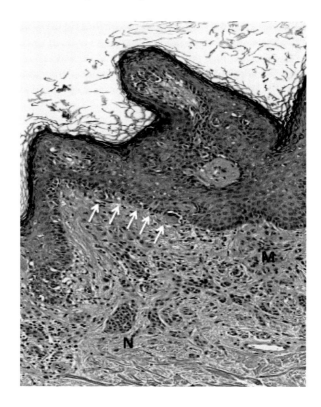

~8.0 % of the lesions biopsied in our series [16]. Diagnoses ranged from ordinary nevi, dysplastic nevi, nevi with atypia, and melanoma. Melanocytic lesions may also have combined features seen in cutaneous epithelial toxicities to keratinocytes and include hyperkeratosis, papillomatosis, and hypergranulosis—wartlike morphology (Fig. 12.3).

BRAFi-associated melanocytic lesions clinically are small pigmented papular lesions. The occurrence of new pigmented lesion or change in color and/or size of existing melanocytic lesion prompts biopsy in patients on BRAFi [23]. Histologically, we have noticed that BRAFi-associated melanocytic lesions tend to have more prominent cytologic atypia of melanocytes. In our experience, more than 75 % of melanocytic lesions biopsied during BRAFi therapy were classified as dysplastic nevi or nevi with atypical features [24]. As noted by others, lesions commonly demonstrated moderate to severe cytologic atypia [15]. The development of second primary cutaneous melanoma in patients treated with BRAFi therapy occurred in ~13–58 % of patients who had biopsy of a melanocytic lesion [13, 24–27]. In contrast second primary cutaneous melanoma in patients with no history of BRAFi therapy occurs in ~0.2–19 % of patients [28–30]. Second primary melanomas in either setting are thin tumors with Breslow depth of ≤1.0 mm, reflecting the importance of skin surveillance in patients with melanoma [10, 21–23, 28–33]. Paradoxical activation of MAPK pathway in *BRAF*^{WT} (wild-type) keratinocytes is the mechanism proffered for BRAFi-associated keratinocytic proliferations [34, 35]. Since >98 % of melanocytic lesions that prompted a biopsy in patient during BRAFi therapy had melanocytic lesions with the absence of *BRAF V600E* mutation, similar paradoxical activation in *BRAF^WT* melanocytes appears to be in force [13, 15, 23, 25–27, 36].

Skin surveillance programs by dermatologists are critical to the management of patients on BRAFi therapy since these patients are vulnerable to develop a spectrum of skin toxicities including the development of a second primary melanoma.

12.2 Dermatologic Toxicities to MEK Inhibitor

The skin toxicity profiles of MEK inhibitors (MEKi) are similar to epidermal growth factor inhibitors (EGFRi) [12, 37]. The most common forms of DT associated with MEKi are the morbilliform and papulopustular eruptions with histologic features of DHR and an acute suppurative folliculitis (Fig. 12.4), respectively [38–40]. *Staphylococcus aureus* colonization of the folliculitis is not uncommon and may require antimicrobial treatment [41, 42].

Since MEK is downstream of BRAF in the MAPK cell signaling pathway, combinatorial therapy with BRAFi+MEKi may benefit melanoma treatment response as well as mitigate skin toxicity profile compared with mono-targeted

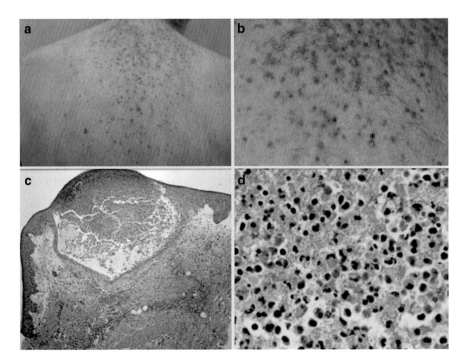

Fig. 12.4 Papulopustular eruption typical of MEKi or EGFRi therapy. (**a**) Multiple, discrete, erythematous papules on the back. (**b**) Lesions appear folliculocentric and some with pustules (*asterisk*). (**c**) and (**d**) Biopsy shows suppurative folliculitis with dilated follicle with dense, acute inflammation composed of neutrophils, eosinophils, and lymphocytes (hematoxylin and eosin, ×40 and ×400, respectively)

agent therapy. Patients treated with combination of BRAFi+MEKi experienced fewer DT, particularly CEP typical of BRAFi therapy [43, 44].

12.3 Dermatologic Toxicities to Immune Checkpoint Antibodies

Immune checkpoint-targeted therapy with monoclonal antibodies (e.g., anti-CTLA-4 and anti-PD-1) designed to restore the host immune function against cancer cells has shown tremendous promise in the treatment of melanoma [5, 9–11]. Although the treatment response in patients treated with targeted immunotherapy was encouraging, immune-related toxicities were an inevitable consequence to therapy [45]. Immune-related toxicities include non-cutaneous reactions involving the gastrointestinal, hepatic, endocrine, pulmonary, renal, and neurologic systems and cutaneous reactions (e.g., pruritus, maculopapular rash, vitiligo) [45, 46].

Patients on immune checkpoint therapy are at increased risk to develop maculopapular rash, pruritus, and vitiligo [45]. Patients who were treated with CTLA-4 inhibitor (ipilimumab) typically developed maculopapular, erythematous, and reticular eruptions on the trunk and extremities [47, 48]. Histologic examination often demonstrated features of a DHR with superficial perivascular lymphocytic infiltrate with eosinophils [47]. The morphology of ipilimumab-associated dermatologic toxicities is reminiscent to drug exanthem or DHR reactions seen with nontargeted medications (e.g., antibiotics) [48, 49].

Maculopapular eruptions are also associated with anti-PD-1 inhibitor (e.g., nivolumab and pembrolizumab); however, in contrast to ipilimumab-associated dermatologic toxicities, we and others have noticed that a subset of patients treated with anti-PD-1 inhibitor more often developed bullous eruptions with histologic and immunofluorescence features of bullous pemphigoid [50]. We have experienced bullous pemphigoid-associated dermatologic toxicities in patients treated with nivolumab and pembrolizumab (Fig. 12.5) [51]. Some of these patients at one time were also treated with ipilimumab and/or other small molecule inhibitor(s). An immunobullous toxicity appears to be less frequent with ipilimumab; however, further skin surveillance and patient monitoring are necessary to examine if there is an association of an immunobullous dermatologic toxicity with a particular immune checkpoint molecule or whether this form of skin toxicity manifests from combinatory effect from multiple immune checkpoint or targeted therapeutic agents.

12.4 Summary

Dermatologic toxicities are a known consequence of melanoma-targeted therapy. As novel therapeutic agents continue to develop and become available for patients with advanced-stage melanoma, the recognition of skin toxicities will be critical.

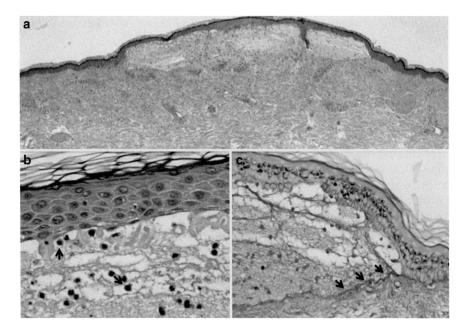

Fig. 12.5 Bullous pemphigoid with immune checkpoint therapy. (**a**) Subepidermal blister cavity with associated mixed inflammatory infiltrate with eosinophils (hematoxylin and eosin, ×20). (**b**) Blister cavity contains edema and inflammatory cells including eosinophils (*arrows*) (hematoxylin and eosin, ×400). (**c**) PAS stain highlights basement membrane zone on the floor of the blister cavity (*arrow*) supporting an immunobullous process (PAS stain, x400). Direct immunofluorescence (not pictured) confirmed linear deposits of IgG and C3 along the basement membrane

Dermatologists and dermatopathologists will be essential in the examination and management of skin toxicities from melanoma-targeted therapy.

References

1. Hauschild A, Agarwala SS, Trefzer U et al (2009) Results of a phase III, randomized, placebo-controlled study of sorafenib in combination with carboplatin and paclitaxel as second-line treatment in patients with unresectable stage III or stage IV melanoma. J Clin Oncol 27(17):2823–2830
2. Patel PM, Suciu S, Mortier L et al (2011) Extended schedule, escalated dose temozolomide versus dacarbazine in stage IV melanoma: final results of a randomised phase III study (EORTC 18032). Eur J Cancer 47(10):1476–1483
3. Kirkwood JM, Manola J, Ibrahim J, Sondak V, Ernstoff MS, Rao U (2004) A pooled analysis of eastern cooperative oncology group and intergroup trials of adjuvant high-dose interferon for melanoma. Clin Cancer Res 10(5):1670–1677
4. Chapman PB, Hauschild A, Robert C et al (2011) Improved survival with vemurafenib in melanoma with BRAF V600E mutation. N Engl J Med 364(26):2507–2516

5. Metcalfe W, Anderson J, Trinh V, Hwu WJ (2015) Anti-programmed cell death-1 (PD-1) monoclonal antibodies in treating advanced melanoma. Discov Med 19(106):393–401
6. Sosman JA, Kim KB, Schuchter L et al (2012) Survival in BRAF V600-mutant advanced melanoma treated with vemurafenib. N Engl J Med 366(8):707–714
7. Jang S, Atkins MB (2013) Which drug, and when, for patients with BRAF-mutant melanoma? Lancet Oncol 14(2):e60–e69
8. Weber JS, D'Angelo SP, Minor D et al (2015) Nivolumab versus chemotherapy in patients with advanced melanoma who progressed after anti-CTLA-4 treatment (CheckMate 037): a randomised, controlled, open-label, phase 3 trial. Lancet Oncol 16(4):375–384
9. Hodi FS, O'Day SJ, McDermott DF et al (2010) Improved survival with ipilimumab in patients with metastatic melanoma. N Engl J Med 363(8):711–723
10. Robert C, Long GV, Brady B et al (2014) Nivolumab in previously untreated melanoma without BRAF mutation. N Engl J Med 372(4):320–330
11. Robert C, Thomas L, Bondarenko I et al (2011) Ipilimumab plus dacarbazine for previously untreated metastatic melanoma. N Engl J Med 364(26):2517–2526
12. Curry JL, Torres-Cabala CA, Kim KB et al (2014) Dermatologic toxicities to targeted cancer therapy: shared clinical and histologic adverse skin reactions. Int J Dermatol 53(3):376–384
13. Dalle S, Poulalhon N, Thomas L (2011) Vemurafenib in melanoma with BRAF V600E mutation. N Engl J Med 365(15):1448–1449, author reply 1450
14. Debarbieux S, Dalle S, Depaepe L, Poulalhon N, Balme B, Thomas L (2013) Second primary melanomas treated with BRAF blockers: study by reflectance confocal microscopy. Br J Dermatol 168(6):1230–1235
15. Gerami P, Sorrell J, Martini M (2012) Dermatoscopic evolution of dysplastic nevi showing high-grade dysplasia in a metastatic melanoma patient on vemurafenib. J Am Acad Dermatol 67(6):e275–e276
16. Curry JL, Tetzlaff MT, Nicholson K et al (2014) Histological features associated with vemurafenib-induced skin toxicities: examination of 141 cutaneous lesions biopsied during therapy. Am J Dermatopathol 36(7):557–561
17. Mays R, Curry J, Kim K et al (2013) Eruptive squamous cell carcinomas after vemurafenib therapy. J Cutan Med Surg 17(6):419–422
18. Pattanaprichakul P, Tetzlaff MT, Lapolla WJ et al (2014) Sweet syndrome following vemurafenib therapy for recurrent cholangiocarcinoma. J Cutan Pathol 41(3):326–328
19. Ramani NS, Curry JL, Kapil J, Rapini RP, Tetzlaff MT, Prieto VG, Torres-Cabala CA (2014) Panniculitis With necrotizing granulomata in a patient on BRAF inhibitor (dabrafenib) therapy for metastatic melanoma. Am J Dermatopathol 37:e96–e99
20. Kim GH, Levy A, Compoginis G (2013) Neutrophilic panniculitis developing after treatment of metastatic melanoma with vemurafenib. J Cutan Pathol 40(7):667–669
21. Monfort JB, Pages C, Schneider P et al (2012) Vemurafenib-induced neutrophilic panniculitis. Melanoma Res 22(5):399–401
22. Yorio JT, Mays SR, Ciurea AM et al (2014) Case of vemurafenib-induced Sweet's syndrome. J Dermatol 41(9):817–820
23. Cohen PR, Bedikian AY, Kim KB (2013) Appearance of new vemurafenib-associated melanocytic nevi on normal-appearing skin: case series and a review of changing or new pigmented lesions in patients with metastatic malignant melanoma after initiating treatment with vemurafenib. J Clin Aesthet Dermatol 6(5):27–37
24. Mudaliar K, Tetzlaff MT, Duvic M et al (2016) BRAF inhibitor therapy-associated melanocytic lesions lack the BRAF V600E mutation and show increased levels of cyclin D1 expression. Hum Pathol 50:79–89
25. Zimmer L, Hillen U, Livingstone E et al (2012) Atypical melanocytic proliferations and new primary melanomas in patients with advanced melanoma undergoing selective BRAF inhibition. J Clin Oncol 30(19):2375–2383
26. Dalle S, Poulalhon N, Debarbieux S et al (2013) Tracking of second primary melanomas in vemurafenib-treated patients. JAMA Dermatol 149(4):488–490

27. Perier-Muzet M, Thomas L, Poulalhon N et al (2014) Melanoma patients under vemurafenib: prospective follow-up of melanocytic lesions by digital dermoscopy. J Invest Dermatol 134(5):1351–1358

28. Goggins WB, Tsao H (2003) A population-based analysis of risk factors for a second primary cutaneous melanoma among melanoma survivors. Cancer 97(3):639–643

29. Vecchiato A, Pasquali S, Menin C et al (2014) Histopathological characteristics of subsequent melanomas in patients with multiple primary melanomas. J Eur Acad Dermatol Venereol 28(1):58–64

30. Murali R, Goumas C, Kricker A et al (2012) Clinicopathologic features of incident and subsequent tumors in patients with multiple primary cutaneous melanomas. Ann Surg Oncol 19(3):1024–1033

31. Murali R, Brown PT, Kefford RF, Scolyer RA, Thompson JF, Atkins MB, Long GV (2012) Number of primary melanomas is an independent predictor of survival in patients with metastatic melanoma. Cancer 118(18):4519–4529

32. Johnson TM, Hamilton T, Lowe L (1998) Multiple primary melanomas. J Am Acad Dermatol 39(3):422–427

33. Chen T, Fallah M, Forsti A, Kharazmi E, Sundquist K, Hemminki K (2015) Risk of next melanoma in patients with familial and sporadic melanoma by number of previous melanomas. JAMA Dermatol 151(6):607–615

34. Hall-Jackson CA, Eyers PA, Cohen P et al (1999) Paradoxical activation of Raf by a novel Raf inhibitor. Chem Biol 6(8):559–568

35. Gibney GT, Messina JL, Fedorenko IV, Sondak VK, Smalley KS (2013) Paradoxical oncogenesis—the long-term effects of BRAF inhibition in melanoma. Nat Rev Clin Oncol 10(7):390–399

36. Haenssle HA, Kraus SL, Brehmer F et al (2012) Dynamic changes in nevi of a patient with melanoma treated with vemurafenib: importance of sequential dermoscopy. Arch Dermatol 148(10):1183–1185

37. Macdonald JB, Macdonald B, Golitz LE, LoRusso P, Sekulic A (2015) Cutaneous adverse effects of targeted therapies: Part II: inhibitors of intracellular molecular signaling pathways. J Am Acad Dermatol 72(2):221–236, quiz 237-228

38. Banerji U, Camidge DR, Verheul HM et al (2010) The first-in-human study of the hydrogen sulfate (Hyd-sulfate) capsule of the MEK1/2 inhibitor AZD6244 (ARRY-142886): a phase I open-label multicenter trial in patients with advanced cancer. Clin Cancer Res 16(5): 1613–1623

39. Flaherty KT, Robert C, Hersey P et al (2012) Improved survival with MEK inhibition in BRAF-mutated melanoma. N Engl J Med 367(2):107–114

40. Anforth R, Liu M, Nguyen B et al (2014) Acneiform eruptions: a common cutaneous toxicity of the MEK inhibitor trametinib. Australas J Dermatol 55(4):250–254

41. Balagula Y, Barth Huston K, Busam KJ, Lacouture ME, Chapman PB, Myskowski PL (2011) Dermatologic side effects associated with the MEK 1/2 inhibitor selumetinib (AZD6244, ARRY-142886). Invest New Drugs 29(5):1114–1121

42. Querfeld C, Duffy K, Magel G, Oble D, Cohen EE, Shea CR (2011) Disseminated follicular eruption during therapy with the MEK inhibitor AZD6244. J Am Acad Dermatol 64(2): e17–e19

43. King AJ, Arnone MR, Bleam MR et al (2013) Dabrafenib; preclinical characterization, increased efficacy when combined with trametinib, while BRAF/MEK tool combination reduced skin lesions. PLoS One 8(7):e67583

44. Flaherty KT, Infante JR, Daud A et al (2012) Combined BRAF and MEK inhibition in melanoma with BRAF V600 mutations. N Engl J Med 367(18):1694–1703

45. Abdel-Rahman O, ElHalawani H, Fouad M (2015) Risk of cutaneous toxicities in patients with solid tumors treated with immune checkpoint inhibitors: a meta-analysis. Future Oncol 11:2471–2484

46. Weber JS, Yang JC, Atkins MB, Disis ML (2015) Toxicities of immunotherapy for the practitioner. J Clin Oncol 33(18):2092–2099

47. Lacouture ME, Wolchok JD, Yosipovitch G, Kahler KC, Busam KJ, Hauschild A (2014) Ipilimumab in patients with cancer and the management of dermatologic adverse events. J Am Acad Dermatol 71(1):161–169

48. Jaber SH, Cowen EW, Haworth LR, Booher SL, Berman DM, Rosenberg SA, Hwang ST (2006) Skin reactions in a subset of patients with stage IV melanoma treated with anti-cytotoxic T-lymphocyte antigen 4 monoclonal antibody as a single agent. Arch Dermatol 142(2): 166–172

49. Pichler WJ, Yawalkar N, Britschgi M et al (2002) Cellular and molecular pathophysiology of cutaneous drug reactions. Am J Clin Dermatol 3(4):229–238

50. Carlos G, Anforth R, Chou S, Clements A, Fernandez-Penas P (2015) A case of bullous pemphigoid in a patient with metastatic melanoma treated with pembrolizumab. Melanoma Res 25(3):265–268

51. Jour G, Glitza IC, Ellis RM et al (2016) Autoimmune dermatologic toxicities from immune checkpoint blockade with anti-PD-1 antibody therapy: a report on bullous skin eruptions. J Cutan Pathol (in press)

Index

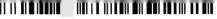

Printed in the United States
By Bookmasters